Gastrointestinal Nematodes of Sheep and Cattle

Biology and Control

Gastrointestinal Nematodes of Sheep and Cattle
Biology and Control

Ian Sutherland
Ian Scott

Foreword by Professor Sir James Armour

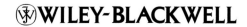

A John Wiley & Sons, Ltd., Publication

Blackwell Publishing was acquired by John Wiley & Sons in February 2007. Blackwell's publishing programme has been merged with Wiley's global Scientific, Technical, and Medical business to form Wiley-Blackwell.

Registered office
John Wiley & Sons Ltd, The Atrium, Southern Gate, Chichester, West Sussex, PO19 8SQ, United Kingdom

Editorial offices
9600 Garsington Road, Oxford, OX4 2DQ, United Kingdom
2121 State Avenue, Ames, Iowa 50014-8300, USA

For details of our global editorial offices, for customer services and for information about how to apply for permission to reuse the copyright material in this book please see our website at www.wiley.com/wiley-blackwell.

Library of Congress Cataloging-in-Publication Data

Sutherland, Ian, 1962-
Gastrointestinal nematodes of sheep and cattle / Ian Sutherland, Ian Scott.
    p. ; cm.
  Includes bibliographical references and index.
  ISBN 978-1-4051-8582-0 (hardback : alk. paper)   1. Sheep—Parasites.   2.   Cattle—Parasites.   3. Nematode.   I.   Scott, Ian, 1967- II.   Title.
  [DNLM: 1.   Nematode Infections—veterinary.   2.   Cattle Diseases.
 3.   Gastrointestinal Disease—veterinary.   4.   Sheep Diseases. SF 810.N4 S966g 2010]
  SF810.N4S88 2010
  636.089′6965—dc22
                                                                                          2009021833
A catalogue record for this book is available from the British Library.

Set in 10.5/12.5 pt Sabon by Macmillan Publishing Solutions, Chennai, India
Printed in Singapore by Markono Print Media Pte Ltd

1   2010

Contents

Foreword

Gastrointestinal nematodes (GIN) are arguably the major cause of ill health and poor productivity in grazing sheep and cattle worldwide, especially in young stock. This has been the situation for many years and persists today despite significant increases in our knowledge base on these parasites.

In this book, Sutherland and Scott provide a global overview of previous and current research on GIN and identify deficiencies in our knowledge base that require attention.

The overview is divided into 12 well-structured chapters, each accompanied by selected references. Key areas covered include parasite biology, pathophysiology and epidemiology, although the largest chapters focus on anthelmintic drugs, resistance to these drugs and host immune responses to GIN. Concentration on these latter subjects is no surprise since treatment and control of these parasites centres on the use of anthelmintics while consumers have been vocal on the need for non-chemical or immunological control methods as an alternative to anthelmintics.

On the subject of anthelmintic resistance, the authors highlight the paradox that although the efficacy of modern anthelmintics is so high and they provide health and production benefits, the only nematodes surviving treatment are likely to be resistant strains from which future generations would be derived. Clearly if continued use of the same anthelmintic was employed, especially if integrated with a rotation involving the so-called clean pastures, then selection for resistance would be enhanced.

Solutions are available to slow down the development of resistance, but the authors rightly point out that the problem is now severe and global, and the discovery and fast-track marketing of new drugs unrelated chemically to existing brands is an urgent priority. Furthermore, any new anthelmintics must be deployed in a manner likely to delay resistance.

The chapter on host immune responses provides a useful overview of the extensive literature on this area. Although not concentrating on prophylaxis by immunisation, progress on identifying protective antigens is presented. Many believe vaccination is the ultimate solution to controlling GIN, particularly the more pathogenic species, and more investment in this approach is required.

There are also interesting chapters on the interaction between nutrition and parasitism and a possible role for selecting breeds or lines within breed which are genetically resistant to GIN.

The authors are to be congratulated on producing a book which is both informative and thought provoking. It is required reading for all students, scientists and veterinarians interested in parasitic disease and livestock production.

Professor Sir James Armour
Emeritus Professor of Veterinary Parasitology
University of Glasgow

Preface

The gastrointestinal nematode parasites of grazing ruminants comprise one of the greatest limitations on food production on a global scale. Allowing for inherent variability, this statement holds true regardless of farming system, climate, geographical region and host species. Productivity losses result from both parasite challenge and parasitism, while regular treatment of the infections is costly in terms of chemicals and labour. While it is difficult to accurately determine the annual cost of the infections, it is worthwhile considering that in the late 1990s, global sales of anthelmintics for grazing livestock alone exceeded US$1 billion.

If anything, the relative cost of gastrointestinal parasitism has become greater in recent decades as the availability of effective broad-spectrum anthelmintics has enabled the intensification of pastoral agriculture. To an extent, it appears the success of the various anthelmintic products developed since the 1960s has created a rod for our own backs, particularly as resistance has arisen to each active family in turn. Furthermore, as consumers increasingly demand a reduction in chemical application to food and fibre producing animals, the pressure increases to control nematode parasites within intensive pastoral systems without recourse to regular drug treatment.

The development of effective, sustainable control options for gastrointestinal parasites has thus far proven difficult, partly due to a lack of fundamental knowledge of parasite biology and the host–parasite relationship, and partly due to the high degree of biological plasticity of the parasites themselves, which have demonstrated time and again an ability to adapt to our attempts at control (and in the early days annihilation).

However, assuming there will be an ongoing global demand for the products of pastoral agriculture, there must also be ongoing research efforts into the development of sustainable control options for gastrointestinal parasites. Ideally, these should be informed by an improved understanding of the biology of the parasites, but also of the likely long-term impacts of parasite management strategies and also how each of the various methods can be combined in integrated control programs. The obvious starting point for any future research strategy is to review what has gone before, in the hope of learning from past successes and mistakes. The aim of this book is to provide a starting point for this process by reviewing all of the major aspects of worm biology, epidemiology and the various worm control strategies which have been introduced or proposed over the past 50 years. While integrated pest control is discussed in a number of chapters, the focus of this book is to describe the individual components.

By necessity, some of the chapters provide a somewhat superficial review of their research area; for example, many books have been written on various aspects of the immunology of gastrointestinal nematode parasitism, or the chemistry and pharmacokinetics of anthelmintics. What we have attempted here, however, is to provide an overview of each area and a historical timeline of research efforts. For that reason, original research material has been referenced wherever possible.

Acknowledgements

The authors would like to thank a number of people who have contributed to this book. A number of AgResearch staff, including Dave Leathwick, Richard Shaw, Tony Pernthaner, Stewart Bisset, Tania Waghorn, Caroline Costall and Sarah Rosanowski have been by turns helpful, patient and encouraging, as have Massey staff such as Bill Pomroy, Heather Simpson, Barbara Adlington and Ann Tunnicliffe. Two of our Australian colleagues, Stephen Love and Brown Besier, were enthusiastic and generous in their assistance, as were Barry Hosking and Colin MacKay of Novartis Animal Health Ltd. Juliet Sutherland deserves special mention for her assistance, and forbearance.

1 Nematode parasites

For pastorally reared livestock, internal parasite infections represent the greatest threat to health and productivity. Parasites generally achieve maximal importance in young (non-immune) animals kept at pasture and returning regularly to areas they have grazed before, and when the climate is generally warm and wet, and winters are mild. Nevertheless, some studies have shown that even where access to pasture is considerably reduced, parasitism can still cause considerable problems and some parasites can adapt to husbandry conditions that would normally be considered incompatible with parasite biology. Of all the helminth parasites of livestock, the gastrointestinal nematodes (GIN) have arguably the greatest overall impact.

The nematodes

In the past, nematodes have been ascribed to various phyla, namely, the Aschelminthes or Nemathelminthes, but are now generally recognised as belonging to their own unique phylum, the Nematoda (Hodda, 2007). The nematodes are biologically quite distinct from other 'helminths' such as the Platyhelminthes (cestodes and trematodes) and Acanthocephala (the thorny-headed worms). Indeed, nematode moulting behaviour has encouraged some to consider them as being more closely related to other moulting organisms (forming the superphylum, the Ecdysozoa) than they are to the other helminth taxa (Aguinaldo *et al.*, 1997). Acceptance for this new arrangement is by no means universal and there are strong arguments against it (reviewed by Hodda, 2007), but taken at face value such a relationship could explain why a drug like ivermectin can have excellent activity against nematodes and arthropods, but none against flukes or tapeworms.

Traditionally, two major classes of nematodes have been recognised (Anderson, 2000; Chitwood, 1950), the Secernentea and the Adenophorea – the vast majority of 'adenophorean' nematodes being aquatic with this class contributing only a handful of vertebrate parasites (e.g. *Trichuris* spp., *Trichinella* spp.). The major parasites of terrestrial vertebrates were placed within the Secernentea and were split amongst the following orders: the Ascaridida, the Oxyurida, the Rhabditida, the Spirurida and finally the Strongylida (the strongylids). This latter order includes the vast majority of nematode species causing gastrointestinal disease in ruminants.

The strongylid order contains several superfamilies, the bulk of ruminant nematode parasites being found in one, the Trichostrongyloidea. The trichostrongyloid nematodes are all rather slender and tend to be small, the majority being around 2 cm or less. With simple, small mouths they are described as mucosal browsers, i.e. feed on small particulate matter, mucus and dissolved molecules on the mucosal surface. A small number of important genera can be found in other superfamilies such as the Ancylostomatoidea and Strongyloidea. Nematodes in both of these superfamilies tend to be stouter than the trichostrongyloids. The Ancylostomatoidea contains the blood-feeding hookworms, whereas the Strongyloidea contains a number of plug-feeding nematodes – nematodes that ingest a plug of host tissue which is liquefied in the buccal capsule by enzymatic action and the liquid material is swallowed.

The important nematode genera and species parasitising ruminant livestock

Climate and geographical location, management factors, the classes of stock present on a farm and the presence or absence of other stock or wildlife that may act as reservoirs of parasites can all have a major impact on the exact balance of species present. It is generally accepted that the major parasites of sheep do not establish that well in cattle and *vice versa*, thus few parasites are common to both when sheep and cattle share the same grazing, whereas many of the major parasites of sheep will establish readily in goats. *Bos taurus* and *Ovis aries* are farmed on all inhabited continents, having arrived there largely as the result of human activity and their parasites have gone with them. Thus a parasite such as *Ostertagia ostertagi* is ubiquitous in cattle in temperate climates, whether this is in North or South America, in Europe and Asia or in Australia and New Zealand.

In the following discussion of the major genera and species of livestock, the parasites will be grouped according to the organ they infest rather than on any taxonomic basis. Unless stated otherwise, it can be assumed that the parasites mentioned are strongylids, from the superfamily Trichostrongyloidea. The list has concentrated on the more economically important parasites and thus has a bias towards GIN of temperate climates. Many nematodes are not discussed, but it should be born in mind that parasites such as *Mecistocirrus digitatus*, though prevalent and important in some parts of the world, have similar biology and behaviour to some of those listed in the following sections – *Haemonchus* spp. in the case of *M. digitatus* (Aken *et al.*, 1997). Likewise, the camelid strongylid, *Camelostrongylus mentulatus*, when it occurs in sheep, is effectively a straight swap for *Teladorsagia* spp. (Hilton *et al.*, 1978).

Abomasal genera

Haemonchus

Main species: *H. contortus, H. placei*

Being the largest of the common abomasal parasites, *Haemonchus* spp. are also the most pathogenic being unusual for trichostrongyloids in feeding on blood (see later). Also regarded as one of the most prolific parasites, females produce up to 10,000 eggs per day. *H. contortus* is primarily a parasite of sheep and goats, but can be found in cattle and some species of deer, whereas *H. placei* is primarily a parasite of cattle. For some time there was a debate as to whether *H. contortus* and *H. placei* were separate species, but there is genetic evidence that this is indeed so (Blouin *et al.*, 1997), and hybrids of the two species may be infertile (Le Jambre, 1995). In New Zealand where *H. placei* has not been recorded, small numbers of *H. contortus* may be found in cattle, but clinical disease is exceptional. A rarer third species, *H. similis*, has been recorded in cattle and deer in North America and Europe. *Haemonchus* spp. generally prefer warm, moist conditions and hence are more of a problem in tropical and subtropical conditions, the free-living stages of the parasites struggle to overwinter in cooler climates. In temperate countries such as the United Kingdom and New Zealand, the prevalence and the risk of disease have traditionally been greater in the warmer southern and northern parts of the respective countries. There are however reports of increasing numbers of cases of ovine haemonchosis occurring in Scotland and Sweden (Sargison *et al.*, 2007; Waller *et al.*, 2005).

Common names of *Haemonchus* spp. include twisted stomach worm, wire worm and Barber's pole worm and one can see why when viewing freshly collected females in which the pale uterus entwines around the red, blood-filled intestine. Adults of all three species are 2–3 cm in length and are therefore easily seen on the mucosal surface during post-mortem examination.

Ostertagia

Main species: *O. ostertagi (O. lyrata)*

O. ostertagi is a cosmopolitan parasite of cattle and is considered the most important parasite of cattle in temperate regions. It is also important in subtropical climates with adequate winter rainfall. Well adapted to cooler climates, *O. ostertagi* survives reasonably well over winter as L3 on pasture or in soil, or as arrested larvae inside the animal. Originally described as a separate species, based on the presence within populations of small numbers of male nematodes with different morphology, *O. lyrata* is now considered as a morphological variant of *O. ostertagi*. A number of studies have examined this, including studies of ribosomal and mitochondrial DNA (Zarlenga *et al.*, 1998), and so far none have refuted the hypothesis that *O. ostertagi* and *O. lyrata* are the same species. Insofar as *O. lyrata* males are usually present in smaller numbers than *O. ostertagi* males, *O. lyrata* is considered the minor morphotype, *O. ostertagi*, the major morphotype.

The adults are slender, brownish-red worms reaching approximately 1 cm in length and can be observed on the mucosal surface, from where they can be difficult to remove, being embedded within the mucus layer. *Ostertagia* spp. females are considered of low fecundity, laying as few as 50 eggs per day.

O. leptospicularis is primarily considered a parasite of cervids, but has occasionally been recovered from cattle and sheep.

Teladorsagia

Main species: *T. circumcincta (T. (Ostertagia) trifurcata, T. davtiani)*
Teladorsagia spp. essentially occupy the niche in sheep and goats that *O. ostertagi* does in cattle, and their behaviour and effects are very similar. For a long time, these organisms were in the genus *Ostertagia* (*O. circumcincta*). As with *O. ostertagi/O. lyrata*, *T. circumcincta/T. trifurcata/T. davtiani* are considered one species with *T. trifurcata* and *T. davtiani*, minor morphotypes. Recent genetic analyses found more variation between different strains of *T. circumcincta*, including a comparison of goat vs. sheep *T. circumcincta*, than existed between the major and minor morphotypes (Grillo *et al.*, 2007, 2008). *T. circumcincta* may thus include a cryptic species, but *T. trifurcata/T. davtiani* are not implicated.

Both *Ostertagia* spp. and *Teladorsagia* spp. are sometimes referred to as the brown stomach worms.

Trichostrongylus

Main species: *T. axei*
The only species of this genus found consistently in the gastric compartment, *T. axei* has been found in cattle, sheep, goats, deer, pigs and horses. It is the smallest of the common abomasal nematodes and is relatively easily overlooked when alongside the others (*Haemonchus, Ostertagia/Teladorsagia*). *T. axei* burrows between the epithelial cells and thus occupies a slightly different niche than the other abomasal GIN species.

Small intestinal genera

Trichostrongylus

Main species: *T. colubriformis, T. vitrinus, T. longispicularis, T. rugatus*
These are relatively small worms, less than 1 cm in length. *T. longispicularis* is primarily a parasite (minor pathogen) of cattle, whereas *T. colubriformis* and *T. vitrinus* are important parasites of sheep and goats. In the warmer

parts of temperate regions moving into subtropical areas, small intestinal *Trichostrongylus* spp. make a greater contribution to ill health in small ruminants, and the infections can exhibit very high egg counts. In a study of South Australian sheep, *T. rugatus* dominated in low rainfall areas, *T. vitrinus* in wetter districts whereas *T. colubriformis* was common throughout the state, but was rarely dominant (Beveridge & Ford, 1982).

Worms in this genus are sometimes referred to as the black scour worms.

Nematodirus

Main species: *N. battus, N. filicollis, N. spathiger, N. helvetianus*
These are sometimes called the thin-necked or thread-necked worms as the anterior part of the female is noticeably narrower than the posterior. This is primarily the result of the very large eggs produced by this parasite. *Nematodirus* spp. are fairly cosmopolitan in distribution. The distribution of *N. battus* is the most restricted being confined to the northern United Kingdom, parts of Northern Europe and Canada, possibly reflecting only a recent cross-over from deer – disease due to *N. battus* was not recorded in sheep before 1951 (Winter, 2002). *N. Helvetianus* is primarily a parasite of cattle, whereas the others are more prevalent in small ruminants. *N. battus* does however infect cattle, particularly young calves. The biology of *Nematodirus* spp. is atypical for the trichostrongyloids. Larvae develop to the ensheathed L3 stage within the egg, hence the larger egg size; development is generally slow, and the eggs of *N. battus* and *N. filicollis* appear to enter a period of developmental arrest and require a period of chilling to trigger hatching (Chapter 3). Thus, for *N. battus* and *N. filicollis*, there may be only one generation of the parasites each year. Infection is passed from one year's lambs or calves to those born the next year, with a negligible role for adult stock – transmission that can be encouraged by the use of specific paddocks for calving/lambing from one year to the next. Disease is seen in the spring and early summer and follows the (synchronous) hatching of a large number of eggs (Sargison, 2004). Deaths of young stock are not uncommon. Immunity to these worms develops rapidly, thus curtailing the period of risk, and a definite age resistance has been observed in sheep, with parasite-naive 8-month old lambs refractory to infection (Winter *et al.*, 1997).

Cooperia

Main species: *C. oncophora, C. punctata, C. pectinata, C. surnabada (C. mcmasteri), C. curticei*
Cooperia spp. are cosmopolitan parasites of cattle and sheep, with *C. curticei* most often recovered from sheep. These species are generally considered to be of only mild pathogenicity, although *C. punctata* and *C. pectinata* may be more damaging, which may relate to a more invasive behaviour of their larvae (Taylor *et al.*, 2007).

Large intestinal genera

Oesophagostomum

Main species: *Oe. radiatum, Oe. columbianum, Oe. venulosum*
Up to 2 cm in length, these strongyloid nematodes are sometimes called nodule worms because of the (inflammatory) nodules that develop around larvae that have burrowed into the submucosa of the host intestine. *Oe. radiatum* is found in cattle worldwide, whereas *Oe. venulosum* and *Oe. columbianum* occur in sheep. *Oe. venulosum* is the more common species of the two sheep species and is the least pathogenic. *Oesophagostomum* spp. are strongyloid, plug-feeding nematodes, but the shallow buccal capsule in the adult renders this stage relatively non-pathogenic. Pathogenicity relates principally to the encystment of larvae in the submucosa of the distal small intestine and the large intestine. These nodules may comprise a significant inflammatory component and may eventually fill with green, eosinophilic pus. Nodules may attain 2–3 cm in diameter and tend to be more pronounced following repeated exposure. Clinical signs, including diarrhoea, often accompany the emergence of the parasites from confinement within the nodules. These parasites prefer warmer conditions, struggling in areas with colder winters.

Chabertia ovina

Ch. ovina is another strongyloid nematode, but in contrast to *Oesophagostomum* spp., *Ch. ovina* has a very large, bell-shaped buccal capsule and is capable of taking a significant bite of the intestinal mucosa. It is therefore considered to be quite pathogenic, but seldom occurs in large numbers. As few as 300 adults may however be enough to cause clinical signs. Disease specifically due to this nematode has been recorded in the winter rainfall areas of Australia and South Africa (Taylor *et al.*, 2007).

Nematode evolution

The oldest known fossil of a nematode is of an insect parasite preserved in 135 million year old amber (Poinar, 2003), but otherwise, as with most small, soft-bodied invertebrates, nematode history cannot be traced through fossil evidence. Nevertheless, researchers have used various tools to hypothesise that the nematodes may date back as long as 1000 million years ago (Hedges, 2002; Meldal *et al.*, 2007; Vanfleteren *et al.*, 1994) and most likely originated in the sulphide-rich sediments present, then and now, at the bottom of all major bodies of water (Bryant, 1994). These benthic deposits are still rich in nematode species today and interestingly share many of the characteristics of the contents of the gastrointestinal tracts of vertebrate animals, being a slurry of organic (and inorganic) material with low oxygen levels. Despite this aquatic ancestry, parasitic nematodes are far more abundant in terrestrial animal hosts than in their marine and freshwater counterparts and the major reason for this is that nematodes, lacking adaptations for swimming, enjoy little contact with the vast majority of pelagic animal species. Nematodes eventually spread to the land, where they have become one of the most abundant organisms in soil. From here, nematodes switched from a free-living existence to a parasitic one, a process thought to have occurred on at least six occasions (Dorris *et al.*, 1999).

Recent reviews of nematode evolution have challenged much of the older classification of nematode taxonomy (Blaxter, 2003; De Ley & Blaxter, 2002, 2004; Hodda, 2007), with a major change affecting the strongylid order, which may now be reduced to the level of superfamily (becoming Strongyloidea) within the order Rhabditida, and the various superfamilies (Trichostrongyloidea, Strongyloidea, etc.) reduced to family level (Trichostrongylidae, Strongylidae). However, since the older nomenclature is commonly used throughout the veterinary literature, this book will continue to reflect the older systematics. The Rhabditida order contains many free-living and microbivorous nematodes and includes one of the most well-studied organisms in biology, *Caenorhabditis elegans* (Dorris *et al.*, 1999; Mitreva *et al.*, 2005), and there are in fact many similarities in morphology and behaviour of the free-living rhabditids and the earlier larval stages of many parasites.

The history of the strongylids as parasites may date as far back as the late Devonian or early Carboniferous (approximately 350 million years), to sometime after the first appearance of amphibians on land (Durette-Desset *et al.*, 1994). The ancestral strongylid parasite was undoubtedly a close relative of a free-living ancestor of contemporary free-livers such as *C. elegans* (Chilton *et al.*, 2006). Pivotal to this origin of strongylid parasitism may have been the relative ease with which the larvae of these newly parasitic forms could penetrate the softer amphibian skin – oral routes of infection evolving only later.

The subsequent history of strongylid evolution is undoubtedly complex, but involved all of the terrestrial vertebrate phyla and rather than following a close path of co-evolution of host and parasite, there have been numerous instances of host-switching, combined with explosive radiations of parasite species taking advantage of radically different new host forms. The evolutionary histories of the nematode fauna of herbivores such as the horses, macropodid marsupials and ruminants offer such examples. The predominant nematode parasites of kangaroos and horses belong to the same superfamily of strongylid nematodes, the Strongyloidea, whereas the dominant parasites of ruminants are trichostrongyloids. Strongyloid parasites of ruminants are nevertheless present in genera such as *Chabertia* and *Oesophagostomum*. The equids, in common with many earlier herbivores (including ruminant ancestors), developed an enlarged caecum as the site for bacterial fermentation of plant material. The development of such a vast digestive organ may have considerably lessened competition between nematode species allowing the great diversification seen in the equine strongyloids (Durette-Desset *et al.*, 1994), and in extant adult equids, the majority of nematode parasites are large intestinal species with much of the rest of the gastrointestinal tract, the small intestine in particular, rather bereft of parasites. In contrast, both the large kangaroo species and the ruminants developed as foregut fermenters with associated changes in anatomy (and an inferred anterior shift in the availability of nutrients) that led to an extensive radiation of nematode species in the stomach and small intestine (Durette-Desset *et al.*, 1994). In the case of the kangaroos, the strongyloid nematodes of the cloacine family were the principal beneficiaries of these profound changes whereas in the ruminants it was the trichostrongyloids which took advantage of the modified niches.

A major contributor to the success of strongylid nematode species was the evolution and spread of the grasses which became widespread in the mid to high planetary latitudes from about 15 million years ago. This period is also associated with a gradual replacement of browsing herbivores by grazing species (Janis *et al.*, 2000). By ingesting herbage closer to the ground and therefore facing more faecal contamination, and because grasses generally support the presence of the free-living stages of nematode parasites to a greater extent than do broadleaf species, grazing animals are typically more exposed to nematode parasitism than are browsers.

The domestication and subsequent movement of livestock has undoubtedly had a major impact on the distribution and prevalence of parasites in these species. Parasites such as *H. contortus*, *H. placei*, *O. ostertagia* and *T. circumcincta* have been transported far beyond the regions where they would have originally evolved. Sheep may first have been domesticated in Mesopotamia, and parasites such as *T. circumcincta* were likely present in their wild ancestors. In contrast, sheep may have become exposed to *H. contortus* only once humans imported them to Africa and into contact with other ruminant species such as antelope (Hoberg *et al.*, 2004).

The transition to parasitism

Of the more than 25,000 recognised species of nematodes, approximately 60% are parasites of plants or animals (De Meeus & Renaud, 2002). The nematodes have thus proven extremely successful in adopting both free-living and parasitic lifestyles. As stated previously, before shifting to parasitic lifestyles, free-living nematodes first successfully adapted to niches in the terrestrial environment. As such they had to develop the ability to cope with highly variable levels of moisture, something that is a major limiter of nematode activity on land. Immediately, one of the benefits, perhaps the most important, of parasitism becomes apparent. In environments prone to drying out, the ability of the host animal to locate water and then conserve it within its own tissues can far exceed those of a small invertebrate. Likewise, the host can be relied upon to be more adept at locating nutrients, presenting nourishment to its resident parasites in the form of either digesta or nutrients already assimilated into host tissues and secretions or held within commensal organisms of the gut microflora. Within the host, nematodes are also (presumably) spared predation by nematophagous organisms, including other nematode species, various metazoans and fungi.

Within the host, parasites also benefit from more stable temperatures. Even within so-called cold-blooded hosts, temperatures will vary less than in the external environment, whilst in avian and mammalian hosts, temperature will vary little. Overall, a parasitic nematode inhabits an environment that is far more stable than do their free-living relatives. The relative protection afforded by the host environment has even allowed parasitic nematodes to become considerably larger than their free-living counterparts (Yeates & Boag, 2006).

Most free-living nematodes are quite small, reaching maximum lengths of only a few millimetres. The small size and simplicity of free-living nematodes is largely a function of the constraints placed on them by the external environment. In moving through the liquid phase surrounding the particulate matter of soil and sediments, both small size and a lack of appendages are favourable physical characteristics. However, removed from these restrictions, some parasites have achieved massive proportions, with the largest nematode ever described (*Placentonema gigantissima*) reaching over 8 m in length in the placentas of whales. A counter-argument to larger size in nematodes being primarily a benefit of parasitism is that it is rather a necessity. Larger females can lay more eggs and this may be an absolute requirement for some nematode species to ensure that at least some of their progeny will encounter and infect a suitable host. *Ostertagia* spp. and *Teladorsagia* spp. in their bovine and ovine hosts, respectively, are arguably amongst the most successful of the world's nematode parasites, despite their smaller size and reputations for being of relatively poor fecundity. This suggests that other factors than egg output *per se* may be far more important in determining the success of a species.

Nematode biology

Morphology

Nematodes are morphologically very similar, sharing a relatively simple body plan, viz. an essentially cylindrical, unsegmented tube. The mouth is terminally situated at the anterior end of the body, whilst the anus emerges on the ventral surface behind the tip of the tale.

The nematode surface

The external surface consists of a collagen-rich cuticle that is secreted by the underlying epidermis (hypodermis). The cuticle is tough and protective, but is known to be permeable to a limited range of molecules such as water and ammonia. The relative inability of the cuticle to stretch and enlarge is thought to be the major reason for moulting during growth, nevertheless some of the larger parasites, such as the ascarids, achieve remarkable rates of elongation even after the final moult. In addition to collagens, the cuticle may contain various other components. The outer surface is usually covered by a glycoprotein-rich surface coat. In addition, the cuticle may also contain water, lipids, various enzymes and haemoglobin-like molecules. As such, the cuticle is very much a 'living tissue'.

Cuticle structure has been shown to vary markedly between different nematode groups. Innervated, finger-like projections (papillae), transverse annulations or longitudinal ridges, wing-like alae and circumferential inflations (dilations) are important features that can be used in the identification of nematode species. For many of the trichostrongyloid nematodes, longitudinal ridges are arranged in a specific pattern known as the synlophe. This is thought to play an important role in allowing nematodes to remain in intimate contact with the mucosal surface.

The composition of the cuticle may also vary according to the life-cycle stage. In adult nematodes, 80% or more of the cuticle may be composed of collagens (Fetterer & Rhoads, 1993), and in a study of expressed sequence tags (ESTs) of (growing) L4 *T. circumcincta*, a large proportion of overall gene expression was for collagens (Nisbet *et al.*, 2008). In free-living stages, the non-collagen protein, cuticlin, is important and probably plays a role in resisting the more noxious environmental conditions (DeGiorgi *et al.*, 1997; Fetterer & Rhoads, 1993). Other studies have identified a number of stage-specific substances. One example is a 35 kDa epicuticular glycan (CarLa) found initially in *T. colubriformis* (Harrison *et al.*, 2003) and subsequently in all of the major GIN species investigated (Shaw, personal communication). CarLa is present in the L3, but not in the L4 or adult stages; neither is the molecule found in *C. elegans*. It is also a major antigen – one of the three surface-associated larval antigens shown to dominate the natural mucosal antibody response directed against the L3 (Maass *et al.*, 2007). In summary, therefore, each parasitic stage – L3, L4, adult – may present a vastly different set of antigenically distinct molecules to the host.

The nematode body

Below the cuticle, the epidermis forms a continuous tube and extends into the interior in four longitudinal cords – two lateral, one dorsal and one ventral. The dorsal and ventral cords contain nerves whereas the lateral cords contain the canals of the excretory system. Beneath the epidermis are longitudinal muscle fibres, arranged in ventral and dorsal blocks.

The internal body cavity of nematodes is described as a pseudocoelom. In many nematodes, but by no means all, the pseudocoelom is fluid-filled and this fluid is under pressure thus providing antagonism to the muscles of the body wall, and contraction of either the dorsal or ventral muscle blocks causes flexion. When the muscles relax, the pressure of the pseudocoelomic fluid allows the worm to then straighten. Contraction/relaxation of the muscles thus produces alternating dorso-ventral flexion allowing nematodes to move in an undulating manner. This basic sinusoidal movement is easily seen in cultured larvae suspended in water, but in more appropriate conditions, e.g. *C. elegans* on the surface of agar, the worms are capable of very fine movements, particularly of the head during feeding, and they can move backwards as well as forwards (Burr & Robinson, 2004).

Maintenance of the pressure of the pseudocoelomic fluid is of great importance to the worms and is thought to be the major role of the nematode excretory system. In the secernentean nematodes, this system comprises the two lateral longitudinal ducts running the length of the body, a transverse duct connecting the two and a further duct connecting the transverse duct to the excretory pore on the ventral surface of the body. This external pore is usually situated anteriorly. In some worm genera, e.g. *Trichostrongylus* spp., the excretory pore is situated in a small depression (notch). Secretory cells may be associated with the excretory system, extending its function beyond just osmoregulation. For example, secreted enzymes may be involved in the extracorporeal digestion of substrates, whilst other substances may be absorbed onto the cuticular surface, contributing to the surface coat.

The gut and feeding

The nematode gut is a straight tube extending from the mouth to the anus. The structure of the mouth is one of the most variable parts of nematode anatomy and is highly adapted to the mode of feeding of individual species/stages. The mouth may be a simple invagination of the cuticle or it may be surrounded by two, three or six lips, or a series of fused sensory papillae (such as the external leaf crown of strongyloid nematodes such as *Oesophagostomum* spp.). The diameter of the oral opening varies considerably; nematodes feeding on fluids, fine particulate matter or bacteria have narrow openings, whereas those feeding on tissues (the plug feeders) have wider mouths. In the case of the latter, this usually gives the anterior end of the worm a blunter appearance rather than a smooth taper, whereas in an organism like *Ch. ovina*, the anterior end is visibly flared. Behind the mouth lies the buccal cavity. In the simple-mouthed trichostrongylids, such as *Ostertagia* spp., *Teladorsagia* spp. and *Trichostrongylus* spp., the buccal cavity is much reduced and the oesophagus (pharynx) begins almost immediately. In *H. contortus*, a 13-µm long and 3-µm wide tooth or lancet arises from the dorsal lining of the buccal cavity. This buccal lancet is used to pierce the vasculature of the host's mucosa to allow blood feeding. In the plug-feeding strongyloids and blood-feeding hookworms, a much broader cavity (capsule) is present that may possess additional adornments such as teeth, gutters and, in the hookworms, cutting plates.

Oral structure can vary between the different stages of the nematode life cycle. Thus the preparasitic, early larval stages of strongylid nematodes have cylindrical buccal cavities adapted for bacterial feeding that are very similar to those of their close relatives, the rhabditids (Figure 1.1).

This rhabditiform arrangement is lost by the (non-feeding) L3 stage. In *H. contortus*, the buccal lancet develops first in the L4 stage, while the relatively shallow, cylindrical buccal capsule found in adult *Oesophagostomum* spp. is different from the more globular (more primitive) version found in the L4.

Behind the mouth is the oesophagus; this muscular structure pumps food into the intestine and as such has to resist the pressure of the pseudocoelomic fluid, which tends to compress the intestine thus resisting filling. A valve is therefore present between the oesophagus and the intestine to prevent regurgitation. The structure and appearance of the oesophagus can vary markedly

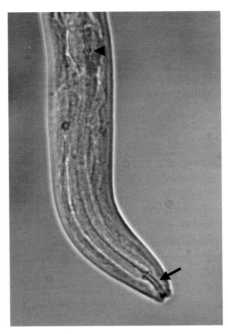

Figure 1.1 The anterior end of a newly hatched L1 *T. circumcincta*. The cylindrical buccal capsule (arrow) and the 'grinder' (arrow head), structures found only in the L1 and L2, are visible. Similar structures can be found in other microbivorous nematodes such as the free-living rhabditid *C. elegans*. Image courtesy of Laura Green and Kevin Pedley.

between different taxonomic groups, but also between different life-cycle stages. For example, adult strongylid nematodes typically have a filariform (from the Latin for thread, *filum*) oesophagus that is relatively straight with only a slight posterior thickening. In others, the posterior swelling is more pronounced and bulb-shaped. In the microbivorous rhabditids, and in the first and second larval stages of strongylid nematodes, the oesophagus is described as rhabditiform and the prominent posterior bulb contains a specialised area – the grinder (Figure 1.1) – in which the cuticle is thickened to allow ingested bacteria to be physically disrupted (Bird & Bird, 1991; Munn & Munn, 2002). In addition to muscle cells, the oesophagus may also contain cells responsible for secreting digestive enzymes.

The intestine consists of a simple epithelial tube, and its cells may be individually discernible or may be arranged in a syncitium. The luminal surface of the cells is covered by prominent microvilli, whilst the outer basal surface bears only a thin basement membrane. The intestinal cells may contain large stores of lipids and proteins: the lipid deposits are very obvious in the L3 of the strongylid nematodes and act as their sole energy supply until they are ingested by a host. Up to 30% of the dry weight of an infective larva may be stored lipid (Bird & Bird, 1991).

Posteriorly, the intestine terminates in the rectum and anus (cloaca in males), where a muscular sphincter is situated to control defecation. Defecation in nematodes can occur surprisingly frequently – every 3–5 min – and can be quite an energetic process with some of the larger ascarids capable of generating (in air) a 60-cm jet of faeces (Bird & Bird, 1991).

The genital tracts of male and female nematodes

Male nematodes are usually smaller than the females, sometimes remarkably so. Most males (all strongylids) have one testis, which is essentially a blind-ending tube terminating at the cloaca. Spermatogenesis is usually confined to the blunt tip of the testis, and mature spermatozoa are stored distally in a more dilated section, the seminal vesicle. The seminal vesicle then merges into the vas deferens, the most terminal part of which is muscular, forming the ejaculatory duct that controls the release of the sperm during copulation. Males typically possess one or two chitinous spicules associated with the terminal portion of the reproductive tract. The spicules are pushed into the vulva of the female during copulation to direct the flow of ejaculate. Usually, but not always, symmetrical, the shape of the spicules varies uniquely according to nematode species and is an important tool in identification. The exception occurs in a small number of species in which different morphological variants of the same species (morphotypes) possess different shaped spicules. A third, usually smaller, chitinous structure, the gubernaculum, may also be present.

A variety of other structures may be associated with reproduction in the male. The tale is usually adorned with sensory papillae and some, e.g. some of the ascarid nematodes, have suckers for attaching to the body of the female. In the strongylid nematodes this function is performed by a very prominent structure, the copulatory bursa – hence the strongylids are sometimes referred to as the 'bursate' nematodes. The copulatory bursa is essentially an expanded area of cuticle forming two lateroventral membranes or lobes with a further dorsal lobe. These structures are strengthened by several integral bursal rays. The dorsal lobe may fuse with the lateroventral ones or be distinct. In the trichostrongyloids, the dorsal lobe is distinct, but is much reduced. The structure of the various lobes and the spacing and patterning of the bursal rays in particular are also important tools used in identification. A homologous structure can be found in male *C. elegans*, and given the relative simplicity of the rest of the body, it is perhaps no surprise that 40% of the cells of a male *C. elegans* are sexually differentiated (Bird & Bird, 1991).

Female nematodes may possess one or two genital tracts, i.e. are monodelphic or didelphic. In didelphic nematodes such as the trichostrongyloids, the two tracts share a common vulva. The position of the vulva may vary considerably. For many trichostrongyloid nematodes the vulva is situated within the mid-portion of the body, but still towards the tail. As a result, one of the two tracts heads anteriorly, whereas the other extends towards the tail – a condition known as amphidelphy. As with the males, meiosis occurs generally at the blind tip of the tract (ovary) adjacent to which is the spermatheca in which spermatozoa are stored after mating. The spermatheca leads to the uterus, which in mature females contains eggs in various stages of development. The number of eggs is another feature that varies between species, larger females producing and storing more eggs. The release of eggs out of the uterus may be control-led by muscular sphincters (the ovejector apparatus). In the strongylid nematodes, these (paired) sphincters are conspicuous and the area between the two sphincters is termed the vagina. The vulva is protected by a cuticular flap in some species – an additional feature used in identification. In some nematodes, the genital tract is entwined around the intestine; this is particularly obvious in *H. contortus*.

The nematode nervous system

The nervous system of *C. elegans* has been extensively studied and is thought to be fairly typical of secernentean worms. Due mostly to its large size, the nervous system of *Ascaris suum* has also been fairly well studied and is broadly similar to that of *C. elegans*. *C. elegans* hermaphrodites have just over 300 neurons in total; males have more (around 380) the bulk of the difference representing the innervation of the copulatory bursa and the 40 or so muscles controlling the tail, spicules and bursa of the male. Despite its much greater size, *A. suum* actually has slightly fewer neurons (about 250).

The nervous system is organised into a number of different ganglia situated mostly in the anterior and posterior ends, and into the dorsal and ventral nerve cords, which run for most of the body length alongside ridges of the epidermis. The larger ventral nerve cord arises from a ring of nerves that surrounds the oesophagus. The somatic musculature is innervated either by the nerve ring (anteriorly) or by motor neurons in the ventral nerve cord. Both the ventral and dorsal muscle blocks are innervated by motor neurons whose cell bodies are wholly within the ventral cord. The dorsal and ventral cords are linked via regular circumferential connections or commissures.

Nematodes possess various sensory structures and are capable of responding to a range of stimuli – chemical, thermal and mechanical, while only a very few nematodes are capable of responding to light. Sense organs are predominantly confined to the cuticle of the anterior and posterior ends (especially in the male), but there are also a number of internal sensory organs as well and the gut is richly endowed with sensory capability.

A large range of chemicals are utilised as neurotransmitters. Acetylcholine, gamma-aminobutyric acid (GABA), glutamate, serotonin (5-HT), and various peptides, especially the FMRFamide-like peptides, have all been demonstrated in nematodes. Other putative neurotransmitters include histamine, nitric oxide (NO) and catecholamines such as dopamine, adrenaline/noradrenaline. The nematode nervous system is the target of several classes of anthelmintic drugs (Chapter 4).

Nematode genetics

One of the fundamental aspects of nematode biology is that despite their relative morphological simplicity, they are in fact genetically and biochemically complex. The completion of the genome project for *C. elegans* revealed a genome size of approximately 100 Mb, representing approximately 20,000 genes, at least half of which may be unique to nematodes (Blaxter, 2003). Comparisons can be made to the estimated 15,000 genes of the fruit fly *Drosophila melanogaster* and the 30,000–40,000 genes of mammals. Work is currently under way to sequence the *H. contortus* genome, which based on flow cytometry results has been estimated at 53 Mb (Leroy *et al.*, 2003). The same technology has been used to estimate the genome of *T. circumcincta* to be slightly larger at 59 Mb. It remains to be seen as to whether the smaller genome sizes of these economically important strongylid parasites are reflected in a smaller number of genes. A smaller genome may simply reflect a reduction in non-coding material. Interestingly, estimates for other nematode parasites reveal much bigger genomes, e.g. 230 Mb for *Ascaris suum* and 350 Mb for the canine hookworm *Ancylostoma caninum* (Abubucker *et al.*, 2008).

Chromosome number in nematodes has been shown to vary quite considerably, from $n = 1$ to 25 (Blaxter, 2000), however, most strongylid organisms examined so far have $n = 6$, as does *C. elegans*, and sex determination is by an XX–XO mechanism (seldom XX–XY), with females having 12 chromosomes in total ($2n$), males 11.

Recent studies show a high level of genetic diversity within populations of various economically important parasite species, likely due to very large effective population sizes (Anderson *et al.*, 1998; Grillo *et al.*, 2007; Prichard, 2001).

Nematode physiology

The mechanisms that nematodes use to generate energy have been shown to vary not just between species, but also between different life-cycle stages. Nematodes utilise aerobic and anaerobic pathways and may switch from one to the other during their development. Aerobic pathways generate more energy (38 moles of ATP for the complete oxidation of 1 mole of glucose, compared to 2 moles of ATP when glucose is fermented to lactate) and allow for the more complete catabolism of carbon skeletons. Lacking a circulatory system and residing in a low oxygen tension environment, nematodes such as the ascarids are too big for oxygen to penetrate interior tissues by diffusion, and thus they respire anaerobically as adults despite being largely aerobic as eggs and earlier larval stages (L1 and L2) (Kita, 1992; Kita *et al.*, 1997). Availability of oxygen is less of a problem for nematodes such as the trichostrongyloids, which are of much smaller diameter and reside much closer to the mucosal surface in an environment with a higher oxygen tensions than that found in the luminal fluid. As a result, nematodes such as *T. circumcincta* and *Nippostrongylus brasiliensis* are likely to be largely aerobic (Fry *et al.*, 1983; Kita *et al.*, 1997; Simcock *et al.*, 2006). Interestingly, *H. contortus* may respire anaerobically, despite its diet of oxyhaemoglobin, fermenting glucose to products such as acetate, succinate and propionate (Roos & Tielens, 1994).

One indication of which pathway is utilised is the main metabolite stored. Anaerobic nematodes/stages tend to store carbohydrate, either as glycogen or as trehalose, whereas aerobic nematodes/stages tend to store lipid.

A number of nematodes have been shown to produce haemoglobin-like molecules – nemoglobins (Blaxter, 1993; Weber & Vinogradov, 2001). Nemoglobins exist in three forms: (1) a monomeric globin domain containing a single haem group found intracellularly in the body wall and oesophageal muscles, (2) a tetramer found extracellularly in the cuticle and (3) an octamer of two-domain subunits also found extracellularly, but in the pseudocoelomic fluid. The intracellular, monomeric nemoglobins may function in a manner similar to mammalian myoglobin, facilitating oxygen capture and usage in the relatively low oxygen tension of the gut. This form may be present in virtually all nematodes including free-livers such as *C. elegans* and its presence has been identified in several strongylid parasites of livestock such as *T. colubriformis* (Frenkel *et al.*, 1992), *O. ostertagi* (DeGraaf *et al.*, 1996), *T. circumcincta* (Nisbet *et al.*, 2008) and, despite its purported anaerobiosis, *H. contortus* (Fetterer *et al.*, 1999). *N. brasiliensis* has the intracellular form and the cuticular form, suggesting that other strongylids may have the cuticular form as well (Blaxter *et al.*, 1994), whereas the larger, pseudocoelomic form has only been detected in the ascarids.

In most parasitic nematodes, expression of the nemoglobin genes increases in the later parasitic stages. Nemoglobins may, however, perform functions other than oxygen utilisation, for example NO detoxification (Barrett & Brophy, 2000), and certainly, although the pseudocoelomic form in *A. suum* binds exceptionally well to oxygen, it does not readily release it, even in a vacuum, and thus likely serves to maintain anaerobic conditions within the nematode rather than facilitate aerobic activity. Possession of nemoglobins is the reason why many nematodes appear reddish in colour e.g. *Ostertagia* and *Teladorsagia* spp., which are sometimes therefore described as the brown stomach worms.

A further reminder of the relative complexity of nematodes is the demonstration of oxidative and reductive pathways that enable nematodes to detoxify harmful chemicals encountered in the host and also in the external environment. Reductive pathways may be more important in parasitic stages given the lower oxygen tensions involved. Indeed, initial attempts to identify oxidative catalysts such as cytochrome P450 were unsuccessful (Barrett, 1997); however, recent experiments suggest that nematodes do possess cytochrome P450 (Kotze *et al.*, 2006). Reductive and hydrolytic pathways are probably more important in the first steps of nematode metabolism (Barrett, 1997), followed by conjugation reactions with glutathione, a reaction catalysed by glutathione transferase. This latter enzyme also plays a role in nematode defence against host-derived reactive oxygen species, alongside superoxide dismutase, catalase and glutathione peroxidase (Callahan *et al.*, 1988).

Interestingly, recent work has suggested that nematode detoxification pathways play some role in allowing the worms to metabolise anthelmintic molecules. Solana and co-workers (Solana *et al.*, 2001) showed that cytosolic and microsomal fractions of *A. suum* were able to sulphoxidate albendazole to the less active sulphoxide; however, only fractions from the trematode *Fasciola hepatica* could oxidise the sulphoxide to the fully inactive sulphone. An additional mechanism that equips nematodes to deal with xenobiotics is the possession of the ATP-binding cassette (ABC) transporters. These molecules actively pump foreign substances out of cells and are well represented in nematodes, including *C. elegans*. *C. elegans* has three families of ABC transporters (Lespine *et al.*, 2008), the P-glycoproteins for which there are at least 14 separate genes, and the HAF and MRP families. Homologues of various *C. elegans* transporters have been found in parasitic nematodes including *H. contortus* and *O. ostertagi*. Recent work has demonstrated that treatment of *H. contortus* with macrocyclic lactone anthelmintics selects the constitutive or inducible overexpression of at least five P-glycoproteins (Prichard & Roulet, 2007).

The dauer larva

In response to adverse environmental factors – declining food availability, increased competition, or desiccation – many free-living nematodes are able to generate an alternate life-cycle stage that is better suited to outlast the period of adversity and resume normal development once conditions improve. This typically involves the development of a third larval stage that is structurally, behaviourally and biochemically distinct from normal L3 (Burnell *et al.*, 2005; Elling *et al.*, 2007). The cuticle of these more 'enduring' (dauer) larvae is modified (is more protective and better able to resist desiccation); the gut is non-functional and movement is usually considerably curtailed. Further development does not proceed whilst conditions remain adverse. Dauer larvae of free-living nematodes also show a pronounced phoretic association with other invertebrates such as dung beetles and use these larger, more mobile organisms as a means of reaching new food supplies. The pathways and processes controlling entry and exit to and from the dauer stage are undoubtedly complex, but include sensory information received as far back as the L1 stage. Such input includes nematode pheromones, which obviously increase in concentration in times of overcrowding.

Many view the infective L3 of GIN as a dauer equivalent and consider the ability to form the dauer stage as an important pre-existing adaptation of free-living nematodes for their eventual transition to parasitism – having a dauer stage facilitating the 'sit and wait' approach necessary for infective stages to persist in the environment prior to encountering and infecting a suitable host. There are however many differences between the true dauer larvae and the infective stages of nematode parasites (Elling *et al.*, 2007), suggesting that the two may have developed independently or that there has at least been considerable divergence in biology since free-livers and parasites last shared a common ancestor.

Anhydrobiosis

Terrestrial nematodes have adapted to cope with highly varying levels of environmental moisture. Obviously, relative humidity is an important factor as it predicts the rate at which soils, faecal material etc. will dry out, but the main variable is the presence or absence of liquid water. As water disappears, nematode activity reduces and they become quiescent; all movement and activity ceases and the worm's tissues begin to dehydrate. For many nematodes, marked water loss proves fatal, although some have developed the ability to survive almost the complete loss of body water (anhydrobiosis). The ability of individual nematodes to undergo anhydrobiosis can be expected to vary widely, with those species that inhabit desiccation-prone environments more likely to evolve this trait than others. Likewise, species vary in their ability to tolerate fast or slow rates of water loss, with the probable majority requiring a slower rate. A slow rate of desiccation is thought to allow nematodes the time to manufacture chemicals such as trehalose and glycerol, which protect membrane integrity in the absence of water. Coiling behaviour helps slow the rate of water loss by reducing surface area, some nematodes aggregating in clumps to achieve the same effect. Likewise, some rely on additional features to slow the rate of desiccation – the presence of the sheath for infective L3 or, for unhatched stages, the eggshell. Several workers have shown that as the cuticles and sheaths of nematodes dry they become less permeable, thus further slowing rates of desiccation (Bird & Bird, 1991).

While anhydrobiotic nematodes are metabolically inactive, recovery from anhydrobiosis can be exceptionally rapid, locomotion returning in as little as 2 hours once liquid water returns.

Lettini and Sukhdeo (2006) examined the ability of four nematode species to undergo anhydrobiosis. Whilst *H. contortus* and *T. colubriformis* L3 could undergo several cycles of desiccation/rehydration, L3 of two rodent strongylids, *Heligmosomoides polygyrus* and *N. brasiliensis*, were killed by a single desiccating event.

The nematode life cycle

Across most nematode groups the life cycle is largely identical, with sexually dioecious adults (occasionally parthenogenic females or self-fertilising hermaphrodites) producing eggs out of which a larval stage emerges that grows via a series of four moults until the adult form is again achieved. Moulting allows the identification of four distinct larval stages (L1–L4). Some texts refer to a fifth larval stage – the L5 – essentially the immature adult, but since no further moult is involved in its further maturation, this term is not used here. Some (plant nematodologists especially) prefer the use of the term juvenile instead of larva, but as pointed out by Bird and Bird (1991) this largely anthropomorphic term has no strict parallel in biology, and by definition, the term juvenile does not implicitly rule out reproductive capability.

Pre-parasitic development

Few nematode parasites can complete their life cycles entirely within the host. Instead, a defined stage of the life cycle will leave the definitive host and pursue further development in the environment, sometimes in one or more additional host species. Development proceeds to another defined life-cycle stage capable of infecting the definitive host. For most strongylid nematodes parasitising livestock, it is the egg, at various stages of development, that exits the host; occasionally, as in lungworms such as *Dictyocaulus viviparus*, it is a newly hatched larva (L1). For most strongylid nematodes, eggs hatch whilst still in the faeces and larval development proceeds as far as the L3. It is this stage that exits the faeces and is infective for the definitive host. For some parasites, the L3 develops within the egg. For this to occur, all of the required nutrients for larval development must have been invested in the egg *in utero*. The L3 may then remain within the egg until the egg is ingested by a suitable host, as occurs with the ascarids, or the L3 may emerge into the environment (e.g. *Nematodirus* spp.). Development of the embryo is fuelled principally by its lipid stores and thus requires oxygen, and levels of dissolved O_2 in gut fluid are probably too low to allow much development before the egg exits the host animal in its faeces. Strongylid eggs appear in freshly voided faeces with the embryo still in the morula stage.

The fully formed L1 may develop in as little as 24 hours and then hatching takes place, presumably once a defined level of development has been achieved. Hatching involves an increase in the permeability of the eggshell, which allows an intake of water into the egg, increased hydration of the L1 and the exit of trehalose out of the egg (Perry, 2002). Emergence of the L1 out of the egg requires the muscular activity that only a fully hydrated larva can generate and is probably assisted by various enzymes including lipases, chitinases and metalloproteinases. In many instances, the eggshell softens prior to hatching and the action of the anterior, or posterior, end of the L1 forces an opening.

At approximately 300-μm long, emerged L1 quickly commence moving and feeding within the faecal material. As stated earlier, the L1 and L2 are both microbivorous, feeding on bacteria present in the faeces.

There are two moults in the pre-parasitic phase of development – the L1 to the L2 and then the L2 to the L3. Moulting is essentially a multi-stage process. After a period of feeding, the larva typically enters a period of inactivity (lethargus). Next, the old cuticle separates from the epidermis (apolysis), which then proceeds to secrete a new cuticle. The next stage (ecdysis) involves rupture of the old cuticle and is followed by the emergence of the subsequent life-cycle stage. Characteristically for many parasitic nematodes, apolysis occurs during the second moult, but ecdysis is delayed, and the larva retains the cuticle of the L2. The L3 is therefore smaller than the L2. For most strongylids the L2 (and hence L3) is between 600 and 1000 μm long.

With its retained sheath, the ensheathed L3 cannot feed and represents a point of arrest in the nematode life cycle – there will be no further development until a host is encountered. The L3 is however still active and begins to migrate away from the faeces into the external environment. The gut of an L3 is non-patent, but the intestinal cells are packed with stored metabolites and are usually clearly visible. The number of intestinal cells can be used to identify the L3 of different species, as can the length of the gap between the tip of the tail of the L3 and the actual termination of the sheath.

With a significant part of the life cycle spent outside the host animal, environmental factors have a major impact on developmental success. Predictably, moisture levels, temperature and the availability of oxygen are the key drivers, affecting not only how quickly eggs hatch and larvae develop, but also how long larvae (and eggs) survive (Chapter 3). In changing from a feeding stage (L2) to the infective stage (ensheathed L3) nematodes change their behaviour dramatically, from actively feeding to migration away from the food source. The factors that trigger this behavioural change are poorly understood, but those that affect its success are better known.

As stated earlier, the presence of liquid water is vital for nematode activity. Free-living larvae move through the fluid phase of the faecal material and once the third larval stage has been achieved, a film of moisture on the surface of the adjacent vegetation is an absolute requirement for migration away from the faeces and onto herbage. The depth of the moisture film, in comparison to the diameter of the nematode, is critical in determining how rapidly nematodes can make progress, too little or too much, and nematode movement slows and eventually stops (Burr & Robinson, 2004). Solid masses of faeces retain moisture even when the adjacent pasture is relatively dry. This plays an important role in facilitating the survival of larvae over shorter dry periods. The hard crust that develops on the dung exterior reduces evaporation, but also prevents larvae from escaping, and mechanical disruption of the faeces may eventually be required to allow larvae to escape. In contrast to normal faeces, watery, diarrhoeic faeces offer little protection against desiccation. Experimentally, nematodes have been shown to be capable of surviving dehydration to a remarkable degree, yet in the field, prolonged desiccation is widely recognised as one of the few phenomena to seriously deplete free-living stages.

Oxygen is required for hatching and larval development. In the solid dung mass, oxygen levels, particularly towards the centre, may in fact be limiting, which slows development. Disruption of the pat increases the availability of oxygen, and in moist and warm conditions, accelerates development. Once the ensheathed L3 has exited the dung, the availability of oxygen increases and is presumably no longer limiting.

At colder temperatures (10°C and below) nematode biology slows dramatically and at some point all development and activity ceases. Within a particular species, genetic variation allows some individuals to be more cold-tolerant – or, conversely, more heat-tolerant – than others, and this allows climate-adapted strains to eventually develop. Experimentally, eggs and larvae remain viable for extended periods at sub-zero temperatures, but survival will eventually be curtailed. Freezing represents the greatest threat, with the formation of ice crystals causing considerable damage to membranes and structures. Nematodes may either be freeze-resistant or freeze-tolerant. Unhatched eggs and some ensheathed L3s may supercool at freezing temperatures, i.e. ice crystals do not form. This is particularly true in the absence of liquid water, which prevents inoculative freezing – the extension of ice crystals by direct contact. The eggshell, and to a lesser extent the extra sheath of infective L3s, can be a barrier to inoculative freezing. Free-living larval stages may achieve a degree of freeze-tolerance by utilising molecules such as trehalose and glycerol as cryoprotectants (Wharton, 2002). Ultimately, however, the more freeze–thaw cycles nematodes undergo, the more likely they are to die.

The optimum temperature for development is generally quoted as being around 25°C. At higher temperatures, metabolic activity increases further, but mortality markedly increases. Thermotolerance has been shown for a number of nematode species (Wharton, 2002) and may be partly mediated by classic heat-shock proteins (HSPs), which can both protect proteins against denaturation and repair damaged proteins. At sub-lethal, warm temperatures, increased activity depletes the stored nutrient reserves of larvae and thus ultimately reduces longevity; the optimum temperature for survival of ensheathed larvae is thus back at around 10°C. The epidemiological significance of the development and survival of eggs to L3 of the major GIN species is discussed in Chapter 3.

The parasitic phase of the life cycle

The parasitic phase of the life cycle can only commence when the L3 encounters the host. For many species, this is a largely passive process – the grazing animal inadvertently ingesting larvae as it feeds. Once in the host, the first step in the transition to the parasitic phase is the completion (ecdysis) of the second moult, i.e. loss of the retained sheath – exsheathment. Exsheathment is triggered by the chemical conditions present in the proximal gastrointestinal tract of the host.

It is generally assumed that exsheathment typically occurs in the part of the gut immediately anterior to the actual site occupied by the adult parasite; thus abomasal parasites exsheath in the rumen, whereas small intestinal species exsheath in the abomasum. However, a considerable proportion of the L3s of small intestinal species may still exsheath in the rumen (Hertzberg *et al.*, 2002). In the rumen, the equilibrium between bicarbonate (HCO_3^-) and carbonic acid (H_2CO_3) at the near neutral pH of rumen fluid, and the relatively high levels of CO_2 are thought to be pivotal to exsheathment. In contrast, in the abomasum, the presence of pepsin/HCl is considered important. As with other moults in the life cycle, exsheathment is an active process involving the activity of enzymes on the cuticle and the physical activity of the larva to achieve egress. A number of enzymes may be contained in the so-called exsheathing fluid secreted by the larva (Lee, 2002). For example, a zinc metalloproteinase has been identified, which attacks a specific annular portion of the sheath of *H. contortus* L3 (Gamble *et al.*, 1989). Its action causes the anterior end of the sheath to break off and the L3 then emerges – other secreted substances may act as lubricants. Amongst the parasite-derived factors influencing exsheathment are eicosanoid metabolites such as leukotrienes (LT). Administration of the lipoxygenase inhibitor diethylcarbamazine to ensheathed L3 of *Oesophagostomum dentatum* caused the complete inhibition of exsheathment (Joachim *et al.*, 2005). This inhibition was reversible by washing or the administration of LT. Exsheathment can be rapidly triggered *in vitro* using solutions of hypochlorite.

Exsheathment generally occurs rapidly and the exsheathed larvae may start to appear in more distal parts of the gut within 24 hours of infection. There is some evidence that persistence of larvae in the rumen for beyond 12–24 hours increases their mortality (Hertzberg *et al.*, 2002).

Upon entering the abomasum, the larvae of species such as *Haemonchus* spp., *Ostertagia* spp. and *Teladorsagia* spp. immediately penetrate into the pits and glands of the mucosa. This may preferentially occur in either the fundic or pyloric areas although in general the fundic mucosa is more frequently targeted. Once confined within the pits/glands the L3 presumably commences feeding, but on what precisely is not known. All undergo at least the next moult to the L4 within this mucosal niche. The L4 of *Haemonchus* is thought to then emerge onto the mucosal surface and completes its development here (Charleston, 1965), whilst *Ostertagia* and *Teladorsagia* spp. remain in the pits/glands to undergo the final moult. Similarly, larvae of small and large intestinal species penetrate into the glands and crypts of the intestines. Some, e.g. *Oesophagostomum* spp., may penetrate through the epithelium to the lamina propria of the submucosa (McCracken & Ross, 1970). This has important immunological considerations since these more invasive larvae arguably expose more of themselves to the host's immune system, whilst the majority of other larvae remain on the other side of the epithelium.

The mucosal phase of development is sometimes referred to as the histotropic or histotrophic phase. These terms suggest a much closer association with the cells of the host than typically occurs and are probably more appropriately applied to the life cycles of parasites such as *Trichuris* spp. and *Trichinella* spp., which do actually penetrate and feed on individual cells.

The reasons GIN enter this mucosal phase are poorly understood. By encysting in the mucosa, larvae may access higher oxygen levels or alternate substrates. Some see mucosal invasion as a relic of the evolutionary past of nematodes, reflecting the ancestral behaviour of nematodes as necessarily migratory following invasion across the skin. An alternative reason may be that by encysting, larvae are able to undergo the lethargus associated with moulting without risking losing their place in the gut; this implies that emerged nematode stages must actively maintain their position and that any reduction in activity, including the paralysis caused by anthelmintics, threatens this. However, the observation that *Haemonchus* is able to undergo the final moult on the mucosal surface must make this open to conjecture.

Hypobiosis

In some circumstances, parasitic development may become arrested. Arrested development (sometimes referred to as inhibited development or hypobiosis) has been defined as *the temporary cessation of development of nematodes at a precise point in early parasitic development when such an interruption contains a facultative element, occurring in certain hosts, certain circumstances or certain times of the year and often affecting only a proportion of the worms* (Michel, 1978). True hypobiosis needs to be carefully distinguished from the apparent delay/interference in development that can manifest as a slower transition between stages or the stunting of eventual adults that can occur when larger numbers of worms are competing for limited resources (Hong *et al.*, 1986) or due to immune interference in development. For many arrest-prone species, but not all, a cessation of growth occurs early in the fourth larval stage, and hypobiotic larvae have little, but variable, metabolic activity. The underlying genetic and physiological mechanisms responsible for parasites either entering or leaving the hypobiotic state are poorly understood. Hypobiosis is discussed more fully in Chapter 3.

Pre-patent periods

The pre-patent period is defined as the time taken from ingestion of larvae/ eggs to when the infection becomes patent, i.e. the first appearance of eggs/ larvae in the host animal's faeces. Given that the conditions parasites encounter in the host are far more stable than those in the environment, development within the host, assuming that the nematodes do not undergo hypobiosis, generally proceeds at a fairly predictable rate and for many of the important GIN, eggs first appear in the faeces of infected animals 2–4 weeks after infection, although for some species, e.g. some *Cooperia* spp., this may occur slightly sooner (Anderson, 2000).

Niches occupied by parasitic nematodes within the vertebrate host

The gut of the vertebrate host consists of numerous niches, which GIN can occupy. In addition to the different organs themselves, there are several available niches within each organ – mucosal tissue, a layer of secreted mucus, and the digesta present within the lumen.

Larger parasites such as the ascarids generally occupy the lumen of the gut. They are better able to resist peristaltic contractions and thus maintain their position in the small intestine. Smaller parasites such as the trichostrongyloids would struggle to do this and if present in the luminal contents would undoubtedly be swept along with the bulk flow of digesta and hence out of their preferred organ and even out of the animal. Instead, the trichostrongyloids are found in much more intimate association with the mucosal surface. Some species such as the abomasal parasites *Teladorsagia* spp., *Ostertagia* spp. and *Haemonchus* spp. can be found within the mucus layer covering the mucosal surface (Figure 1.2).

In contrast, *T. axei* pushes between the epithelial cells of the superficial mucosa and persists in the tunnels it creates.

Interestingly, whilst *Teladorsagia* spp., *Ostertagia* spp. and *Haemonchus* spp. all have obvious synlophes, *T. axei* does not. It may be that the synlophe assists in allowing those nematodes that have it to better embed themselves within the mucus. The mucus layer of the abomasum is, however, of finite

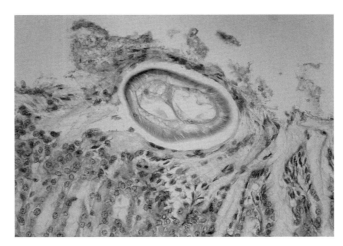

Figure 1.2 Section of abomasal fundic mucosa from a sheep infected with *T. circumcincta*. A cross section of an adult nematode can be seen on the mucosal surface and appears embedded in a tunnel of mucus and cellular debris.

dimensions. Since it is seldom preserved with routine histological methods, there is little information on the depth of the mucus layer within the abomasa of ruminants, but studies in humans have estimated a depth of approximately 100 µm for the basal, firmly adherent mucus layer in the gastric fundus, with a similar depth of loosely adherent mucus above this, and the total mucus depth increases to closer to 300 µm in the human pylorus (Atuma *et al.*, 2001). It is likely that similar dimensions are involved in the ovine and bovine stomach, and thus the depth of the mucus layer is broadly similar to the diameter of the trichostrongyloid nematodes that infest it – effectively the worms are tunnelling within the mucus layer itself. This raises the question of whether larger nematode species could be accommodated at all.

In the small intestine, the other species of *Trichostrongylus*, e.g. *T. colubriformis*, which also lack a synlophe, reside for at least part of their length in tunnels within the epithelium (Figure 1.3), whereas synlophe-bearing genera such as *Nematodirus* and *Cooperia* adopt an entirely different strategy. These nematodes appear to entwine themselves around the villi (Durette-Desset, 1985) using the ridges of the synlophe to grip the villous epithelium, and it is of note that specimens of both *Nematodirus* spp. and *Cooperia* spp. are often visibly coiled when freshly recovered from small intestinal washes.

The different intestinal species also vary in their precise location along the gut with *Trichostrongylus* spp. considered to prefer a more anterior niche in comparison to *Cooperia* spp. or *Nematodirus* spp. (Davey, 1938; Sommerville, 1963; Tetley, 1937). Interestingly, the luminal pH of the anterior small intestine continues to be acidic for some distance away from the pylorus. Eventually, the pH is brought to near normal by the secretion of bicarbonate. Davey (1938) cited pH and the presence of bile salts as two factors influencing predilection sites.

When 30,000 *T. vitrinus* and *T. colubriformis* L3 were co-administered to sheep, *T. vitrinus* preferentially established in the most anterior part of the gut,

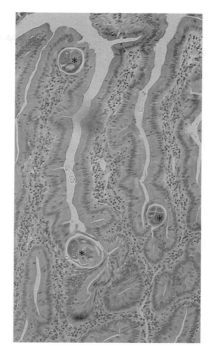

Figure 1.3 Section of proximal small intestine of a goat infected with *T. colubriformis*. Cross sections of adult nematodes (*) can be seen between the epithelial cells of the villi.

displacing *T. colubriformis* posteriorly (Roy *et al.*, 2004). In addition, fewer *T. colubriformis* established, however, at lower larval doses, this competition was not evident. In contrast, when *T. vitrinus*, *T. colubriformis* and *T. rugatus* were co-administered, *T. colubriformis* and *T. vitrinus* did not compete and established in equal numbers in the anterior small intestine, but *T. rugatus* was displaced (Beveridge *et al.*, 1989). In calves infected with *C. oncophora* (Armour *et al.*, 1987), the majority of worms were present in the duodenum, but in at least one animal there was a posterior shift of the population with the bulk of the nematodes in the more distal small intestine, with approximately equal numbers of worms in the jejunum and ileum.

A posterior shift in worm population has also been reported in association with anthelmintic use in instances of anthelmintic resistance. In one study (Bogan *et al.*, 1988) worm counts were performed on sheep infected with *C. curticei*, some of which had been treated with ivermectin. Efficacy of treatment was calculated 7 and 14 days post-treatment at 61 and 90%, respectively. In performing the worm counts, the small intestine had been divided into four equal quarters, and whilst most worms were present in the first half of the gut of the untreated control animals, post-ivermectin, more worms were recovered from the third and fourth quarters. The hypothesis advanced was that the ivermectin successfully paralysed the resistant parasites, which therefore lost their grip of the mucosa and were swept down the gut, but once they had recovered motility, they were able to re-establish contact with the mucosa.

The particular niche occupied by the various species of GIN may ultimately influence which immune responses will be more effective in expelling individual GIN species. Nawa *et al.* (1994) compared the immune expulsion by rats of *Strongyloides* spp., which are burrowing nematodes, and *N. brasiliensis*, a nematode that wraps itself around villi utilising a very well-developed synlophe. Whilst mast cell function was seen as pivotal for expulsion of *Strongyloides* spp., hyperplasia of goblet cells was required for the elimination of *N. brasiliensis*. If similar mechanisms operate in the ruminant small intestine, the immune mechanisms required to expel *Trichostrongylus* spp. may be quite different from those required to deal with *Cooperia* spp.

The lifespan of parasitic nematodes

The lifespan of free-living nematodes such as *C. elegans* is relatively short, most dying within 1–2 months. Temperature has a marked effect on survival with increased lifespan at cooler temperatures (32 days at 16°C vs. 11 days at 25.5°C) (Klass, 1977). Some free-living species, such as the vinegar eels, *Turbatrix aceti*, achieve much longer lifespans. Vogel (1974) maintained *T. aceti* at 15°C for over 200 days, whereas at 30°C this reduced to 70 days. Interestingly, dietary restriction prolongs lifespan in nematodes (Sutphin & Kaeberlein, 2008), whilst reducing fecundity. Thus it might be expected that well-fed parasitic species, kept at the high temperatures of their mammalian hosts, would also be relatively short-lived, yet the longest nematode lifespans recorded are for parasitic species. Human hookworms have been recorded as living for as long as 15 years (Gems, 2002), whereas the filarial parasite, *Dirofilaria immitis*, the canine heartworm, may live as long as 7 years. In contrast, some parasites continue to have fairly short life expectancies. Many of the important GIN species of livestock probably live only for a few months. An important determinant of how long nematodes can persist in the host is, of course, host immunity. Many of the adults of the ascarid parasites are rejected once the host has reached approximately 6–12 months of age even though the host developed the ability to reject or limit the development of newly acquired larvae much earlier. For young grazing ruminants, immunity may not limit the lifespan of some of the first nematodes to establish, but it will certainly eliminate others that are acquired subsequently.

Knowing the lifespan of parasites can be important for several reasons. For example, in the context of the development of anthelmintic resistance, long-lived survivors of a drench may be capable of releasing resistant progeny for a prolonged period. Or, in the case of immune status, an ability to prevent the establishment of the L3 of short-lived parasite species may be relatively more important than removing the mature adults. It remains unclear as to what extent the relative pathogenicity of the individual GIN species determines the length of survival, or indeed how quickly protective immunity may develop. These concepts are discussed in more detail in the subsequent chapters.

References

ABUBUCKER, S., MARTIN, J., YIN, Y. *et al.* (2008). The canine hookworm genome: Analysis and classification of *Ancylostoma caninum* survey sequences. *Molecular and Biochemical Parasitology*, **157**, 187–192.

AGUINALDO, A. M. A., TURBEVILLE, J. M., LINFORD, L. S. *et al.* (1997). Evidence for a clade of nematodes, arthropods and other moulting animals. *Nature*, **387**, 489–493.

AKEN, D. V., VERCRUYSSE, J., DARGANTES, A. P., LAGAPA, J. T., RAES, S. & SHAW, D. J. (1997). Pathophysiological aspects of *Mecistocirrus digitatus* (Nematoda: Trichostrongylidae) infection in calves. *Veterinary Parasitology*, **69**, 255–263.

ANDERSON, R. C. (2000). *Nematode Parasites of Vertebrates: Their Development and Transmission*, CABI Publishing, New York.

ANDERSON, T. J. C., BLOUIN, M. S. & BEECH, R. N. (1998). Population biology of parasitic nematodes: Applications of genetic markers. *Advances in Parasitology*, **41**, 219–283.

ARMOUR, J., BAIRDEN, K., HOLMES, P. H. *et al.* (1987). Pathophysiological and parasitological studies on *Cooperia oncophora* infections in calves. *Research in Veterinary Science*, **42**, 373–381.

ATUMA, C., STRUGALA, V., ALLEN, A. & HOLM, L. (2001). The adherent gastrointestinal mucus gel layer: Thickness and physical state *in vivo*. *American Journal of Physiology-Gastrointestinal and Liver Physiology*, **280**, G922–G929.

BARRETT, J. (1997). Helminth detoxification mechanisms. *Journal of Helminthology*, **71**, 85–89.

BARRETT, J. & BROPHY, P. M. (2000). *Ascaris* haemoglobin: New tricks for an old protein. *Parasitology Today*, **16**, 90–91.

BEVERIDGE, I. & FORD, G. E. (1982). The trichostrongyloid parasites of sheep in South Australia and their regional distribution. *Australian Veterinary Journal*, **59**, 177–179.

BEVERIDGE, I., PULLMAN, A. L., PHILLIPS, P. H., MARTIN, R. R., BARELDS, A. & GRIMSON, R. (1989). Comparison of the effect of infection with *Trichostrongylus colubriformis*, *Trichostrongylus vitrinus* and *Trichostrongylus rugatus* in Merino lambs. *Veterinary Parasitology*, **32**, 229–245.

BIRD, A. F. & BIRD, J. (1991). *The Structure of Nematodes*, Academic Press, San Diego.

BLAXTER, M. (2000). Genes and genomes of *Necator americanus* and related hookworms. *International Journal for Parasitology*, **30**, 347–355.

BLAXTER, M. L. (1993). Nemoglobins – divergent nematode globins. *Parasitology Today*, **9**, 353–360.

BLAXTER, M. L. (2003). Nematoda: Genes, genomes and the evolution of parasitism. *Advances in Parasitology*, **54**, 101–195.

BLAXTER, M. L., INGRAM, L. & TWEEDIE, S. (1994). Sequence, expression and evolution of the globins of the parasitic nematode *Nippostrongylus brasiliensis*. *Molecular and Biochemical Parasitology*, **68**, 1–14.

BLOUIN, M. S., YOWELL, C. A., COURTNEY, C. H. & DAME, J. B. (1997). *Haemonchus placei* and *Haemonchus contortus* are distinct species based on mtDNA evidence. *International Journal for Parasitology*, **27**, 1383–1387.

BOGAN, J. A., MCKELLAR, Q. A., MITCHELL, E. S. & SCOTT, E. W. (1988). Efficacy of ivermectin against *Cooperia curticei* infection in sheep. *American Journal of Veterinary Research*, **49**, 99–100.

BRYANT, C. (1994). Ancient biochemistries and the evolution of parasites. *International Journal for Parasitology*, **24**, 1089–1097.

BURNELL, A. M., HOUTHOOFD, K., O'HANLON, K. AND VANFLETEREN, J. R. (2005). Alternate metabolism during the dauer stage of the nematode *Caenorhabditis elegans. Experimental Gerontology*, **40**, 850–856.

BURR, A. H. J. & ROBINSON, A. F. (2004). Locomotion behaviour. In *Nematode Behaviour* (eds Gaugler, R. & Bilgrami, A. L.), CABI Publishing, New York.

CALLAHAN, H. L., CROUCH, R. K. & JAMES, E. R. (1988). Helminth anti-oxidant enzymes – a protective mechanism against host oxidants. *Parasitology Today*, **4**, 218–225.

CHARLESTON, W. A. G. (1965). Pathogenesis of experimental haemonchosis with special reference to development of resistance. *Journal of Comparative Pathology and Therapeutics*, **75**, 55–67.

CHILTON, N. B., HUBY-CHILTON, F., GASSER, R. B. & BEVERIDGE, I. (2006). The evolutionary origins of nematodes within the order Strongylida are related to predilection sites within hosts. *Molecular Phylogenetics and Evolution*, **40**, 118–128.

CHITWOOD, B. G. (1950). Nemic relationships. In *Introduction to Nematology* (eds Chitwood, B. G. & Chitwood, M. B.), University Park Press, Baltimore.

DAVEY, D. G. (1938). Studies on the physiology of the nematodes of the alimentary canal of sheep. *Parasitology*, **30**, 278–295.

DE LEY, P. & BLAXTER, M. L. (2002). Systematic position and phylogeny. In *The Biology of Nematodes* (ed. Lee, D. L.), Taylor and Francis, London.

DE LEY, P. & BLAXTER, M. L. (2004). A new system for Nematoda: Combining morphological characters with molecular trees, and translating clades into ranks and taxa. *Proceeding of the Fourth International Congress of Nematology*, **2**, 633–653.

DE MEEUS, T. & RENAUD, F. (2002). Parasites within the new phylogeny of eukaryotes. *Trends in Parasitology*, **18**, 247–251.

DEGIORGI, C., DELUCA, F., DIVITO, M. & LAMBERTI, F. (1997). Modulation of expression at the level of splicing of cut-1 RNA in the infective second-stage juvenile of the plant parasitic nematode *Meloidogyne artiellia. Molecular and General Genetics*, **253**, 589–598.

DEGRAAF, D. C., BERGHEN, P., MOENS, L. *et al.* (1996). Isolation, characterization and immunolocalization of a globin-like antigen from *Ostertagia ostertagi* adults. *Parasitology*, **113**, 63–69.

DORRIS, M., DE LEY, P. & BLAXTER, M. L. (1999). Molecular analysis of nematode diversity and the evolution of parasitism. *Parasitology Today*, **15**, 188–193.

DURETTE-DESSET, M. C. (1985). Trichostrongyloid nematodes and their vertebrate hosts: Reconstruction of the phylogeny of a parasitic group. *Advances in Parasitology*, **24**, 239–306.

DURETTE-DESSET, M. C., BEVERIDGE, I. & SPRATT, D. M. (1994). The origins and evolutionary expansion of the strongylida (Nematoda). *International Journal for Parasitology*, **24**, 1139–1165.

ELLING, A. A., MITREVA, M., RECKNOR, J. *et al.* (2007). Divergent evolution of arrested development in the dauer stage of *Caenorhabditis elegans* and the infective stage of *Heterodera glycines. Genome Biology*, **8**, R211.1–19.

FETTERER, R. H. & RHOADS, M. L. (1993). Biochemistry of nematode cuticle – relevance to parasitic nematodes of livestock. *Veterinary Parasitology*, **46**, 103–111.

FETTERER, R. H., HILL, D. E. & RHOADS, M. L. (1999). Characterization of a hemoglobin-like protein from adult *Haemonchus contortus. Journal of Parasitology*, **85**, 295–300.

FRENKEL, M. J., DOPHEIDE, T. A. A., WAGLAND, B. M. & WARD, C. W. (1992). The isolation, characterisation and cloning of a globin-like, host-protective antigen from the excretory–secretory products of *Trichostrongylus colubriformis*. *Molecular and Biochemical Parasitology*, **50**, 27–36.

FRY, M., BAZIL, C. & JENKINS, D. C. (1983). A comparison of mitochondrial electron transport in the intestinal parasitic nematodes *Nippostrongylus brasiliensis* and *Ascaridia galli*. *Comparative Biochemistry and Physiology B-Biochemistry & Molecular Biology*, **75**, 451–460.

GAMBLE, H. R., PURCELL, J. P. & FETTERER, R. H. (1989). Purification of a 44 kilodalton protease which mediates the ecdysis of infective *Haemonchus contortus* larvae. *Molecular and Biochemical Parasitology*, **33**, 49–58.

GEMS, D. (2002). Ageing. In *The Biology of Nematodes* (ed. Lee, D. L.), Taylor and Francis, London.

GRILLO, V., JACKSON, F., CABARET, J. & GILLEARD, J. S. (2007). Population genetic analysis of the ovine parasitic nematode *Teladorsagia circumcincta* and evidence for a cryptic species. *International Journal for Parasitology*, **37**, 435–447.

GRILLO, V., CRAIG, B. H., WIMMER, B. &GILLEARD, J. S. (2008). Microsatellite genotyping supports the hypothesis that *Teladorsagia davtiani* and *Teladorsagia trifurcata* are morphotypes of *Teladorsagia circumcincta*. *Molecular and Biochemical Parasitology*, **159**, 59–63.

HARRISON, G. B. L., PULFORD, H. D., HEIN, W. R., SEVERN, W. B. & SHOEMAKER, C. B. (2003). Characterization of a 35-kDa carbohydrate larval antigen (CarLA) from *Trichostrongylus colubriformis*: A potential target for host immunity. *Parasite Immunology*, **25**, 79–86.

HEDGES, S. B. (2002). The origin and evolution of model organisms. *Nature Reviews Genetics*, **3**, 838–849.

HERTZBERG, H., HUWYLER, U., KOHLER, L., REHBEIN, S. & WANNER, M. (2002). Kinetics of exsheathment of infective ovine and bovine strongylid larvae *in vivo* and *in vitro*. *Parasitology*, **125**, 65–70.

HILTON, R. J., BARKER, I. K. & RICKARD, M. D. (1978). Distribution and pathogenicity during development of *Camelostrongylus mentulatus* in abomasum of sheep. *Veterinary Parasitology*, **4**, 231–242.

HOBERG, E. R., LICHTENFELS, J. R. & GIBBONS, L. (2004). Phylogeny for species of *Haemonchus* (Nematoda: Trichostrongyloidea): Considerations of their evolutionary history and global biogeography among Camelidae and Pecora (Artiodactyla). *Journal of Parasitology*, **90**, 1085–1102.

HODDA, M. (2007). Phylum Nematoda. *Zootaxa*, 1668, 265–293.

HONG, C., MICHEL, J. F. & LANCASTER, M. B. (1986). Populations of *Ostertagia circumcincta* in lambs following a single infection. *International Journal for Parasitology*, **16**, 63–67.

JANIS, C. M., DAMUTH, J. & THEODOR, J. M. (2000). Miocene ungulates and terrestrial primary productivity: Where have all the browsers gone? *Proceedings of the National Academy of Sciences of the United States of America*, **97**, 7899–7904.

JOACHIM, A., RUTTKOWSKI, B. & DAUGSCHIES, A. (2005). Ecdysis of *Oesophagostomum*: Possible involvement of eicosanoids and development of a bioassay. *Parasitology Research*, **95**, 391–397.

KITA, K. (1992). Electron transfer complexes of mitochondria in *Ascaris suum*. *Parasitology Today*, **8**, 155–159.

KITA, K., HIRAWAKE, H. & TAKAMIYA, S. (1997). Cytochromes in the respiratory chain of helminth mitochondria. *International Journal for Parasitology*, **27**, 617–630.

KLASS, M. R. (1977). Aging in nematode *Caenorhabditis elegans* – major biological and environmental factors influencing lifespan. *Mechanisms of Ageing and Development*, **6**, 413–429.

KOTZE, A. C., DOBSON, R. J. & CHANDLER, D. (2006). Synergism of rotenone by piperonyl butoxide in *Haemonchus contortus* and *Trichostrongylus colubriformis in vitro*: Potential for drug-synergism through inhibition of nematode oxidative detoxification pathways. *Veterinary Parasitology*, **136**, 275–282.

LE JAMBRE, L. F. (1995). Relationship of blood loss to worm numbers, biomass and egg production in *Haemonchus* infected sheep. *International Journal for Parasitology*, **25**, 269–273.

LEE, D. L. (2002). Cuticle, moulting and exsheathment. In *The biology of Nematodes* (ed. Lee, D. L.), Taylor and Francis, London.

LEROY, S., DUPERRAY, C. & MORAND, S. (2003). Flow cytometry for parasite nematode genome size measurement. *Molecular and Biochemical Parasitology*, **128**, 91–93.

LESPINE, A., ALVINERIE, M., VERCRUYSSE, J., PRICHARD, R. K. & GELDHOF, P. (2008). ABC transporter modulation: A strategy to enhance the activity of macrocyclic lactone anthelmintics. *Trends in Parasitology*, **24**, 293–298.

LETTINI, S. E. & SUKHDEO, M. V. K. (2006). Anhydrobiosis increases survival of trichostrongyle nematodes. *Journal of Parasitology*, **92**, 1002–1009.

MAASS, D. R., HARRISON, G. B. L., GRANT, W. N. & SHOEMAKER, C. B. (2007). Three surface antigens dominate the mucosal antibody response to gastrointestinal L3-stage strongylid nematodes in field immune sheep. *International Journal for Parasitology*, **37**, 953–962.

MCCRACKEN, R. M. AND ROSS, J. G. (1970). The histopathology of *Oesophagostomum dentatum* infections in pigs. *Journal of Comparative Pathology*, **80**, 619–623.

MELDAL, B. H. M., DEBENHAM, N. J., DE LEY, P. *et al.* (2007). An improved molecular phylogeny of the Nematoda with special emphasis on marine taxa. *Molecular Phylogenetics and Evolution*, **42**, 622–636.

MICHEL, J. F. (1978). Topical themes in the study of arrested development. *Facts and Reflections III. (Workshop on 'Arrested Development of Nematodes in Sheep and Cattle', Centr. Vet. Inst., Lelystad, The Netherlands, 18–19 May, 1978).* 7–17.

MITREVA, M., BLAXTER, M. L., BIRD, D. M. & MCCARTER, J. P. (2005). Comparative genomics of nematodes. *Trends in Genetics*, **21**, 573–581.

MUNN, E. A. & MUNN, P. D. (2002). Feeding and digestion. In *The Biology of Nematodes* (ed. Lee, D. L.), Taylor and Francis, London.

NAWA, Y., ISHIKAWA, N., TSUCHIYA, K. *et al.* (1994). Selective effector mechanisms for the expulsion of intestinal helminths. *Parasite Immunology*, **16**, 333–338.

NISBET, A. J., REDMOND, D. L., MATTHEWS, J. B. *et al.* (2008). Stage-specific gene expression in *Teladorsagia circumcincta* (Nematoda: Strongylida) infective larvae and early parasitic stages. *International Journal for Parasitology*, **38**, 829–838.

PERRY, R. N. (2002). Hatching. In *The Biology of Nematodes* (ed. Lee, D. L.), Taylor and Francis, London.

POINAR, G. (2003). Trends in the evolution of insect parasitism by nematodes as inferred from fossil evidence. *Journal of Nematology*, **35**, 129–132.

PRICHARD, R. K. (2001). Genetic variability following selection of *Haemonchus contortus* with anthelmintics. *Trends in Parasitology*, **17**, 445–453.

PRICHARD, R. K. & ROULET, A. (2007). ABC transporters and beta-tubulin in macrocyclic lactone resistance: Prospects for marker development. *Parasitology*, **134**, 1123–1132.

ROOS, M. H. & TIELENS, A. G. M. (1994). Differential expression of 2 succinate dehydrogenase subunit-B genes and a transition in energy metabolism during the development of the parasitic nematode *Haemonchus contortus*. *Molecular and Biochemical Parasitology*, **66**, 273–281.

ROY, E. A., HOSTE, H. & BEVERIDGE, I. (2004). The effects of concurrent experimental infections of sheep with *Trichostrongylus colubriformis* and *T. vitrinus* on nematode distributions, numbers and on pathological changes. *Parasite-Journal De La Societe Francaise De Parasitologie*, **11**, 293–300.

SARGISON, N. (2004). Differential diagnosis of diarrhoea in lambs. *In Practice*, **26**, 20–27.

SARGISON, N. D., WILSON, D. J., BARTLEY, D. J. & PENNY, C. D. (2007). Haemonchosis and teladorsagiosis in a Scottish sheep flock putatively associated with the overwintering of hypobiotic fourth stage larvae. *Veterinary Parasitology*, **147**, 326–331.

SIMCOCK, D. C., BROWN, S., NEALE, J. D., PRZEMECK, S. M. C. & SIMPSON, H. V. (2006). L-3 and adult *Ostertagia (Teladorsagia) circumcincta* exhibit cyanide sensitive oxygen uptake. *Experimental Parasitology*, **112**, 1–7.

SOLANA, H. D., RODRIGUEZ, J. A. & LANUSSE, C. E. (2001). Comparative metabolism of albendazole and albendazole sulphoxide by different helminth parasites. *Parasitology Research*, **87**, 275–280.

SOMMERVILLE, R. I. (1963). Distribution of some parasitic nematodes in alimentary tract of sheep, cattle and rabbits. *Journal of Parasitology*, **49**, 593–599.

SUTPHIN, G. L. & KAEBERLEIN, M. (2008). Dietary restriction by bacterial deprivation increases life span in wild-derived nematodes. *Experimental Gerontology*, **43**, 130–135.

TAYLOR, M. A., COOP, R. L. & WALL, R. L. (2007). *Veterinary Parasitology*, Blackwell Publishing, Oxford.

TETLEY, J. A. (1937). Distribution of Nematodes in the small intestine of the sheep. *New Zealand Journal of Science and Technology*, **18**, 805–817.

VANFLETEREN, J. R., VAN DE PEER, Y., BLAXTER, M. L. *et al.* (1994). Molecular genealogy of some nematode taxa as based on cytochrome c and globin amino acid sequence. *Molecular Phylogenetics and Evolution*, **3**, 92–101.

VOGEL, K. G. (1974). Temperature and length of life in *Turbatrix aceti*. *Nematologica*, **20**, 361–362.

WALLER, P. J., RUDBY-MARTIN, L., LJUNGSTROM, B. L. & RYDZIK, A. (2005). The epidemiology of nematode parasites of sheep in Sweden, with particular reference to overwinter survival strategies. *Svensk Veterinartidning*, **57**, 11–20.

WEBER, R. E. & VINOGRADOV, S. N. (2001). Nonvertebrate hemoglobins: Functions and molecular adaptations. *Physiological Reviews*, **81**, 569–628.

WHARTON, D. A. (2002). Nematode survival strategies. In *The Biology of Nematodes* (ed. Lee, D. L.), Taylor and Francis, London.

WINTER, M. D. (2002). *Nematodirus battus* 50 years on – a realistic vaccine candidate? *Trends in Parasitology*, **18**, 298–301.

WINTER, M. D., WRIGHT, C. & LEE, D. L. (1997). The effect of dexamethasone on resistance of older lambs to infection with *Nematodirus battus*. *Journal of Helminthology*, **71**, 133–138.

YEATES, G. W. & BOAG, B. (2006). Female size shows similar trends in all clades of the phylum Nematoda. *Nematology*, **8**, 111–127.

ZARLENGA, D. S., HOBERG, E. P., STRINGFELLOW, F. & LICHTENFELS, J. R. (1998). Comparisons of two polymorphic species of *Ostertagia* and phylogenetic relationships within the ostertagiinae (Nematoda: Trichostrongyloidea) inferred from ribosomal DNA repeat and mitochondrial DNA sequences. *Journal of Parasitology*, **84**, 806–812.

2 Pathophysiology of nematode infections

The adverse effects of gastrointestinal nematode (GIN) parasites on productivity are diverse. As stated in Chapter 1, parasitic infection is generally of greatest importance in young animals reared at pasture. Parasitism affects both feed intake and feed utilisation, and its major impact is therefore on growth rates. Reductions of liveweight gain in growing stock have been recorded as being as high as 60–100% (Abbott *et al.*, 1986; Fox *et al.*, 1989a; Sykes & Coop, 1976, 1977; Sykes *et al.*, 1977), yet actual weight loss can occur in severe clinical disease. The impact of parasitism can however extend beyond interference in musculoskeletal growth. The production of wool and milk and reproductive performance may also be affected (Fernandez-Abella *et al.*, 2006a; Sanchez *et al.*, 2004; Steel *et al.*, 1982). Evidently, the adverse effects of parasitism extend to the activities of adult, immune stock as well as those of the young, naïve animal. Severe clinical parasitism can result in sick, moribund animals some of which will die, often despite anthelmintic treatment. For the rest of the flock or herd, chronic, subclinical parasitism is the norm, even in the face of regular prophylactic use of anthelmintics. The question can be posed as to when animal performance in pastoral systems is ever maximal. The cost of failure to control parasites should be measured not just in terms of productivity but also in the well-being of animals, parasitism representing a significant threat to animal welfare.

Are parasites always harmful?

There has been considerable debate concerning how harmful parasites can afford to be in the context of host–parasite co-evolution (Ewald, 1995). For parasites such as the GIN of livestock, a prevailing view was that they should have as little effect on host health as possible – a weakened host would be more vulnerable to predation, thus prematurely curtailing parasite activity (egg output). A counter argument can however be made that slightly more aggressive parasites can out-compete more benign individuals, if for instance, they are able to convert more of the host's resources into the production of their own progeny. This is particularly relevant for shorter lived parasites, for which host longevity offers less advantage.

In general, grazing ruminants and their GIN parasites appear to have reached an acceptable balance which enabled survival and growth of both host and parasite; this however has almost certainly been upset by the intensification of modern pastoral agriculture. In modern farming enterprises, livestock are host to far higher worm burdens than prior to domestication.

Movement of animals, changes in farming practices and land-use have also resulted in the exposure of host animals to previously unknown species. This may result in the development of a more adverse host–parasite relationship. As an example, *Oesophagostomum venulosum* and *Oe. columbianum* are both known to occur in sheep, and the biology of such closely related parasites must be broadly similar, yet the former is relatively non-pathogenic, whereas *Oe. columbianum* is known to provoke the development of a severe inflammatory response. The likely explanation is that sheep have only more latterly acquired *Oe. columbianum* as a parasite – other ruminant species being the natural hosts – and its more severe pathology is indicative of a less well adapted host–parasite relationship (Stewart & Gasbarre, 1989). When host switching occurs, an element akin to serendipity operates and the new parasite may not prove all that harmful. For example, when the camelid parasite, *Camelostrongylus mentulatus*, crossed into sheep, the sheep acquired a parasite that appears no more pathogenic than is *Teladorsagia circumcincta*, with which *Camelostrongylus mentulatus* can be considered to compete for the same niche (Hilton *et al.*, 1978).

Defining 'harm'

The cost of parasitism to an animal can be considered as the sum of the effects of all parasite species and stages present. This is particularly pertinent in grazing livestock, which are typically infected with a broad range of nematode (and non-nematode) parasites, present in more than one organ. Disease can thus be referred to as parasitic gastroenteritis (PGE), reflecting the presence of numerous species in the abomasal (gastric) and enteric compartments. Nematodes are however known to vary considerably in terms of pathogenicity, and in some instances, one organism dominates the clinical picture allowing conditions such as ostertagiosis in cattle and haemonchosis in both cattle and sheep to be recognised as distinct clinical entities.

The cost of infection is also the sum of the direct and indirect effects of parasites and parasitism. Direct effects principally relate to the parasite's metabolic requirements, which are met in total by the host in one form or another. It must be borne in mind however that as (ectothermic) invertebrate organisms, the metabolic rate of nematode tissue should, gram per gram, be far below that of their warm-blooded mammalian hosts, and for most livestock

GIN species, parasite biomass is negligible in comparison to the host; this implies that disease is seldom likely to result solely from competition for nutrients. Nevertheless, it is recognised that some nematodes, e.g. *Haemonchus* spp. have higher requirements and thus exact a higher direct cost. Other nematodes, such as *Chabertia ovina* and the hookworms (e.g. *Bunostomum* spp.) are also recognised as being directly damaging and burdens need not be that great to threaten the life of the host.

In contrast, the indirect effects of parasitism arise not so much from nematode activity, but from their mere presence, and stem principally from the host's response to invasion and its adverse consequences. Of particular significance is the inflammation that develops within the gut. Innate and, later, adaptive immune and inflammatory processes arise once the presence of the invader is recognised, but unfortunately, many of these responses have damaging effects on the host's own tissues. Inflammation and immunity can appear inextricably linked and diverse cell types, inflammatory mediators and protective mechanisms are involved (see Chapter 12). This is not to imply that inflammation itself is necessarily protective, since pronounced inflammation can occur in the absence of effective immunity, but as a general rule, immunity almost invariably involves some degree of inflammation. As an example, the eosinophil has well-described anti-parasite effects yet also has a prominent role in inflammation (see later).

Whilst worm biomass is still an important predictor of the magnitude of indirect damage, a second element now becomes very important – host responsiveness. Hosts vary in how strongly they react to the presence of pathogens. Whilst some appear to react less and may thus appear 'tolerant' of parasite presence (i.e. 'resilient') – others may be more reactive and consequently suffer more severe disease (Chapter 11). Some animals – those most susceptible to both the parasites themselves and their effects – struggle to mount effective immune responses and thus can harbour larger burdens for prolonged periods of time, consequently suffering marked and ongoing inflammation.

Those animals that mount effective immune responses appear divided into two groups: (1) those that reject parasites efficiently and thus suffer less and (2) those whose anti-parasite responses, though effective, incur a greater measure of self-harm. There is reasonable experimental evidence that these various host 'responder' types do exist (Bisset *et al.*, 2001), at least in sheep, and the explanation most likely lies in the balance of pro-inflammatory and protective responses mounted by the host. Whilst animals tend to utilise the same range of mechanisms, the magnitude of the contribution of the individual components may vary considerably. The concept of host responsiveness is very important in any consideration of resilience/resistance (see Chapter 11).

For many of the trichostrongyloid parasites affecting livestock, the bulk of the harm caused arises indirectly. This applies to parasites such as *Ostertagia ostertagi*, *T. circumcincta* and *Trichostrongylus colubriformis*. Whilst each may have some direct effects (e.g. damage caused by the physical emergence of *Ostertagia/Teladorsagia* from nodules in the abomasal mucosa), the harm arising indirectly almost certainly predominates (see later). Likewise, whilst a parasite like *Haemonchus contortus* can have significant direct effects (related to blood loss), this worm is also capable of indirectly affecting the physiology of the abomasum in a manner similar to *Ostertagia/Teladorsagia* spp.

As stated in the previous chapter, the different stages of the nematode lifecycle can be biochemically, and hence antigenically, distinct. In a primary infection of previously parasite-naive animals, with parasites such as O. *ostertagi* and *T. circumcincta*, there appears little response to the presence of L3 other than some localised changes affecting glands occupied by larvae. The bulk of the pathology and organ dysfunction arises later in conjunction with the L4 and then with adult stages. This at least in part may reflect the relatively small biomass of L3, but over time, the host can become more responsive to L3, and in 'sensitised' animals, more severe pathology can arise following ingestion of L3 (see later).

Since the structure and function of the various organs of the GI tract vary markedly, parasitism of each will be considered separately.

The abomasum

The ruminant abomasum functions similarly to the stomachs of monogastric species but with some important differences. This organ produces four main exocrine secretions – hydrogen ions, pepsinogen, mucus and digestive lysozyme. In contrast to monogastric species, in which acid secretion occurs temporarily, the abomasal contents of (parasite-free) ruminants are maintained at a low pH (between 2 and 3, sometimes less) at all times of the day. The secretion of the other digestive elements is also thought to be at a fairly constant rate. Pepsinogen is a zymogen (an inactive precursor) and is converted at low pH to the active proteolytic enzyme pepsin. Pepsin is however known to have greatest efficacy against proteins of animal origin such as collagen and is most important as a digestive enzyme in animals in which mastication is limited or absent (Hersey, 1987). It is perhaps no surprise therefore that some studies have shown marked variation in the production of pepsinogen by sheep, with some animals appearing to secrete very little (Scott *et al.*, 1998b, 1999). In contrast, one of the major adaptations made by ruminants to a fully herbivorous lifestyle is the adoption of lysozyme as a digestive enzyme. This is not unique to ruminants but has been observed in a small number of other, leaf-eating species, such as langur monkeys and the hoatzin (a bird) (Dobson *et al.*, 1984; Ruiz *et al.*, 1994; Stewart *et al.*, 1984, 1987). Lysozymes are a group of enzymes that disrupt the peptidoglycan molecules present in the cell walls of gram-positive bacteria. Most animals possess a single lysozyme gene, and the enzyme is present in a variety of secretions, e.g. tears and saliva, in which the function of the lysozyme is protective, i.e., to lyse bacteria before they have time to colonise the epithelial surface. Ruminants, however, have multiple digestive lysozyme genes and these are expressed in the abomasum. These lysozymes are adapted to function at a lower pH (approximately 5) and are resistant to peptic activity. By using digestive lysozymes, ruminants can better tap into the nutrients, otherwise trapped within bacteria exiting the rumen.

The last major component of exocrine secretion is mucus. Secreted mucin molecules, buffered by bicarbonate, form a gel-like layer on the mucosal surface that serves as an important barrier preventing autodigestion of the underlying mucosa by the other exocrine secretions, in ruminants much as it does in other species. The mucus layer is the major niche in the abomasum for parasites like *Ostertagia* spp. and *Teladorsagia* spp. (Chapter 1).

In the fundic mucosa, the surface epithelium invaginates into a number of pits. From the base of the pits arise usually two or three blind-ending tubular glands which penetrate deeper into the mucosa. The pits and the mucosal surface predominantly comprise cells that secrete mucus (NB, in the bovine, the surface mucous cells have also been shown to secrete pepsinogen), whilst a broader range of cells exists in the glands. Higher up in the neck region of the gland are the mucous neck cells, cells that can secrete both mucins and pepsinogen and are therefore considered to be relatively immature. The neck also contains some of the acid-secreting parietal cells. Parietal cells may also be found in the mid-region and base of the glands, but the activity of the deepest cells may be less than that of those higher up. The other main cells of the gland base are the chief cells and the endocrine cells. The chief cells are the major source of pepsinogen whilst endocrine cells release histamine and have a major input into the activity of parietal cells. The pylorus has a roughly similar structure but lacks chief and parietal cells; its cells predominantly produce mucins but some pepsinogen as well (Scott *et al.*, 1999). Less work has been done to ascertain which cells secrete lysozyme, but since mucins and pepsinogen occupy the same granules in mucous cells, mucous neck cells and chief cells, it is feasible that the same granules contain lysozyme as well.

Ostertagiosis has been characterised as a hyperplastic gastritis (Murray *et al.*, 1970), with important changes occurring in the epithelial cell populations described above – in parallel with a pronounced inflammatory reaction. Similar changes occur in teladorsagiosis in sheep (Armour *et al.*, 1966; Scott *et al.*, 1998a, 2000) and in some instances in haemonchosis, particularly when large doses of infective larvae have been given experimentally to sheep (Bueno *et al.*, 1982b; Christie, 1970; Nicholls *et al.*, 1987; Simpson *et al.*, 1997). The numbers of mature parietal and chief cells are generally reduced, and the number of cells with a mucous cell phenotype is increased. Mucous cell hyperplasia (sometimes referred to as metaplasia) initially occurs focally, affecting pits and glands adjacent to the one occupied by the developing larva – although the hyperplasia subsequently becomes more generalised – presumably triggered in response to the presence of the adults on the mucosal surface. The earlier focal changes are seen as small, raised, pale nodules on the mucosal surface (Figure 2.1).

Frequently, the centre of the nodule is depressed giving an umbilicated appearance that is indicative of the hyperplasia being confined to the adjacent glands and not the one occupied by the larva. The umbilicated appearance however intensifies once the larva emerges and the dilated gland it once occupied collapses.

At the same time that some parietal cells are lost, the activity of any remaining cells may be severely reduced, and overall, the pH of the abomasal contents rises to near neutral. Following single infections with larvae, this major

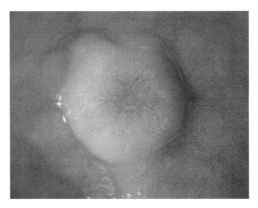

Figure 2.1 Nodule present on the surface of the fundic mucosa of a sheep infected 10 days previously with *T. circumcincta*. Approximately 5 mm across, the nodules form via the penetration of gastric glands by an L3, followed by hyperplasia of the surrounding pits and glands. The centre of the nodule is depressed, leading to an umbilicated appearance.

elevation in pH seems to occur at around the time that the nematodes emerge from their confinement within the gastric glands. The precise timing may vary, with pH rising later, around 20 days after infection, in calves infected with *O. ostertagi* (Jennings *et al.*, 1966) in comparison to lambs infected with *T. circumcincta* (Lawton *et al.*, 1996; Scott *et al.*, 1998a, 2000), reflecting the earlier emergence of *T. circumcincta*, just after the final moult as early as 8 days after infection. In contrast, *H. contortus* emerges and pH rises even earlier, soon after the moult to the L4, approximately 2–4 days after infection (Charleston, 1965; Nicholls *et al.*, 1987). After remaining elevated for a variable period, pH gradually returns to normal, and in many studies of teladorsagiosis, the recovery of abomasal secretion is underway by the time eggs appear in the faeces.

Elevated abomasal pH is also a characteristic feature of field infections and has been observed in both cattle, in both Type I and Type II ostertagiosis, and in sheep (Anderson *et al.*, 1965). Clearly, field infections involve the gradual intake of infective larvae in contrast to inoculation with a single dose, but it can be reasonably assumed that the severity of the pH change and the associated pathology will vary according to the level of the accumulated burden and individual variation in responsiveness. Elevated pH is not classically associated with clinical cases of haemonchosis (Charleston, 1965), but in heavier infections, some derangement of abomasal function is certainly demonstrable (Simpson *et al.*, 1997).

Other abnormalities occur roughly in parallel with elevated pH. The serum concentrations of gastrin and pepsinogen increase, whilst serum albumin levels are generally lowered (McKellar, 1993). Gastrin is secreted by G-cells in the pyloric mucosa and has an important role in the regulation of acid secretion, principally by affecting histamine release by endocrine (Enterochromaffin-like [ECL]) cells in the fundus. For a long time, the primary cause of increased serum gastrin concentrations was assumed to be the failure of the parietal cells to secrete acid; however, the concentrations of gastrin observed during infection can be far in excess of what would be seen if the abomasal contents were simply alkalinised. Inflammation in the pyloric tissue may play a much greater role (Weigert *et al.*, 1996) by directly stimulating gastrin release from G-cells.

Increased serum pepsinogen concentrations have long been associated with increases in vascular and epithelial permeabilities (Armour *et al.*, 1966; Jennings *et al.*, 1966; Murray, 1969), i.e., pepsinogen is thought to 'leak' into the vasculature. However, it has been shown that elevated serum levels can persist beyond the period of demonstrable leakage of other macromolecules such as albumin (Holmes & Maclean, 1971). Some have argued therefore that pepsinogen may be released by chief cells directly into the circulation. There is some evidence to suggest that this could take place, since calves treated with omeprazole (a parietal cell inhibitor) developed a hypergastrinaemia in response to suppression of parietal cell activity, and also developed elevated blood pepsinogen concentrations, due presumably to the effect of higher gastrin levels on chief cells, but without any attendant increases in permeability (Fox *et al.*, 1989b).

In some studies, elevated serum pepsinogen concentrations developed even when other parameters of abomasal function, such as abomasal pH or serum gastrin levels, remained relatively unchanged (McKellar *et al.*, 1987; Scott *et al.*, 2000). Conversely, pepsinogen concentration may remain low as other parameters increase (Coop *et al.*, 1977; Hertzberg *et al.*, 2000; Lawton *et al.*, 1996; Simpson *et al.*, 1997). An explanation for the latter observation almost certainly lies in the marked variation in pepsinogen production, mentioned earlier. Animals that produce little of the enzyme will have little available for uptake into the circulation.

The production of pepsinogen, by animals that produce it in reasonable amounts, continues during parasitism, despite the decline in the number of mature chief cells. Pepsinogen has a short half-life as can be seen in the many studies in which elevated levels drop rapidly, e.g. after drenching (Scott *et al.*, 2000) or treatment with the anti-muscarinic drug atropine (Mostofa & McKellar, 1989) and elevated levels imply continuity of secretion. Pepsinogen has been localised immunohistochemically to the hyperplastic mucous cell population that replaces the normal gland cells (Scott *et al.*, 1999).

Previous work has shown that the transfer of adult *T. circumcincta* into the abomasa of previously parasite-naive sheep rapidly results in increases in abomasal fluid pH and increases in the serum concentrations of gastrin and pepsinogen (Anderson *et al.*, 1985; Lawton *et al.*, 1996; Scott *et al.*, 2000). Similar results have been observed with transplants of adult *O. ostertagi* in cattle (McKellar *et al.*, 1986, 1987), and adult *H. contortus* in sheep (Simpson *et al.*, 1997). These findings suggested that the effects of parasitism might be mediated directly by chemicals (excretory/secretory products or ES) released by the parasites themselves. Support for this argument was seen by the demonstration that immersion of the parasites in a solution of low pH rapidly results in their death (Eiler *et al.*, 1981; Simpson *et al.*, 1999) and at face value it seems reasonable to suggest that the nematodes may directly increase abomasal pH to enhance their survival.

The results of studies into a role for ES in inhibiting parietal cell activity are equivocal at best. Eiler *et al.* (1981) successfully inhibited *in vivo* acid secretion by rat stomachs using a somatic extract of *O. ostertagi*. In a later study, *H. contortus* ES inhibited the activity of dispersed rabbit gastric glands (Merkelbach *et al.*, 2002), but at least in this experiment, the effect could largely be attributed to the concentration of ammonia present in the ES (presumably as the nematode's main nitrogenous waste product). The same thing occurred when *T. circumcincta* ES was tested using the same methodology (Scott, unpublished). One major difficulty associated with establishing the effect of ES on acid secretion has been the failure to develop a successful *in vitro* methodology using bovine or ovine tissue/cells. Dispersed ovine gastric glands, prepared using the standard methodology for preparing viable and responsive rabbit glands, proved too poorly responsive to allow any meaningful investigation of potential ES effects (Merkelbach *et al.*, 2002).

Extrapolation of *in vitro* studies to the situation in the intact animal should, however, always be made with caution. In *in vitro* experiments, ES may gain access to cell receptors that ordinarily they are prevented from reaching – the apical membranes of the epithelial cells of the gastric glands having been shown to be highly and unusually impermeable to a variety of agents (Waisbren *et al.*, 1994). Obviously, any increase in epithelial permeability caused by inflammation would alter this, but one can question what role is left for ES to play in an organ already badly affected by an inflammatory response. Likewise, any suggestion that ES can have a selective cytotoxic effect on parietal cells can be tempered by the observation that ES in some studies promoted the growth and division of some epithelial cell types rather than any loss (Huby *et al.*, 1995).

Ostertagiosis is similar to several other gastric diseases with widely differing aetiologies – any insult to the stomach tends to result in reduced output of acid and an increase in mucus secretion. This suggests that the observed cellular and physiological changes represent a host mechanism that is not necessarily specific for parasites. One common factor in many of these diseases is the presence of inflammation. The failure to secrete acid can therefore be viewed as one of the cardinal signs of inflammation, namely 'loss of function'. In fact, there is ample evidence that any increase in the pH of the abomasal contents is actually deleterious to parasite survival. Following single infections with larvae, rapid loss of worms coincides with the period of maximally elevated pH (Murray *et al.*, 1970). When pH returns to more normal levels, further worm loss is curtailed. In cattle that received transplants of adult *O. ostertagi* and in which pH did not increase, the majority of the transplanted worms could still be found 2–3 weeks later (McKellar *et al.*, 1986). By pharmacologically increasing abomasal pH using the H_2-receptor antagonist cimetidine, Hall and Oddy (1984) achieved the complete elimination of all resident *H. contortus* and about 80% of *T. circumcincta*, although a direct anthelmintic action for cimetidine could not be ruled out.

What may be happening is that as abomasal pH increases, the parasites are encouraged to leave the mucus layer and move into the luminal contents (Figure 2.2).

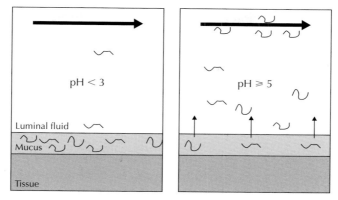

Figure 2.2 Diagram to represent the hypothesis concerning the effect of pH on the distribution of abomasal nematodes such as *T. circumcincta*. The box on the left represents a normally functioning abomasum in which the pH of the luminal contents is less than 3, and in which the majority of nematodes are confined to the mucus layer covering the mucosa. In the box on the right, the pH has risen due to hyposecretion of acid and more worms leave the mucus and enter the contents (small arrows), but may as a result be ejected from the organ along with the bulk flow of digesta (large arrow).

Unfortunately, once here, they are very likely caught in the bulk flow of digesta and may be rapidly ejected. This was illustrated in the study of Hertzberg *et al.* (2000), who examined acid secretion in six sheep fitted with abomasal cannulae and infected with *Ostertagia leptospicularis*. Although based on data from a limited number of animals and at one time-point (18 days post-infection), there was an extremely strong correlation ($R^2 = 0.93$, $P = 0.0019$ – our analysis, not theirs) between abomasal pH and the number of worms recovered in abomasal fluid samples.

Further evidence of the influence of pH on worm distribution was seen in a recent comparison of two groups of sheep, both infected with *T. circumcincta*, but with one group immunocompromised by the administration of dexamethasone. When pH was elevated (mean 5.1), approximately 50% of the worms were recovered from the luminal contents, whereas in the steroid-treated group, in which pH remained more normal (mean 2.8), the vast majority (80%) of the population was found to be closely adherent to the mucosal surface (Scott, unpublished). There was no overall difference between the total worm burdens of the two groups, but since the animals were killed just after worm emergence had taken place, it can be argued that although the worms were in the process of moving out of the mucus layer, into the contents, they had not been in their new location long enough to have been expelled; it is noted that it took several days of elevated pH in response to cimetidine treatment for the worms to be expelled in the study of Hall and Oddy (1984). In the infected, non-steroid-treated animals, there was increased expression of the pro-inflammatory cytokine interleukin-1beta (IL-1β) (Scott, unpublished) – IL-1β being the most potent known inhibitor of acid secretion by parietal cells (Robert *et al.*, 1991). In contrast, the steroid-treated sheep that maintained abomasal acidity had lower levels of IL-1β expression.

This suggests that any inhibitors of acid secretion are more likely to be of host, rather than parasite origin.

The small intestine

The small intestine is divided anatomically into the (anterior) duodenum, (middle) jejunum and (posterior) ileum. One significant characteristic of the duodenum is the presence of mucus-secreting sub-mucosal glands (Brunner's glands). These glands disappear in the jejunum, where the villi also tend to be longer. In the ileum, there are a number of unencapsulated lymphoid nodules, or Peyer's patches, in the mucosa. Along the length of the intestine, the majority of the epithelial cells covering villi are specialised absorptive cells (enterocytes), amongst which are interspersed mucus-secreting goblet cells.

About 20% of the total digestion of the organic material contained in pasture-based diets occurs in the small intestine. As in monogastric species, the small intestine is an important site for protein digestion in ruminants. For pasture-fed ruminants, protein leaving the rumen is a mixture of dietary proteins that were not degraded by microbial action in the rumen, and microbial proteins; between the two, they represent approximately two-thirds of ingested protein, with the majority of the rest being broken down into ammonia, the bulk of which is converted to urea and eliminated in urine. There is little carbohydrate digestion in the ruminant small intestine – what little does take place being of polysaccharides of microbial origin.

The distal small intestine is probably more important for the digestion and absorption of proteins, since the acidic conditions in the proximal gut are unsuitable for the activity of many of the proteolytic enzymes secreted by the intestinal cells and the pancreas. Eventually, secretion of bicarbonate brings pH up to a point at which these enzymes (and abomasal lysozyme) can function.

The majority of GIN living in the small intestine preferentially occupies the most anterior 3–6 m, the duodenum and the anterior portion of the jejunem (Barker, 1975b; Rahman & Collins, 1990; Sommerville, 1963) and typically, the pathology triggered by parasite presence is confined to the parasitised section.

The pathology is broadly similar across a range of worm species and generally consists of villous atrophy – villi become stunted, sometimes club-shaped or absent altogether – combined with hyperplasia of the crypt glands (Barker, 1973, 1975a; Beveridge *et al.*, 1989; Garside *et al.*, 2000). At the same time, there is usually an increased cellularity of the lamina propria, as inflammatory and immune cells infiltrate the mucosa. In heavy infections (e.g. following doses of 100,000 L3s of *T. colubriformis* or *T. vitrinus*), in addition to the complete loss of villi, there may also be areas of erosion of the residual epithelium, *T. vitrinus* causing more severe lesions (Beveridge *et al.*, 1989).

A number of mediators have been implicated in the development of pathology in the small intestine, including NO and the neurotransmitter substance P(SP). In mice deficient in the enzyme inducible NO synthase (iNOS), infection with *Trichinella spiralis* failed to trigger the development of significant pathology (Lawrence *et al.*, 2000). Immunoneutralisation of SP, or use of a specific SP receptor antagonist, limited pathology in *T. spiralis*-infected mice (Agro & Stanisz, 1993; Kataeva *et al.*, 1994). These results reinforce the role of the host response as being responsible for much of the damage caused by the presence of parasites.

The large intestine

About 10–15% of the total digestion of the consumed feed occurs in the large intestine (caecum and colon) of ruminants, and there is additional microbial fermentation, accounting for about 10% of total volatile fatty acid (VFA) production. Absorption of water is also an important function of the large intestine.

Many parasites of the hindgut preferentially occupy the caecum and proximal colon. Parasite presence is usually associated with inflammation of the caecal mucosa (typhlitis) and/or colon (colitis), and mucosal changes are similar to those observed in the stomach, with hyperplasia of epithelial cells usually prominent. The feeding behaviour of many large intestinal parasites, *Ch. ovina* for example, tends to be more directly damaging than that of abomasal and small intestinal species. Likewise, the presence and emergence of larvae of e.g. *Oesophagostomum* spp. can be associated with damage and inflammation of varying severities. The emergence of these larvae creates a defect in the intestinal mucosa, which may allow penetration of bacteria into the tissues, exacerbating parasite-induced inflammation. In pigs, a direct correlation has been shown between the presence of the invasive parasite *Trichuris suis* and colitis caused by the bacterium *Campylobacter jejuni* (Abner *et al.*, 2002).

The impact of parasites on overall gut function

Infection with GIN causes a variety of pathophysiological effects in and outside the gut, the summation of which is that the infected animal enters a state of relative protein deficiency (Stear *et al.*, 2003). This fact is supported by the observation that disease can generally be alleviated by feeding supplementary protein (Chapter 10). The major factor affecting performance is the anorexia associated with parasitism (Fox, 1993, 1997; Greer, 2008; McKellar, 1993; Sykes, 1994). In many studies, reductions in voluntary food intake account for the majority (up to 90%) of the difference in weight gain between infected and worm-free animals. The extent of the anorexia can vary considerably, but shows a general relationship to worm burden, and in some circumstances animals can be completely anorexic. At lower levels of parasitism, reduced feed intake may be the only major clinical feature of infection. In addition to anorexia, animals also show reduced feed conversion efficiency – the inability to efficiently utilise the nutrients that they consume. This reduced ability to utilise nutrients stems not just from impaired digestion, but also from changes in the animal's overall metabolism (see below). In terms of interference in digestion and absorption, the effects of parasitism were summarised by Hoste (2001) as follows.

- Reduced absorptive area due to loss of mature villi.
- A decrease in absorptive capacity of remaining enterocytes, especially, as many are now immature.
- A reduction in enzyme activities, particularly of brush-border enzymes.
- Reduced contact time between digesta and mucosa.

Diarrhoea is one of the main clinical findings in ostertagiosis in cattle (both type I and type II disease), and in PGE in sheep. In the latter species, particularly when wool of significant length is present, this can lead to a build up of faecal material known as breech soiling or dags (Figure 2.3).

Not only are dags a visible sign of worm infections, but can result in an increased incidence of blowfly strike (Morris, 2000). It is noted that breech soiling is not recognised as typically occurring in haemonchosis. Experimentally, diarrhoea has been observed in calves with primary infections of *O. ostertagi* (see below), but is not typically seen in similar studies of *T. circumcincta* in sheep, although the pelleted faeces of sheep may soften.

The exact causes of diarrhoea in GIN parasitism remain poorly understood. In gastrointestinal infections in ruminants, the marked reductions in feed intake that can accompany parasitism may in fact reduce the rate of passage of ingesta in the gut. This was seen in calves infected with *O. ostertagi* (Fox *et al.*, 1989a) and would appear to mitigate against the likelihood of diarrhoea developing. In contrast, in sheep infected with *H. contortus*, there was an increase in flow rate in the duodenum that was associated with increased faecal water (Bueno *et al.*, 1982a).

In calves infected with *O. ostertagi*, Jennings *et al.* (1966) demonstrated increases in the numbers of viable aerotolerant bacteria in the abomasal

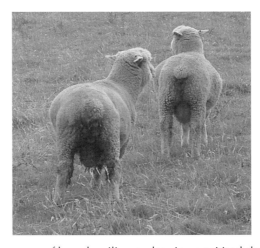

Figure 2.3 The appearance of breech soiling or dags in parasitised sheep.

contents at the time when pH was elevated and linked this finding with the appearance of diarrhoea at about the same time. Other studies have also observed increases in bacterial numbers, particularly of anaerobes, in the abomasa of *H. contortus-* or *T. circumcincta*-infected sheep (Nicholls *et al.*, 1987; Simcock *et al.*, 1999), but make no mention of animals becoming diarrhoeic.

Palmer and Greenwood-Van Meerveld (2001) reviewed a lot of the data from studies in laboratory animal species with respect to the potential for neuroimmune modulation of gut function during enteric parasitism. There is *in vitro* and *in vivo* evidence of altered propulsive behaviour in nematode-infected gut caused in part by altered functioning of the enteric nervous system (ENS). These changes can result in short- and long-term changes in neuromuscular function leading to enhanced net oral–anal propulsion of digesta. Increases in the mass of smooth muscle layers are common and can occur in the presence or absence of marked inflammatory responses. There is also a significant interaction between the ENS and cells of the immune/inflammatory response. Stead and co-workers (Stead *et al.*, 1991, 1987) demonstrated an increased number of mast cells lying in direct contact with enteric neurons, and mast cell products may stimulate nerve activity directly (Wang *et al.*, 1995). The longitudinal muscle of rat intestine may make abnormally exaggerated responses to normal agonists during the enteric phase of infection with *T. spiralis*, but this hypercontractile state does not develop in athymic rats, indicating that the mechanism is T-cell dependant. In contrast, circular muscle may enter a state of hypocontractility. Increases in fluid-propelling activity were seen at an earlier stage of the infection in jejunal segments from immune guinea pigs secondarily challenged with *T. spiralis* (Alizadeh *et al.*, 1989).

In non-ruminant, animals, a striking feature of myoelectric activity in the interdigestive period is the migrating myoelectric complex (MMC). The MMC controls the stereotypical behaviour of the fasting gut, sweeping cellular debris and residual digesta distally, and controlling the bacterial flora (Szurszewski, 1969). In ruminants, the MMC is uninterrupted by feeding, unlike in monogastric species, and therefore maintains an almost continuous passage of digesta along the intestine (Grivel & Ruckebusch, 1972). In dogs and rats infected with *T. spiralis*, the MMC were severely disrupted. Atypical, rapidly propagating myoelectric events supervened that explained, at least partly, the accelerated transit of digesta. This abnormal myoelectrical activity was accompanied by net intestinal water and electrolyte secretion (Lee *et al.*, 1997; Palmer *et al.*, 1984; Schanbacher *et al.*, 1978). Athymic rats infected with *Nippostrongylus brasiliensis* had elevated basal rates of ion secretion, indicating that T-cell independent mechanisms are also involved (McKay *et al.*, 1995). In sheep experimentally infected with *T. axei* and *Ch. ovina*, disturbances of myoelectrical activity in the gut accompanied the onset of diarrhoea approximately 3 weeks after infection (Bueno *et al.*, 1975). In general, myoelectric disturbances appear to correlate with a range of clinical signs including vomiting, the sensation of pain, diarrhoea and anorexia.

Some studies have examined the possibility that parasite secretions may directly affect gut function. *N. brasiliensis* adults release a 34 kDa protein capable of mimicking the physiological effects of mammalian vasoactive intestinal polypeptide (VIP), an important transmitter in the ENS. This parasite-derived VIP-like molecule reduced the frequency and amplitude of contractions of isolated intestinal segments from uninfected rats (Foster & Lee, 1996). These findings support the hypothesis of biological 'holdfasts', whereby parasites seek to diminish the chances of their expulsion by reducing the muscular activity of the host's gut. Similar roles have been suggested for the morphine produced by *Ascaris suum* (Goumon *et al.*, 2000) and the acetylcholinesterases produced by many nematode parasites, including *T. colubriformis* and *Nematodirus* spp. (Huby *et al.*, 1995, 1999). More recent views of the activity of these substances, however, favour roles in regulation of epithelial growth and permeability, immunomodulation or the nematodes' own internal signalling pathways rather than as holdfasts (Hoste, 2001; Palmer & Greenwood-Van Meerveld, 2001).

Compensatory mechanisms may ameliorate the impact of parasitism in a confined area of the gut. Other, usually more distal, non-parasitized parts of the gut offer considerable reserve capacity. Villous hypertrophy has been demonstrated in the ileum of infected rabbits and sheep (Hoste *et al.*, 1988, 1993; Roy *et al.*, 1996), and overall increases in the length of the intestine have been recorded as well (Scofield, 1980; Singhvi & Crompton, 1982). In abomasal infections of previously parasite-naive lambs with *T. circumcincta*, there were marked increases in the wet weights of abomasa (Scott *et al.*, 1998a). Whilst hypertrophy of the mucosa and tissue oedema account for at least some of this increase, a marked increase in overall organ size in infected animals is readily apparent to anyone comparing an abomasum from a parasite-naive animal with one from an infected lamb (Figure 2.4).

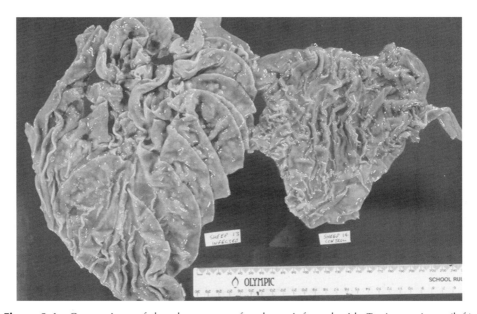

Figure 2.4 Comparison of the abomasum of a sheep infected with *T. circumcincta* (left), with that of an uninfected control animal (right) showing the marked increase in organ size caused by the presence of the parasites. Image: Courtesy of W. Pomroy.

A limitation on this reserve capacity for digestion is that expression of certain specific enzymes/carriers may be restricted to particular regions of the gut (Hoste, 2001), yet evidence points to a considerable reserve of secreted and brush-border enzymes such that enzyme function and absorptive area are not the main limiters of animal performance during parasitism.

Inflammatory lesions in the gut are associated with loss of plasma proteins. Likewise, it must be remembered that haematophagous parasites consume plasma, as well as red blood cells. Plasma losses of 90 ml and 500 ml per day were reported respectively in sheep and calves infected with *T. circumcincta* or *O. ostertagi* (Parkins & Holmes, 1989). Bremner reported plasma losses of 1300 ml per day in calves infected with the large intestinal parasite *Oesophagostomum radiatum* (Bremner, 1969) and similar levels were reported in calves infected with the relatively non-pathogenic *Cooperia oncophora* (Armour *et al.*, 1987), although losses in the uninfected control animals in this latter study (700 ml per day) were higher than might be expected for unexplained reasons. Evidence suggests that much of this lost protein can be recovered in the distal gut, but for that lost in infections in the large intestine, some of it may inevitably hit the ground in faeces. Declines in plasma protein concentration can manifest in some instances as oedema and ascites; sub-mandibular oedema or 'bottle-jaw' being a commonly reported clinical finding in cases of haemonchosis and Type II ostertagiosis especially (Taylor *et al.*, 2007).

Steroid-treatment of lambs infected with both *T. colubriformis* and *T. circumcincta* reduced the extent of appetite suppression, but did not prevent loss of albumin into the gut (Vaughan *et al.*, 2006); however, the authors of this study did not show whether steroid-treatment had been completely effective in abrogating the host immune response. Further loss of protein into the gut is in the form of secretions, especially mucus, and sloughed epithelial cells. Likewise, the hypertrophy, of muscle layers and of the mucosae, and the proliferation of immune and inflammatory cells all occur at the expense of other tissues. In summary, the gut becomes a nutrient (protein) sink, critically diverting resources from other metabolic activities – e.g. growth, lactation, wool production and reproduction. In one study of sheep infected with *T. colubriformis*, the infected gut sequestered an extra 24% of available leucine (Yu *et al.*, 2000).

Effects beyond the gut

During GIN infections, the effects of parasitism extend beyond the gut to affect multiple body systems. The anabolic activities of the liver and immune system in particular, are increased, whilst the rates of synthesis of new tissues in the musculoskeletal system, namely bone and muscle, and the bone marrow, are typically reduced (Colditz, 2008; Fox, 1993; Greer, 2008; Holmes, 1985; Hoste, 2001; McKellar, 1993; Sykes & Coop, 1977). Metazoan cells require growth signals, e.g. interleukins, somatotrophins and insulin, to regulate their uptake of nutrients, suggesting some measure of central control. Interestingly, in general inflammatory states, cells become resistant at a molecular level to the anabolic effects of a range of mediators and hormones and this results in decreased nutrient utilisation by a variety of somatic tissues. This tends to suggest that the effects of infection spill over from the gut to affect diverse body systems, but that nutrient deprivation *per se* is only partially involved. The production of a range of hormones involved with growth and metabolism has been examined during parasitism, but with no clear picture yet emerging (McKellar, 1993).

An impairment of bone growth can be attributed to reduced deposition of calcium and phosphorus. This may be mediated in part by reduced serum phosphate concentrations; reductions of up to 50% having been observed in *T. colubriformis*-infected sheep (Greer, 2008). Of potentially greater significance is the role of cytokine-stimulated osteoclast activity – osteoporosis being a common extra-intestinal manifestation of inflammatory bowel disease in humans (Ardizzone *et al.*, 2008; Tilg *et al.*, 2008). Conjecturally, the reduced erythropoiesis manifest in infections, leading to some degree of anaemia even in the absence of haematophagous parasites – may be triggered similarly by 'overspill' of pro-inflammatory cytokines from the inflamed gut, rather than simply being the result of a dearth of nutrients.

Effects on adult stock

The extra-intestinal effects of parasitism are particularly seen in adult stock. Adult cattle and sheep are skeletally mature; this fact and their more complete immunity to parasites led to the general assumption that they were largely free of any adverse consequences of parasitism. There is however a reasonable amount of evidence suggesting that the activities of adult animals, particularly the production of milk and reproductive performance, may be impaired. The results of earlier studies into the effect of parasites on milk production in dairy cows were largely equivocal, some studies suggesting responses to treatment, while others not (Sanchez *et al.*, 2004). The commonest way of studying parasitism in adult dairy cattle has been to apply anthelmintic treatment to part of a herd and compare milk production between treated and untreated animals. Earlier studies utilised a variety of anthelmintic products, many of which were relatively short-acting, and because of problems with milk withholding times, many studies involved application of treatment in the dry period. With the advent of nil milk withholding times for a number of macrocyclic lactone (ML) products (e.g. eprinomectin), a number of recent studies have applied these products early in lactation, usually at calving, and more consistent increases in milk production have been recorded. Two recent meta-analyses have been conducted that calculated the benefit of treatment of lactating cattle at 0.63 kg milk/cow/day (Gross *et al.*, 1999) and 0.35 kg milk/cow/day (Sanchez *et al.*, 2004). These figures represent an average derived from all the studies considered and are likely to be underestimates since they include a lot of the earlier trial work – a consideration of only those trials that used MLs in early lactation would likely yield a higher figure.

At least part of the production response can be explained by the observation that treated animals may graze for longer and have reduced idling times (time spent neither grazing nor ruminating)(Forbes *et al.*, 2004, 2007). Although another study failed to demonstrate similar changes in grazing behaviour (Gibb *et al.*, 2005), increases in milk production were still present suggesting that at least part of the increase in milk yield was due to improved digestive efficiency.

Similarly, a number of studies have demonstrated effects of parasitism on reproductive performance. In ewes infected with *T. circumcincta* (Jeffcoate *et al.*, 1988), ovulation rates were lower but did not translate into reduced reproductive performance. In a similar study (Fernandez-Abella *et al.*, 2006b), lower numbers of developing follicles in challenged ewes did not subsequently translate into lower numbers of *corpora lutea*. In contrast, in a second study, the same authors (Fernandez-Abella *et al.*, 2006a) observed reduced ovulation rates, increased embryo losses and subsequent reduced fecundity in ewes challenged with *H. contortus* L3. Recently, calved heifers treated with eprinomectin exhibited shorter calving to conception intervals, and more became pregnant at the first post-calving insemination (McPherson, 2000).

Since parasites do not establish in large numbers in adult animals, with the exception of the periparturient period in sheep, these studies clearly demonstrate the cost to productivity of maintaining anti-parasite immunity. The cost to an adult sheep of maintaining immunity in the face of parasite challenge has been estimated at 15% of productivity (Sykes, 1994). In adult cattle, a significant correlation has been observed between the amount of anti-*Ostertagia* antibody in milk measured by ELISA and the magnitude of the response to ML treatment at calving (Charlier *et al.*, 2007). This adds further support to the involvement of immune processes in suppressing productivity.

Anorexia

The exact cause of anorexia in parasitism remains elusive. The potential roles of a number of mediators, e.g. gastrin, cholecystokinin and leptin, have been examined, but no firm conclusions can be drawn other than suggesting at least some role for some of the mediators. Reasonable support for a role of gastrin in suppressing appetite was seen in calves treated with omeprazole (Fox *et al.*, 1989b). The calves developed a hypergastrinaemia and had food intakes reduced by 40%. In a study of lambs infected with *T. circumcincta*, animals suffered elevated abomasal pH and increases in the serum concentrations of gastrin, and were also anorectic (Simcock *et al.*, 1999). There was a weak correlation between serum gastrin concentration and inappetance; however, the correlation between abomasal pH and inappetance was slightly stronger. This suggests that whatever drives the increase in pH may also be responsible for both increases in gastrin and anorexia. Whilst gastrin could conceivably play some role in the anorexia associated with abomasal parasitism, it is unlikely to be involved with purely enteric infections.

Evidence for an immune/inflammatory basis for anorexia can be seen in immunosuppression experiments in which corticosteroid-treated sheep maintain more normal intakes (Greer *et al.*, 2005). One can question therefore whether the anorexia of parasitism is just a manifestation of normal sickness behaviour. The classic components of sickness behaviour are fever, anorexia and depression. Sickness behaviour represents a set of highly conserved responses made by a host following invasion by pathogenic organisms and manifests most classically following invasion by viruses and bacteria (Dantzer, 2004; Johnson, 2002; Konsman *et al.*, 2002). Sickness behaviour is usually an acute phase response to invasion and has host-protective function, at least in the short term – animals that are allowed to become pyrexic or anorexic being more likely to survive. These changes represent motivated behaviour since affected individuals in a sense are choosing to be fevered, to not eat and to reduce physical activity. They are not just passive responses, i.e. an animal too physically weak to eat.

In sensing the presence of nematodes in the gut, animals may be reacting in a highly conserved fashion by becoming anorexic. The problem stems not from recognising nematode presence, but, unlike the situation with most viral and bacterial invaders, the failure of the immune system to rapidly clear the nematode infection means that the stimulus for the development of anorexia is ongoing. Anorexia thus becomes chronic in duration much as it does with certain other chronic conditions, the consumption of tuberculosis – the cachexia of neoplastic disease.

Three pro-inflammatory cytokines are thought pivotal to sickness behaviour, interleukins 1-beta and 6 and tumour necrosis factor-alpha (TNF-α). As referred to earlier, increased expression of IL-1β has been associated with nematode parasitism (Khan & Collins, 1994; Li *et al.*, 1998, 2007). Although fever is not traditionally recognised as a clinical sign in parasitism, the reason for this may lie in the balance of expression of the various pro-inflammatory cytokines. In sheep infected with *T. circumcincta*, the increased expression of IL-1β appeared to be in considerable excess of both IL-6 and TNF-α (Scott, unpublished). The observation that IL-1β is pivotal for the development of an efficient anti-parasite immune response (Helmby & Grencis, 2004) offers at least some explanation as to why immune animals frequently appear to suffer negative impacts – perhaps a little IL-1β is beneficial, but too much can have deleterious effects.

Eosinophils and GIN disease

Eosinophils are a hallmark of inflammation stimulated by metazoan parasites, and they almost certainly evolved in vertebrate animals as a means of combating and eliminating such parasites, yet their presence in tissues is almost invariably associated with harmful consequences. Eosinophils have been shown to produce a range of agents that could adversely affect the function and survival of host tissues (Behm & Ovington, 2000; Rothenberg & Hogan, 2006; Rothenberg *et al.*, 2001). The damaging role of eosinophils in diseases such as asthma is well established (Hamelmann & Gelfand, 2001; Rothenberg & Hogan, 2006).

One interesting observation concerning the influx of eosinophils in disease is their distribution in tissues. In animals given a primary infection, the majority of cells remain confined to the region of the mucosa closest to the muscularis and therefore at some distance from the parasites that attracted them. This has been observed in infections of sheep with *H. contortus* (Balic *et al.*, 2000) and with adult and larval *T. circumcincta* (Scott *et al.*, 2000, unpublished) and suggests that in previously parasite-naive animals, eosinophils are recruited into tissues, but seem unable to directly attack the parasites. Whether they are still active in these circumstances remains to be seen, but in one experiment, large numbers of infiltrating eosinophils were associated with quite significant sub-mucosal oedema (Scott, unpublished). In animals with prior experience of parasitsm, eosinophils appear much more directed and have been implicated in killing newly encysted *H. contortus* L3 (Balic *et al.*, 2002, 2006), while *in vitro*, in the presence of antibody, eosinophils caused significant mortality of *H. contortus* L3 (Rainbird *et al.*, 1998).

Figure 2.5 shows a section of abomasal mucosa from a sheep that had been 'immunised' by a series of sub-cutaneous injections of *T. circumcincta* L3s. The animal was subsequently given an oral dose of larvae and was killed 48 hours later. As can be seen, there is a pronounced eosinophilic infiltrate surrounding the L3, and there also appears to have been a marked hyperplastic response in the mucosa in general.

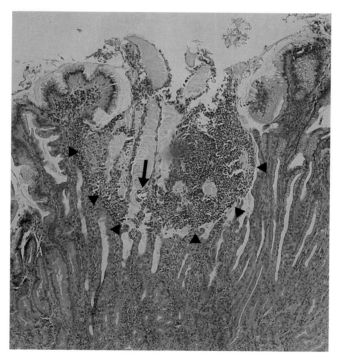

Figure 2.5 A section of abomasal mucosa from a sheep given a series of sub-cutaneous injections of *T. circumcincta* L3s. The animal was subsequently given an oral dose of larvae and was killed 48 hours later. A section of an L3 can be seen in the tissue (arrow) and is surrounded by large numbers of eosinophils (arrowheads). There is also a marked hyperplasia of the surrounding glands.

The exact mechanism underlying eosinophil recruitment remains unresolved. The rapidity of eosinophil influx in formerly parasite-naive animals – as early as six hours after the transplant of adult *T. circumcincta* (Scott unpublished) – may provide evidence for the *in vivo* activity of an eosinophil chemotactic factor similar to that identified for *O. ostertagi* (Klesius *et al.*, 1985) and recently demonstrated *in vitro* for *T. circumcincta* (Wildblood *et al.*, 2005). Alternatively, the signal for eosinophil invasion may be host-derived, through the involvement of mast cells, epithelial cells, or complement (Behm & Ovington, 2000; Kagnoff & Eckmann, 1997; Meeusen & Balic, 2000). Eosinophilia, in primary infections at least, may represent a pronounced innate response – a response more typically associated with parasitic infection of unnatural or non-permissive hosts (Meeusen & Balic, 2000). Is this further evidence that the host–parasite relationship has been abnormally skewed, with marked pathology following exposure of animals to far higher burdens than they are used to?

Further insight into the damaging role of eosinophils comes from the study of winter scours in Merino sheep in south-eastern Australia (Larsen & Anderson, 2000; Larsen *et al.*, 1994, 1995, 1999). In areas with high-winter rainfall, persistent diarrhoea and breech soiling has been observed in a sub-set of ewes in winter and spring and is associated with a 'hypersensitivity' response to high intakes of trichostrongylid larvae off pasture. All ewes are fully immune since patent infections do not establish, but only a proportion scour. One difference between those that do scour and those that do not is the presence of large numbers of eosinophils in the tissues of the former. Those that do not scour are thought to have rejected incoming larvae straight away, possibly involving anti-parasite factors present in mucus (see Chapter 12), but in scouring animals, the larvae have been able to penetrate the tissue triggering eosinophil invasion (Balic *et al.*, 2006).

References

ABBOTT, E. M., PARKINS, J. J. & HOLMES, P. H. (1986). The effect of dietary protein on the pathogenesis of acute ovine haemonchosis. *Veterinary Parasitology*, **20**, 275–289.

ABNER, S. R., HILL, D. E., TURNER, J. R. *et al.* (2002). Response of intestinal epithelial cells to *Trichuris suis* excretory-secretory products and the influence on *Campylobacter jejuni* invasion under *in vitro* conditions. *Journal of Parasitology*, **88**, 738–745.

AGRO, A. & STANISZ, A. M. (1993). Inhibition of murine intestinal inflammation by anti-substance P antibody. *Regional Immunology*, **5**, 120–126.

ALIZADEH, H., WEEMS, W. A. & CASTRO, G. A. (1989). Long term influence of enteric infection on jejunal propulsion in guinea pigs. *Gastroenterology*, **97**, 1461–1468.

ANDERSON, N., ARMOUR, J., JARRETT, W. F. H., JENNINGS, F. W., RITCHIE, J. S. D. & URQUHART, G. M. (1965). A field study of parasitic gastritis in cattle. *Veterinary Record*, **77**, 1196–1204.

ANDERSON, N., HANSKY, J. & TITCHEN, D. A. (1985). Effects on plasma pepsinogen, gastrin and pancreatic-polypeptide of *Ostertagia* spp. transferred directly into the abomasums of sheep. *International Journal for Parasitology*, **15**, 159–165.

ARDIZZONE, S., PUTTINI, P. S., CASSINOTTI, A. & PORRO, G. B. (2008). Extra-intestinal manifestations of inflammatory bowel disease. *Digestive and Liver Disease*, **40** (Suppl 2), S253–S259.

ARMOUR, J., JARRETT, W. F. H. & JENNINGS, F. W. (1966). Experimental *Ostertagia circumcincta* infections in sheep – Development and pathogenesis of a single infection. *American Journal of Veterinary Research*, **27**, 1267–1278.

ARMOUR, J., BAIRDEN, K., HOLMES, P. H., PARKINS, J. J., PLOEGER, H., SALMAN, S. K. & MCWILLIAM, P. N. (1987). Pathophysiological and parasitological studies on *Cooperia oncophora* infections in calves. *Research in Veterinary Science*, **42**, 373–381.

BALIC, A., BOWLES, V. M. & MEEUSEN, E. N. T. (2000). The immunobiology of gastrointestinal nematode infections in ruminants. *Advances in Parasitology*, **45**, 181–241.

BALIC, A., BOWLES, V. M. & MEEUSEN, E. N. T. (2002). Mechanisms of immunity to *Haemonchus contortus* infection in sheep. *Parasite Immunology*, **24**, 39–46.

BALIC, A., CUNNINGHAM, C. P. & MEEUSEN, E. N. T. (2006). Eosinophil interactions with *Haemonchus contortus* larvae in the ovine gastrointestinal tract. *Parasite Immunology*, **28**, 107–115.

BARKER, I. K. (1973). Scanning electron microscopy of duodenal mucosa of lambs infected with *Trichostrongylus colubriformis*. *Parasitology*, **67**, 307–314

BARKER, I. K. (1975a). Intestinal pathology associated with *Trichostrongylus colubriformis* infection in sheep – Histology. *Parasitology*, **70**, 165–171

BARKER, I. K. (1975b). Location and distribution of *Trichostrongylus colubriformis* in small intestine of sheep during prepatent period, and development of villous atrophy. *Journal of Comparative Pathology*, **85**, 417–426.

BEHM, C. A. & OVINGTON, K. S. (2000). The role of eosinophils in parasitic helminth infections: Insights from genetically modified mice. *Parasitology Today*, **16**, 202–209.

BEVERIDGE, I., PULLMAN, A. L., PHILLIPS, P. H., MARTIN, R. R., BARELDS, A. & GRIMSON, R. (1989). Comparison of the effects of infection with *Trichostrongylus colubriformis*, *Trichostrongylus vitrinus* and *Trichostrongylus rugatus* in Merino lambs. *Veterinary Parasitology*, **32**, 229–245.

BISSET, S. A., MORRIS, C. A., MCEWAN, J. C. & VLASSOFF, A. (2001). Breeding sheep in New Zealand that are less reliant on anthelmintics to maintain health and productivity. *New Zealand Veterinary Journal*, **49**, 236–246.

BREMNER, K. C. (1969). Pathogenic factors in experimental bovine oesophagostomosis. 3. Demonstration of protein-losing enteropathy with 51Cr-albumin. *Experimental Parasitology*, **24**, 364–374.

BUENO, L., DAKKAK, A. & FIORAMONTI, J. (1982a). Gastroduodenal motor and transit disturbances associated with *Haemonchus contortus* infection in sheep. *Parasitology*, **84**, 367–374.

BUENO, L., DORCHIES, P. & RUCKEBUSCH, Y. (1975). Disturbances of gut motility with *Trichostrongylus* in sheep – Electromyographic study. *Comptes Rendus Des Seances De La Societe De Biologie Et De Ses Filiales*, **169**, 1627–1632.

BUENO, L., HONDE, C., LUFFAU, G. & FIORAMONTI, J. (1982b). Origin of the early digestive disturbances induced by *Haemonchus contortus* infection in lambs. *American Journal of Veterinary Research*, **43**, 1194–1199.

CHARLESTON, W. A. G. (1965). Pathogenesis of experimental haemonchosis in sheep with special reference to development of resistance. *Journal of Comparative Pathology and Therapeutics*, **75**, 55–67.

CHARLIER, J., DUCHATEAU, L., CLAEREBOUT, E. & VERCRUYSSE, J. (2007). Predicting milk-production responses after an autumn treatment of pastured dairy herds with eprinomectin. *Veterinary Parasitology*, **143**, 322–328.

CHRISTIE, M. G. (1970). Fate of very large doses of *Haemonchus contortus* and their effect on conditions in ovine abomasums. *Journal of Comparative Pathology*, **80**, 89–100

COLDITZ, I. G. (2008). Six costs of immunity to gastrointestinal nematode infections. *Parasite Immunology*, **30**, 63–70.

COOP, R. L., SYKES, A. R. & ANGUS, K. W. (1977). Effect of a daily intake of *Ostertagia circumcincta* larvae on body-weight, food-intake and concentration of serum constituents in sheep. *Research in Veterinary Science*, **23**, 76–83.

DANTZER, R. (2004). Cytokine-induced sickness behaviour: A neuroimmune response to activation of innate immunity. *European Journal of Pharmacology*, **500**, 399–411.

DOBSON, D. E., PRAGER, E. M. & WILSON, A. C. (1984). Stomach lysozymes of ruminants. 1. Distribution and catalytic properties. *Journal of Biological Chemistry*, **259**, 1607–1616.

EILER, H., BABER, W., LYKE, W. A. & SCHOLTENS, R. (1981). Inhibition of gastric hydrochloric acid secretions in the rat given *Ostertagia ostertagi* (a gastric parasite of cattle) extracts. *American Journal of Veterinary Research*, **42**, 498–502.

EWALD, P. W. (1995). The evolution of virulence – A unifying link between parasitology and ecology. *Journal of Parasitology*, **81**, 659–669.

FERNANDEZ-ABELLA, D., CASTELLS, D., PIAGGIO, L. & DELEON, N. (2006a). Study of embryo and fetal mortalities in sheep. I. Effect of different parasitic levels and their interaction with nutrition on embryo losses and fecundity. *Produccion Ovina*, **18**, 25–31.

FERNANDEZ-ABELLA, D., HERNANDEZ, Z. & VILLEGAS, N. (2006b). Effect of gastrointestinal nematodes on ovulation rate of merino Booroola heterozygote ewes [Fec(B) Fec(+)]. *Animal Research*, **55**, 545–550.

FORBES, A. B., HUCKLE, C. A. & GIBB, M. J. (2004). Impact of eprinomectin on grazing behaviour and performance in dairy cattle with sub-clinical gastrointestinal nematode infections under continuous stocking management. *Veterinary Parasitology*, **125**, 353–364.

FORBES, A. B., HUCKLE, C. A. & GIBB, M. J. (2007). Evaluation of the effect of eprinomectin in young dairy heifers sub-clinically infected with gastrointestinal nematodes on grazing behaviour and diet selection. *Veterinary Parasitology*, **150**, 321–332.

FOSTER, N. & LEE, D. L. (1996). Vasoactive intestinal polypeptide-like and peptide histidine isoleucine-like proteins excreted/secreted by *Nippostrongylus brasiliensis*, *Nematodirus battus* and *Ascaridia galli*. *Parasitology*, **113**, 287–292.

FOX, M. T. (1993). Pathophysiology of infection with *Ostertagia ostertagi* in cattle. *Veterinary Parasitology*, **46**, 143–158.

FOX, M. T. (1997). Pathophysiology of infection with gastrointestinal nematodes in domestic ruminants: Recent developments. *Veterinary Parasitology*, **72**, 285–297.

FOX, M. T., GERRELLI, D., PITT, S. R., JACOBS, D. E., GILL, M. & GALE, D. L. (1989a). *Ostertagia ostertagi* infection in the calf – Effects of a trickle challenge on appetite, digestibility, rate of passage of digesta and liveweight gain. *Research in Veterinary Science*, **47**, 294–298.

FOX, M. T., GERRELLI, D., SHIVALKAR, P. & JACOBS, D. E. (1989b). Effect of omeprazole treatment on feed-intake and blood gastrin and pepsinogen levels in the calf. *Research in Veterinary Science*, **46**, 280–282.

GARSIDE, P., KENNEDY, M. W., WAKELIN, D. & LAWRENCE, C. E. (2000). Immunopathology of intestinal helminth infection. *Parasite Immunology*, **22**, 605–612.

GIBB, M. J., HUCKLE, C. A. & FORBES, A. B. (2005). Effects of sequential treatments with eprinomectin on performance and grazing behaviour in dairy cattle under daily-paddock stocking management. *Veterinary Parasitology*, **133**, 79–90.

GOUMON, Y., CASARES, F., PRYOR, S. *et al.* (2000). *Ascaris suum*, an intestinal parasite, produces morphine. *Journal of Immunology*, **165**, 339–343.

GREER, A. W. (2008). Trade-offs and benefits: Implications of promoting a strong immunity to gastrointestinal parasites in sheep. *Parasite Immunology*, **30**, 123–132.

GREER, A. W., MCANULTY, R. W., STANKIEWICZ, M. & SYKES, A. R. (2005). Corticosteroid treatment prevents the reduction in food intake and growth in lambs infected with the abomasal parasite *Teladorsagia circumcincta*. *Proceedings of the New Zealand Society of Animal Production*, **65**, 9–12.

GRIVEL, M. L. & RUCKEBUSCH, Y. (1972). Propagation of segmental contractions along small intestine. *Journal of Physiology-London*, **227**, 611–625.

GROSS, S. J., RYAN, W. G. & PLOEGER, H. W. (1999). Anthelmintic treatment of dairy cows and its effect on milk production. *Veterinary Record*, **144**, 581–587.

HALL, C. A. & ODDY, V. H. (1984). Effect of cimetidine on abomasal pH and *Haemonchus* and *Ostertagia* species in sheep. *Research in Veterinary Science*, **36**, 316–319.

HAMELMANN, E. & GELFAND, E. W. (2001). IL-5-induced airway eosinophilia – The key to asthma? *Immunological Reviews*, **179**, 182–191.

HELMBY, H. & GRENCIS, R. K. (2004). Interleukin-1 plays a major role in the development of Th2-mediated immunity. *European Journal of Immunology*, **34**, 3674–3681.

HERSEY, S. J. (1987). Pepsinogen secretion. In *Physiology of the Gastrointestinal Tract* (ed. Johnson, L. R.), Raven Press, New York.

HERTZBERG, H., GUSCETTI, F., LISCHER, C., KOHLER, L., NEIGER, R. & ECKERT, J. (2000). Evidence for a parasite-mediated inhibition of abomasal acid secretion in sheep infected with *Ostertagia leptospicularis*. *Veterinary Journal*, **159**, 238–251.

HILTON, R. J., BARKER, I. K. & RICKARD, M. D. (1978). Distribution and pathogenicity during development of *Camelostrongylus mentulatus* in abomasums of sheep. *Veterinary Parasitology*, **4**, 231–242.

HOLMES, P. H. (1985). Pathogenesis of trichostrongylosis. *Veterinary Parasitology*, **18**, 89–101.

HOLMES, P. H. & MACLEAN, J. M. (1971). Pathophysiology of ovine ostertagiasis. A study of changes in plasma protein metabolism following single infections. *Research in Veterinary Science*, **12**, 265–271.

HOSTE, H. (2001). Adaptive physiological processes in the host during gastrointestinal parasitism. *International Journal for Parasitology*, **31**, 231–244.

HOSTE, H., KERBOEUF, D. & PARODI, A. L. (1988). *Trichostrongylus colubriformis* – Effects on villi and crypts along the whole small intestine in infected rabbits. *Experimental Parasitology*, **67**, 39–46.

HOSTE, H., MALLET, S. & FORT, G. (1993). Histopathology of the small intestinal mucosa in *Nematodirus spathiger* infection in rabbits. *Journal of Helminthology*, **67**, 139–144.

HUBY, F., HOSTE, H., MALLET, S., FOURNEL, S. & NANO, J. L. (1995). Effects of the excretory/secretory products of six nematode species, parasites of the digestive tract, on the proliferation of HT29-D4 and HGT-1 cell lines. *Epithelial Cell Biology*, **4**, 156–162.

HUBY, F., MALLET, S. & HOSTE, H. (1999). Role of acetylcholinesterase (AChE) secreted by parasitic nematodes on the growth of the cell line from epithelial origin HT29-D4. *Parasitology*, **118**, 489–498.

JEFFCOATE, I. A., HOLMES, P. H., FISHWICK, G., BOYD, J., BAIRDEN, K. & ARMOUR, J. (1988). Effects of trichostrongyle larval challenge on the reproductive performance of immune ewes. *Research in Veterinary Science*, **45**, 234–239.

JENNINGS, F. W., ARMOUR, J., LAWSON, D. D. & ROBERTS, R. (1966). Experimental *Ostertagia ostertagi* infections in calves – Studies with abomasal cannulas. *American Journal of Veterinary Research*, **27**, 1249–1257.

JOHNSON, R. W. (2002). The concept of sickness behavior: A brief chronological account of four key discoveries. *Veterinary Immunology and Immunopathology*, **87**, 443–450.

KAGNOFF, M. F. & ECKMANN, L. (1997). Epithelial cells as sensors for microbial infection. *Journal of Clinical Investigation*, **100**, S51–S55.

KATAEVA, G., AGRO, A. & STANISZ, A. M. (1994). Substance-P-mediated intestinal inflammation: Inhibitory effects of CP 96,345 and SMS 201-995. *Neuroimmunomodulation*, **1**, 350–356.

KHAN, I. & COLLINS, S. M. (1994). Expression of cytokines in the longitudinal muscle myenteric plexus of the inflamed intestine of rat. *Gastroenterology*, **107**, 691–700.

KLESIUS, P. H., HAYNES, T. B. & CROSS, D. A. (1985). Chemotactic factors for eosinophils in soluble extracts of L3 stages of *Ostertagia ostertagi*. *International Journal for Parasitology*, **15**, 517–522.

KONSMAN, J. P., PARNET, P. & DANTZER, R. (2002). Cytokine-induced sickness behaviour: Mechanisms and implications. *Trends in Neurosciences*, **25**, 154–159.

LARSEN, J. W. A. & ANDERSON, N. (2000). The relationship between the rate of intake of trichostrongylid larvae and the occurrence of diarrhoea and breech soiling in adult Merino sheep. *Australian Veterinary Journal*, **78**, 112–116.

LARSEN, J. W. A., ANDERSON, N. & VIZARD, A. L. (1999). The pathogenesis and control of diarrhoea and breech soiling in adult Merino sheep. *International Journal for Parasitology*, **29**, 893–902.

LARSEN, J. W. A., ANDERSON, N., VIZARD, A. L., ANDERSON, G. A. & HOSTE, H. (1994). Diarrhoea in Merino ewes during winter – Association with trichostrongylid larvae. *Australian Veterinary Journal*, **71**, 365–372.

LARSEN, J. W. A., VIZARD, A. L. & ANDERSON, N. (1995). Production losses in Merino ewes and financial penalties caused by trichostrongylid infections during winter and spring. *Australian Veterinary Journal*, **72**, 58–63.

LAWRENCE, C. E., PATERSON, J. C. M., WEI, X. Q., LIEW, F. Y., GARSIDE, P. & KENNEDY, M. W. (2000). Nitric oxide mediates intestinal pathology but not immune expulsion during *Trichinella spiralis* infection in mice. *Journal of Immunology*, **164**, 4229–4234.

LAWTON, D. E. B., REYNOLDS, G. W., HODGKINSON, S. M., POMROY, W. E. & SIMPSON, H. V. (1996). Infection of sheep with adult and larval *Ostertagia circumcincta*: Effects on abomasal pH and serum gastrin and pepsinogen. *International Journal for Parasitology*, **26**, 1063–1074.

LEE, C. W., SARNA, S. K., SINGARAM, C. & CASPER, M. A. (1997). Ca²⁺ channel blockade by verapamil inhibits GMCs and diarrhea during small intestinal inflammation. *American Journal of Physiology-Gastrointestinal and Liver Physiology*, **273**, G785–G794.

LI, C. K. F., SETH, R., GRAY, T., BAYSTON, R., MAHIDA, Y. R. & WAKELIN, D. (1998). Production of proinflammatory cytokines and inflammatory mediators in human intestinal epithelial cells after invasion by *Trichinella spiralis*. *Infection and Immunity*, **66**, 2200–2206.

LI, R. W., SONSTEGARD, T. S., VAN TASSELL, C. P. & GASBARRE, L. C. (2007). Local inflammation as a possible mechanism of resistance to gastrointestinal nematodes in Angus heifers. *Veterinary Parasitology*, **145**, 100–107.

MCKAY, D. M., BENJAMIN, M., BACAESTRADA, M., DINCA, R., CROITORU, K. & PERDUE, M. H. (1995). Role of T-lymphocytes in secretory response to an enteric nematode parasite – Studies in athymic rats. *Digestive Diseases and Sciences*, **40**, 331–337.

MCKELLAR, Q., DUNCAN, J. L., ARMOUR, J., LINDSAY, F. E. F. & MCWILLIAM, P. (1987). Further studies on the response to transplanted *Ostertagia ostertagi* in calves. *Research in Veterinary Science*, **42**, 29–34.

MCKELLAR, Q., DUNCAN, J. L., ARMOUR, J. & MCWILLIAM, P. (1986). Response to transplanted *Ostertagia ostertagi* in calves. *Research in Veterinary Science*, **40**, 367–371.

MCKELLAR, Q. A. (1993). Interactions of *Ostertagia* species with their bovine and ovine hosts. *International Journal for Parasitology*, **23**, 451–462.

MCPHERSON, W. B., SLACEK, B., FAMILTON, A., GOGOLEWSKI, R. P. & GROSS, S. J. (2000). The impact of eprinomectin treatment on dairy cattle reproductive performance. *Proceedings of the Australian and New Zealand Combined Dairy Veterinarian's Conference*, Port Vila, Vanuatu.

MEEUSEN, E. N. T. & BALIC, A. (2000). Do eosinophils have a role in the killing of helminth parasites? *Parasitology Today*, **16**, 95–101.

MERKELBACH, P., SCOTT, I., KHALAF, S. & SIMPSON, H. V. (2002). Excretory/secretory products of *Haemonchus contortus* inhibit aminopyrine accumulation by rabbit gastric glands *in vitro*. *Veterinary Parasitology*, **104**, 217–228.

MORRIS, M. C. (2000). Ethical issues associated with sheep fly strike research, prevention, and control. *Journal of Agricultural & Environmental Ethics*, **13**, 205–217.

MOSTOFA, M. & MCKELLAR, Q. A. (1989). Effect of an antimuscarinic drug on the plasma pepsinogen activity of sheep infected with *Ostertagia circumcincta*. *Research in Veterinary Science*, **47**, 208–211.

MURRAY, M. (1969). Structural changes in bovine ostertagiasis associated with increased permeability of bowel wall to macromolecules. *Gastroenterology*, **56**, 763–772.

MURRAY, M., JENNINGS, F. W. & ARMOUR, J. (1970). Bovine ostertagiasis – Structure, function and mode of differentiation of bovine gastric mucosa and kinetics of worm loss. *Research in Veterinary Science*, **11**, 417–427.

NICHOLLS, C. D., HAYES, P. R. & LEE, D. L. (1987). Physiological and microbiological changes in the abomasums of sheep infected with large doses of *Haemonchus contortus*. *Journal of Comparative Pathology*, **97**, 299–308.

PALMER, J. M. & GREENWOOD-VAN MEERVELD, B. (2001). Integrative neuro-immunomodulation of gastrointestinal function during enteric parasitism. *Journal of Parasitology*, **87**, 483–504.

PALMER, J. M., WEISBRODT, N. W. & CASTRO, G. A. (1984). Trichinella spiralis – Intestinal myoelectric activity during enteric infection in the rat. *Experimental Parasitology*, **57**, 132–141.

PARKINS, J. J. & HOLMES, P. H. (1989). Effects of gastrointestinal helminth parasites on ruminant nutrition. *Nutrition Research Reviews*, **2**, 227–246.

RAHMAN, W. A. & COLLINS, G. H. (1990). The establishment and development of *Trichostrongylus colubriformis* in goats. *Veterinary Parasitology*, **35**, 195–200.

RAINBIRD, M. A., MACMILLAN, D. & MEEUSEN, E. N. T. (1998). Eosinophil-mediated killing of *Haemonchus contortus* larvae: Effect of eosinophil activation and role of antibody, complement and interleukin-5. *Parasite Immunology*, **20**, 93–103.

ROBERT, A., OLAFSSON, A. S., LANCASTER, C. & ZHANG, W. R. (1991). Interleukin-1 is cytoprotective, antisecretory, stimulates PGE2 synthesis by the stomach and retards gastric emptying. *Life Sciences*, **48**, 123–134.

ROTHENBERG, M. E. & HOGAN, S. P. (2006). The eosinophil. *Annual Review of Immunology*, **24**, 147–174.

ROTHENBERG, M. E., MISHRA, A., BRANDT, E. B. & HOGAN, S. P. (2001). Gastrointestinal eosinophils. *Immunological Reviews*, **179**, 139–155.

ROY, E. A., HOSTE, H., FULLER, P., TATARCZUCH, L. & BEVERIDGE, I. (1996). Development of morphological changes and ileal glucagon gene expression in the small intestine of lambs infected with *Trichostrongylus colubriformis*. *Journal of Comparative Pathology*, **115**, 441–453.

RUIZ, M. C., DOMINGUEZBELLO, M. G. & MICHELANGELI, F. (1994). Gastric lysozyme as a digestive enzyme in the hoatzin (*Opisthocomus hoazin*), a ruminant-like folivorous bird. *Experientia*, **50**, 499–501.

SANCHEZ, J., DOHOO, I., CARRIER, J. & DESCOTEAUX, L. (2004). A meta-analysis of the milk-production response after anthelmintic treatment in naturally infected adult dairy cows. *Preventive Veterinary Medicine*, **63**, 237–256.

SCHANBACHER, L. M., NATIONS, J. K., WEISBRODT, N. W. & CASTRO, G. A. (1978). Intestinal myoelectric activity in parasitized dogs. *American Journal of Physiology*, **234**, R188–R195.

SCOFIELD, A. M. (1980). Effect of infection with *Nippostrongylus brasiliensis* on intestinal absorption of hexose in rats. *International Journal for Parasitology*, **10**, 375–380.

SCOTT, I., DICK, A., IRVINE, J., STEAR, M. J. & MCKELLAR, Q. A. (1999). The distribution of pepsinogen within the abomasa of cattle and sheep infected with *Ostertagia* spp. and sheep infected with *Haemonchus contortus*. *Veterinary Parasitology*, **82**, 145–159.

SCOTT, I., HODGKINSON, S. M., KHALAF, S. *et al.* (1998a). Infection of sheep with adult and larval *Ostertagia circumcincta*: Abomasal morphology. *International Journal for Parasitology*, **28**, 1383–1392.

SCOTT, I., KHALAF, S., SIMCOCK, D. C. *et al.* (2000). A sequential study of the pathology associated with the infection of sheep with adult and larval *Ostertagia circumcincta*. *Veterinary Parasitology*, **89**, 79–94.

SCOTT, I., STEAR, M. J., IRVINE, J., DICK, A., WALLACE, D. S. & MCKELLAR, Q. A. (1998b). Changes in the zymogenic cell populations of the abomasa of sheep infected with *Haemonchus contortus*. *Parasitology*, **116**, 569–577.

SIMCOCK, D. C., JOBLIN, K. N., SCOTT, I. *et al.* (1999). Hypergastrinaemia, abomasal bacterial population densities and pH in sheep infected with *Ostertagia circumcincta*. *International Journal for Parasitology*, **29**, 1053–1063.

SIMPSON, H. V., LAWTON, D. E. B., SIMCOCK, D. C., REYNOLDS, G. W. & POMROY, W. E. (1997). Effects of adult and larval *Haemonchus contortus* on abomasal secretion. *International Journal for Parasitology*, **27**, 825–831.

SIMPSON, H. V., SIMPSON, B. H., SIMCOCK, D. C., REYNOLDS, G. W. & POMROY, W. E. (1999). Abomasal secretion in sheep receiving adult *Ostertagia circumcincta* that are prevented from contact with the mucosa. *New Zealand Veterinary Journal*, **47**, 20–24.

SINGHVI, A. & CROMPTON, D. W. T. (1982). Increase in size of the small intestine of rats infected with *Moniliformis* (Acanthocephala). *International Journal for Parasitology*, **12**, 173–178.

SOMMERVILLE, R. I. (1963). Distribution of some parasitic nematodes in alimentary tract of sheep, cattle and rabbits. *Journal of Parasitology*, **49**, 593–599.

STEAD, R. H., KOSECKAJANISZEWSKA, U., OESTREICHER, A. B., DIXON, M. F. & BIENENSTOCK, J. (1991). Remodeling of B-50 (GAP-43)-immunoreactive and NSE-immunoreactive mucosal nerves in the intestines of rats infected with *Nippostrongylus brasiliensis*. *Journal of Neuroscience*, **11**, 3809–3821.

STEAD, R. H., TOMIOKA, M., QUINONEZ, G., SIMON, G. T., FELTEN, S. Y. & BIENENSTOCK, J. (1987). Intestinal mucosal mast cells n normal and nematode-infected rat intestines are in intimate contact with peptidergic nerves. *Proceedings of the National Academy of Sciences of the United States of America*, **84**, 2975–2979.

STEAR, M. J., BISHOP, S. C., HENDERSON, N. G. & SCOTT, I. (2003). A key mechanism of pathogenesis in sheep infected with the nematode *Teladorsagia circumcincta*. *Animal Health Research Reviews*, **4**, 45–52.

STEEL, J. W., JONES, W. O. & SYMONS, L. E. A. (1982). Effects of a concurrent infection of *Trichostrongylus colubriformis* on the productivity and physiological and metabolic responses of lambs infected with *Ostertagia circumcincta*. *Australian Journal of Agricultural Research*, **33**, 131–140.

STEWART, C. B., DOBSON, D. E. & WILSON, A. C. (1984). Lysozyme as a major digestive enzyme in a colobine monkey. *American Journal of Physical Anthropology*, **63**, 222–222.

STEWART, C. B., SCHILLING, J. W. & WILSON, A. C. (1987). Adaptive evolution in the stomach lysozymes of foregut fermenters. *Nature*, **330**, 401–404.

STEWART, T. B. & GASBARRE, L. C. (1989). The veterinary importance of nodular worms (*Oesophagostomum* spp). *Parasitology Today*, **5**, 209–213.

SYKES, A. R. (1994). Parasitism and production in farm. *Animal Production*, **59**, 155–172.

SYKES, A. R. & COOP, R. L. (1976). Intake and utilization of food by growing lambs with parasitic damage to small intestine caused by daily dosing with *Trichostrongylus colubriformis* larvae. *Journal of Agricultural Science*, **86**, 507–515.

SYKES, A. R. & COOP, R. L. (1977). Chronic parasitism and animal efficiency. *ARC Research Review*, **3**, 41–46.

SYKES, A. R., COOP, R. L. & ANGUS, K. W. (1977). Influence of chronic *Ostertagia circumcincta* infection on skeleton of growing sheep. *Journal of Comparative Pathology*, **87**, 521–529.

SZURSZEWSKI, J. H. (1969). A migrating electric complex of canine small intestine. *American Journal of Physiology*, **217**, 1757–1763.

TAYLOR, M. A., COOP, R. L. & WALL, R. L. (2007). *Veterinary Parasitology*, Blackwell Publishing, Oxford.

TILG, H., MOSCHEN, A. R., KASER, A., PINES, A. & DOTAN, I. (2008). Gut, inflammation and osteoporosis: Basic and clinical concepts. *Gut*, **57**, 684–694.

VAUGHAN, A. L., GREER, A. W., MCANULTY, R. W. & SYKES, A. R. (2006). Plasma protein loss in lambs during a mixed infection of *Trichostrongylus colubriformis* and *Teladorsagia circumcincta* – A consequence of the immune response? *Proceedings of the New Zealand Society of Animal Production*, **66**, 83–87.

WAISBREN, S. J., GEIBEL, J. P., MODLIN, I. M. & BORON, W. F. (1994). Unusual permeability properties of gastric gland cells. *Nature*, **368**, 332–335.

WANG, L., STANISZ, A. M., WERSHIL, B. K., GALLI, S. J. & PERDUE, M. H. (1995). Substance P induces ion secretion in mouse small intestine through effects on enteric nerves and mast cells. *American Journal of Physiology-Gastrointestinal and Liver Physiology*, **269**, G85–G92.

WEIGERT, N., SCHAFFER, K., SCHUSDZIARRA, V., CLASSEN, M. & SCHEPP, W. (1996). Gastrin secretion from primary cultures of rabbit antral G cells: stimulation by inflammatory cytokines. *Gastroenterology*, **110**, 147–154.

WILDBLOOD, L. A., KERR, K., CLARK, D. A. S., CAMERON, A., TURNER, D. G. & JONES, D. G. (2005). Production of eosinophil chemoattractant activity by ovine gastrointestinal nematodes. *Veterinary Immunology and Immunopathology*, **107**, 57–65.

YU, F., BRUCE, L. A., CALDER, A. G. *et al.* (2000). Subclinical infection with the nematode *Trichostrongylus colubriformis* increases gastrointestinal tract leucine metabolism and reduces availability of leucine for other tissues. *Journal of Animal Science*, **78**, 380–390.

3 Epidemiology of gastrointestinal nematodes in grazing ruminants

While the life cycle of the gastrointestinal nematode (GIN) is considered to be 'simple' or 'direct', it is clear that the epidemiology of the diseases – strictly speaking, the 'epizootiology' – is anything but simple.

The success of some parasite species may be based on the longevity of infection; examples include filarial worms and schistosomes, both of which can persist in their host and produce offspring for several years. In some circumstances, GIN of grazing ruminants may persist in the host for several months, although this is not normally in an active egg-laying state. For these worms, success is instead based on the potential of the infective third-stage larvae (L3) to persist on pasture for extended periods or for enough parasites to persist within host animals when the external conditions are unsuitable for survival.

Ecology of GINs – pasture

Arguably the single greatest factor which makes GIN of grazing livestock difficult to control is their ability to develop and then survive for long periods on pasture (Callinan, 1978; Gibson & Everett, 1972; Gordon, 1948; Hsu & Levine, 1977; O'Connor et al., 2006; Smeal et al., 1980; Williams & Bilkovich, 1971). Retaining the second-stage sheath, allied with the prior deposition of lipid reserves, means L3 are able to survive harsh conditions while persisting on pasture for extended periods.

All of the free-living stages, from the egg through to the L3, are however, influenced in a variety of ways by climate. This is most easily reviewed by dividing the free-living life stages into two distinct periods: the development of the egg to the L3 and the subsequent survival and translation of the L3 to either death or ingestion by a suitable host animal (Levine, 1963).

Egg to L3 development

The impact of temperature on the ability of eggs to embryonate and then hatch has been extensively studied. It is perhaps unsurprising that the various GIN species have evolved somewhat different responses to temperature and that these differences largely reflect the climatic conditions in the areas each species is best adapted to. For example, the sheep nematode *Teladorsagia circumcincta* can develop at lower temperatures than *Trichostrongylus colubriformis* (Leathwick *et al.*, 1999), while both can develop at lower temperatures than *Haemonchus contortus* (Donald, 1968; Gibson & Everett, 1972; Gordon, 1973; Jasmer *et al.*, 1986). The ability of eggs to withstand cold temperatures is an obvious restriction on the latitudes or microclimates in which each of the species is endemic. The eggs of *T. circumcincta*, regarded as a temperate parasite, can still hatch after periods of exposure to cold which almost completely kill eggs of the tropically-adapted parasite *H. contortus* (Jasmer, 1986; McKenna, 1998). Indeed, unembryonated *H. contortus* eggs have been shown to be the most cold-intolerant life cycle stage of the parasite, with viability dropping to around zero after a week inside faecal pellets maintained at 4°C (Todd *et al.*, 1976).

The situation with *Nematodirus* spp. is somewhat different. These worms have evolved to embryonate and reach the L3 stage prior to hatching, and a period of chilling, while not absolutely necessary, does increase development and hatching (Van Dijk & Morgan, 2008). Optimal development and hatching of *Nematodirus battus* occurred at 11–13°C, significantly lower than for other GIN species (Van Dijk & Morgan, 2008).

Less work has been carried out for the major GIN species of cattle than in species which infect sheep. It has been established, however, that *Ostertagia ostertagi* can hatch at temperatures of 4°C (Pandey, 1972) and develop at 5°C, although the eggs may also hatch at a range of temperatures between 5°C and 37.5°C (Gibson, 1981).

Optimal success of egg to L3 development occurred at a constant 23°C for *T. circumcincta*, with the upper and lower limits in which development was possible being 16–30°C; optimal development of *T. colubriformis* occurred between 25°C and 28°C, with limits of 22–33°C (O'Connor, 2006). Conversely, the percentage of eggs successfully making it through to become L3 was significantly greater at 5°C for *T. circumcincta* than it was for *T. colubriformis* (Rossanigo & Gruner, 1995).

It is intuitive that the availability of sufficient moisture is also crucial to successful embryonation and hatching of GIN eggs. However, while there have been a number of studies to determine the success of development through to L3, there is no available information on the need for necessary moisture for successful hatching *per se*.

Adequate temperature and moisture are crucial in the speed and success of development of L1 to L3. Laboratory culture techniques commonly place faecal samples, regardless of the species present (or isolated parasites in culture medium) at 25–27°C for 6–7 days to ensure optimal recovery of L3. During this period, cultures should not be allowed to dry out. It is hardly surprising that similar conditions in the field allow the greatest developmental success. Laboratory studies have also compared the effect of faecal moisture content of egg to L3 development. There was significantly better recovery of L3 of *H. contortus* if faeces was incubated at 100% relative humidity (RH) compared to samples incubated at 85% RH (Hsu & Levine, 1977), although by contrast, the same study suggested that this humidity did not have to be maintained at a constant rate, and could cycle between 100% and 70% RH, at a constant temperature of 23°C (Hsu & Levine, 1977). The optimal RH values for *T. circumcincta* and *T. colubriformis* at 23°C were 60% and 65%, respectively (Hsu & Levine, 1977).

While the lower temperature threshold, i.e. the temperature at which development can begin, strongly influences the geographical and temporal distribution of GIN species, it is also noted that temperatures in faecal masses can become significantly higher than ambient. When this happens, variability in the ability of species to develop at the upper temperature threshold becomes important (Vlassoff *et al.*, 2001).

Effect of host

The immune status of the host may exert a significant effect on the ability of eggs to develop to L3, with reduced viability observed in eggs derived from adult sheep compared to those derived from naïve lambs (Jørgensen *et al.*, 1998). Allied to the observations that egg to L3 development may be inhibited at lower temperatures, this may imply that egg production from adult stock during winter, particularly in relatively cold climates, may not result in significant pasture contamination over this period.

Survival of L3

The ability of L3 to survive for extended periods is of enormous practical benefit to veterinary parasitologists. The ready availability of larvae for artificial infection is advantageous when compared to working with other parasites in which continuous infection cycles are necessary. However, this advantage is more than outweighed by the impact of extended survival on GIN epizootiology.

The retention of the second-stage larval (L2) sheath assists the L3 to be very resistant to the extremes of temperature and to desiccation, thus enabling extended survival in the laboratory and in the field. Stored in tap water at 8°C in the laboratory, L3 can remain infective for periods over 12 months, although there are suggestions that this period is longer for *T. circumcincta* than for *H. contortus*.

The duration of L3 survival is influenced by numerous factors, such as sward height (Rose & Small, 1984) and the micro- and macroclimate (O'Connor *et al.*, 2006; Sakwa *et al.*, 2003). The location of the L3 in the environment is also important, with observations that viable L3 can be recovered from soil and faecal pellets for lengthy periods following deposition (Morley & Donald, 1980).

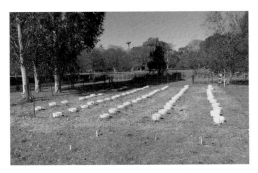

Figure 3.1 'Plot' trial designed to determine larval development and survival in a real 'on-farm' situation. Photo courtesy of Tania Waghorn.

Given the various factors which have been shown to influence parasite hatching, development and survival, and the certainty that these factors will vary with time, location and nematode species, accurate predictions of worm numbers on pasture are difficult, with empirical measurements requiring a large number of replicates which are then harvested over time. An example of such a 'plot trial', set upon a farm in New Zealand, is shown in Figure 3.1.

Translation of infective larvae

One of the paradigms of GIN epidemiology is that the L3 exhibit a negative geotaxis, i.e. that they migrate vertically on grass and make themselves more available for passive ingestion by animals. It has been proposed that the parasites develop through to L3 in faecal material, then migrate out and up (Andersen *et al.*, 1970). The obvious mental image is of the L3 embarking on a perilous journey to the highest peak, desperate to be eaten. Unfortunately, the evidence supporting such a method of host-finding behaviour, however attractive it may appear, is at best conflicting. In fact, once the paradigm is challenged, a flaw quickly becomes apparent: mass migration of L3 would make the known long-term survival of parasite populations on pasture less likely.

The reality of parasite migration and ingestion – referred to as 'translation' (Armour, 1980) – appears to be more prosaic. As stated above, L3 can be recovered from soil for lengthy periods following deposition (Morley & Donald, 1980), implying a lack of a strong negative geotaxis or at least an inability to act on the impulse. A number of studies have reported quantitative comparisons of L3 numbers recovered from soil or grass, with the data displaying significant variability. The percentage of L3 in soil compared to recovery from herbage ranged from 25–30% (Callinan, 1978, 1979) to 68% (Rees, 1950) and 80% (Callinan & Westcott, 1986).

In each of these studies, it was obvious that soil contained significant numbers of L3.

Furthermore, of those L3 recovered from herbage, by far the greatest majority were close to the ground (Callinan & Westcott, 1986; Rogers, 1940; Silangwa &

Todd, 1964). The implication, therefore, is that L3 may not find it particularly easy to migrate vertically for significant distances. The ability of L3 to migrate is strongly influenced by climatic factors such as temperature, humidity and the intensity of light. Extremes of temperature, particularly low, inhibited the migration of L3 (Rees, 1950; Silangwa & Todd, 1964), as did low RH (Callinan & Westcott, 1986; Rees, 1950). There is a relationship between these two variables – even at high RH, low temperatures inhibited migration (Rees, 1950). Low levels of light intensity of less than 3×10^5 lux were found to be optimal for migration (Rogers, 1940); this low intensity would be expected at dawn or dusk. Taken together, it would seem that warm, humid conditions in early morning and late evening are the most suitable for the vertical movement of L3.

However, even when conditions are optimal for migration, only a small percentage of L3 actually moves vertically along herbage (Silangwa & Todd, 1964). Part of the reason for this is the necessity for conditions to be wet enough for moisture to be visible on grass, but not so wet that the L3 have to break through the surface of the water in order to migrate vertically. The surface tension of water has been calculated as 10^4–10^6 times that of gravity (Crofton, 1954), more than enough to inhibit vertical movement; however, this would not necessarily inhibit movement *per se*. Indeed, Crofton (1954) demonstrated that L3 move randomly, assuming favourable conditions, and accumulated where conditions were suitable. Furthermore, he claimed that L3 moved in a single direction, including vertically, along narrow streams of water.

The lack of a negative geotaxis was confirmed in a recent study using *H. contortus* L3 (Sciacca *et al.*, 2002). In this study, L3 were placed on either plates of vertical cones of agar and their movement recorded; no difference was observed between those L3 placed on the flat or vertical structures.

Grazing behaviour and the avoidance of parasites

One of the unavoidable aspects of pastoral grazing systems is the interaction between the need to eat and the need to defaecate. In some instances, animals may defecate more or more often in particular areas, such as rest areas or common latrines (Marsh & Campling, 1970). However, in the relatively intensive grazing systems common in the major agricultural regions, it is common for animals to graze in proximity to faecal material (Gruner & Sauve, 1982). As the numbers of L3 are more likely to be concentrated in and around faecal material, there would appear to be at least two good reasons to avoid the contamination. However, due to the processes involved in digestion, nutrients are relatively concentrated in animal faeces, resulting in high levels of phosphorus, nitrogen and potassium in areas contaminated with faeces and therefore increased pasture growth (Hutchings *et al.*, 2000). This is an obvious dilemma for grazing animals, and while there is an observable avoidance of faecal material (Cooper *et al.*, 2000; Hutchings *et al.*, 1998), this can be overcome if sward height is either sufficiently high or nutritious (Bazely, 1990; Hutchings *et al.*, 2000). The reduced availability of feed in non-contaminated areas, whether due to overgrazing or changes in the season, will also drive animals to graze more closely to faecal material, increasing the number of L3 ingested (Cooper *et al.*, 2000). So, not only does the ingestion of L3 increase, but the plane of nutrition is likely to be reduced (see Chapter 10).

This relationship has been studied in the feral Soay sheep populations on the Scottish Hebridean island of St. Kilda. The Soay sheep were introduced to the area in the Bronze Age (Jewell, 1995) and in recent years have provided an excellent resource for researchers studying the interactions between grazing animals, nutrition and parasitism. In this system, sheep numbers undergo cycles of population growth and contraction, at least some of which has been attributed to parasitism (Gulland, 1992). When animal numbers are high, faecal deposition – with nematode eggs – is relatively high, placing pressure on grazing areas. Eventually, as the availability of clean pasture becomes scarce, animals are forced to ingest higher numbers of L3, at the same time as the plane of nutrition is reduced. In the absence of routine or strategic drenching, sheep mortality eventually occurs (Gulland, 1992). Thereafter, as animal numbers decline, so does faecal deposition and grazing pressure, leading to relatively lower levels of parasitism.

Patterns of infection

While there is significant variability between geographical area, and between nematode species, some generalities can be assigned to the pattern of infections of stock with GIN. If lambing/calving occurs in early spring, then egg output from lactating females (see below) will give rise to a spring peak of L3. A further cohort of L3 may have survived over winter on pasture (assuming climatic conditions are favourable); these cohorts of L3 may be ingested by young stock, giving rise to the first generation of worms which accumulate over summer. It is then that the eggs from the worms parasitising the young stock develop to L3 and become the source of the autumn/winter populations on pasture. This population is further amplified through a further generation/s in the young stock. By late autumn/winter, climatic conditions become less favourable for egg development and survival of L3, and the populations both on pasture and in the animals decrease in size (Vlassoff, 1982; Vlassoff *et al.*, 2001). This process is variable, and in some climates or years, conditions may significantly limit the size of the spring peak of pasture contamination (Vlassoff, 1976).

A number of studies of cattle parasites in the northern hemisphere describe a 'concertina effect' (Armour, 1980) in which O. ostertagi eggs deposited in spring eventually appeared as L3 around 1–3 months later (Michel, 1969), but that eggs deposited later in the season took longer to develop. This information led to the conclusion that in the British Isles, only one generation of these parasites occurred per annum (Michel, 1969). The conclusion that GIN has a similar seasonality, with a limited number of generations, was supported by numerous studies from around the world (Anderson, 1971; Williams & Knox, 1976; Yazwinski & Gibbs, 1975). Conflicting evidence suggests that several generations of parasites may occur per annum, although this is confined to those areas in which both temperatures and humidity are high (Donald, 1964; Le Jambre & Ratcliffe, 1971).

A notable exception to the seasonality of the majority of GIN species is the pattern of infection with *Nematodirus* spp. These parasites originated in cold climates (Hoberg, 2005) and have evolved to infect young lambs in early spring. While L3 can be found on pasture all year round (Leathwick and Sutherland, unpublished), stock quickly becomes immune, so the pattern of infection is more limited than for most GIN species.

Overdispersion of parasites

Parasite burdens tend to be overdispersed within host populations. In other words, a few of the hosts harbour more of the parasites. This is very marked in a number of host–parasite systems, such as the human helminthoses, and is also the case for GIN of grazing livestock, although to a lesser degree. The two major factors responsible for overdispersion of parasites are (a) the ability of the parasites to establish and (b) exposure to the infective stages. There is a significant level of variability in the competency of the immune response to GIN infection between individuals in a flock/herd, which is discussed in detail in Chapters 11 and 12. This variability of immune status is reflected in the numbers of parasites able to establish, persist or produce offspring. While the immune status may therefore explain why overdispersion occurs, the epizootiology of the GIN explains why it occurs to a lesser extent than other host–parasite systems – it is intuitive that individual members of a flock/herd of grazing livestock will have a relatively uniform exposure to L3 on pasture, even allowing for differences in intake and live-weight between animals.

There are potentially practical aspects to the observation that overdispersion occurs in GIN. Being able to selectively drench those animals responsible for the majority of pasture contamination, as well as those animals potentially most at risk of productivity losses, may reduce costs while ensuring sufficient susceptible genotypes escape treatment (see Chapter 8). However, in enterprises with large numbers of stock, it is difficult to envisage this being workable in practice.

Epidemiology of 'parasitism'

In endemic areas, production loss due to GIN is related to such factors as stocking density, pasture contamination and susceptibility of stock.

These factors have been described by various authors (Armour, 1980; Gordon, 1948).

1 an increase in the infective mass.
2 alteration in the susceptibility of stock.
3 the introduction of susceptible stock onto an infected area.

In non-endemic areas, production loss can occur via

4 the introduction of infected stock.

Each of the first three factors is influenced by a multitude of other factors, some of which will be discussed in depth later in the chapter.

An increase in the infective mass

The increase in infective mass for GIN refers to the level of pasture contamination with L3. More specifically, it should refer to the number of L3 ingested per kilogram of intake. This distinction is important, as directly counting the number of L3 in a particular area does not provide a measure of the number likely to be ingested; because the distribution of L3 increases significantly with proximity to the transitional zone between pasture and soil, animals will ingest more L3 as sward height is reduced. For the purpose of clarity, let us therefore define the relationship between pasture contamination and the number of L3 ingested as 'effective pasture contamination'.

Assuming a suitable climate for pasture growth, the stocking density of grazing animals will be the major driver of 'effective pasture contamination'. This can be divided further: the greater the stocking density, the greater will be the total egg production and therefore pasture contamination (not necessarily 'effective'); also, the greater the stocking density, the more likely it is that sward height will be reduced – unless animals are moved regularly to prevent 'overgrazing', this will also put more pressure on animals to graze in areas contaminated with faeces, and therefore is likely to have relatively higher numbers of L3. A further contributing factor to productivity losses in this scenario is that heavy, or overgrazing, carries with it the implication that animals are not receiving the optimum level/quality of nutrition (see Chapter 10).

The impact of increased stocking density will be relatively more severe if animals are susceptible to infection, i.e. have not yet developed an effective protective immunity or have lost a proportion of their immunity (Vlassoff, 1976). In grazing ruminants, not accounting for breed differences, animals are considered susceptible to infection until several weeks or months post-weaning (see Chapter 12 for a discussion on the mechanisms of immunity to parasites). During this period, ingested parasites which establish and breed have the opportunity to produce large numbers of eggs. This varies with species; highly fecund species such as *Haemonchus* spp. produce relatively greater numbers of eggs than, for example, *Ostertagia/Teladorsagia* spp. (Coyne *et al.*, 1991).

It is, therefore, easy to envisage a difference in egg output if one compares an area containing only adult, immune stock with an area containing only young, naive stock. In lamb- or calf-only enterprises, worm control programmes have to be considered differently from breeding units containing a mixture of immune phenotypes. Furthermore, given that a few GIN are equally capable of infecting and reproducing in small and large ruminants, areas in which more than one species is grazed will present a relatively lower parasite threat to each species. It has, therefore, become common practice in many areas to graze sheep and cattle together.

There is a characteristic seasonality in pasture contamination with GIN, which reflects how suitable climatic conditions are for the development and survival of L3 (Tetley, 1941, 1949, 1959). In many grazing systems, this coincides either with animals being turned out onto pasture (Borgsteede, 1977) or when young, naive stock become infected and eventually pass large numbers of eggs onto pasture (Cameron & Gibbs, 1966; Vlassoff, 1973, 1976). Even when lambs are drenched on a regular basis, they remain major contributors to pasture contamination (Vlassoff *et al.*, 2001).

Alteration in the susceptibility of stock

The development of protective immunity to GIN in grazing ruminants occurs as a continuum, and it is not possible to place a threshold on when animals cease to be 'naïve' and become 'immune'. There is also significant variability in how animals respond to different species of GIN. For example, it is common for adult sheep to be completely refractory to infection with *T. colubriformis* but still harbour low numbers of *T. circumcincta*. In general, however, as the expression of acquired immunity develops, the ability of GIN to establish and cycle is reduced.

The 'spring rise' in faecal egg count (FEC), leading to pasture contamination, can be correlated to lactation in breeding ewes (Brunsdon, 1964; Crofton, 1958) and is now commonly known as the periparturient rise (Salisbury & Arundel, 1970) or more recently, the periparturient relaxation of immunity (PPRI) (Armour, 1980). Indeed, taking lambs away from their mothers soon after birth negates the PPRI (O'Sullivan & Donald, 1970), presumably by removing the significant energy requirements involved in lactation (see Chapter 10). While the exact causes of the PPRI remain unclear, there is a well-established association between the effect and circulating levels of prolactin, which begin to increase around 5 weeks before parturition, then decline until weaning (Kelly & Lineen, 1973). The PPRI may allow arrested larvae to resume their development (see below) or it may allow ingested L3 to establish (Donald *et al.*, 1982). However it is mediated, it is clear that the PPRI is a potential source of pasture contamination of L3 which can be ingested by young, naïve stock. However, it has also been established that the PPRI may not always occur, and even if it does, its impact can vary greatly due to factors such as animal genotype. In a study on the replacement of drench survivors in lactating Romney and Coopworth ewes treated with anthelmintic, very few parasites were able to establish and produce eggs (Leathwick *et al.*, 1999). This was significantly different from the situation in more susceptible sheep such as Merinos (Donald *et al.*, 1982) and was proposed to account for the differences in New Zealand and Australian models regarding the development of drug resistance in which the contribution of the lactating animal was significantly less in the former than in the latter (Leathwick *et al.*, 1999).

Climate will also affect the relative contribution of the PPRI to pasture contamination. In areas in which the prevailing climate favours larval development and survival, L3 may survive over winter and be ingested by the next season's young stock. In temperate and parasite-friendly New Zealand, a long-term field study (Jørgensen *et al.*, 1998) established that in 2 out of 3 years there was no significant contribution of the ewe to subsequent parasite populations in their lambs. In drier/hotter or alternatively significantly colder areas, however, the development and survival of L3 is reduced, and those parasites able to survive within a host and then resume development in spring are likely to make a relatively greater contribution to pasture contamination. Similarly, in areas where transmission of parasites occurs mainly in autumn and winter, the contribution of those parasites able to survive in the host over summer is likely to be proportionally greater (Eysker, 1993).

Arrested development and hypobiosis

While some L3 are capable of surviving on pasture until susceptible hosts become available, this is limited by climate, and therefore by geographical region and annual weather patterns. In areas in which survival is limited by climate, pasture contamination which coincides with susceptible (mainly young) stock may therefore be derived largely from those parasites which have survived for extended periods within a host animal (Sargison *et al.*, 2007).

The GIN have evolved a means of arresting development within the host as inhibited fourth-stage larvae (L4), with development resuming in response to a cue such as hormonal changes or alterations in the components of the immune system during the PPRI. This process, also termed hypobiosis, has been observed in several worm species of both sheep (Blitz & Gibbs, 1972; Connan, 1974; Langrova *et al.*, 2008; Waller *et al.*, 1981; Waller & Thomas, 1983) and cattle (Armour & Duncan, 1987; Michel *et al.*, 1974). Arrested development occurs at a specific point in the development of parasites and can account for unexpected clinical disease in livestock which have not grazed contaminated pasture for some time (Armour & Duncan, 1987).

Various factors have been implicated as triggers for ingested L3 to begin their development, but then arrest in host epithelium as L4. Host immune status is one such trigger (Herlich & Merkal, 1963; Michel *et al.*, 1979), particularly in older, more immune animals; the involvement of the immune system appears obvious given the observations of resumed development during the PPRI (Armour & Duncan, 1987; Michel *et al.*, 1979). The density dependence of parasites may also influence the onset of arrested development, supported by evidence of resumed development as resident adult worm burdens decrease or are removed by anthelmintic which is not effective against the inhibited L4.

Several studies have demonstrated a seasonal/climatic influence on arrested development in which factors such as temperature and day length trigger subsequently ingested L3 to arrest (Armour & Bruce, 1974; Langrova & Jankovska, 2004; Langrova *et al.*, 2008; Michel *et al.*, 1974, 1975; Watkins & Fernando, 1984). It is assumed that resumed development of these worms is, however, also related to host immune status.

Introduction of susceptible stock onto an infected area

The sudden introduction of susceptible stock onto pasture contaminated with GIN L3 can result in the rapid onset of clinical disease without the requirement for a generational increase in numbers. Obviously, this is heavily dependent on a range of factors such as host genotype, nutritional status and the relative abundance of worm species.

An example of susceptible stock suffering as a result of the sudden ingestion of L3 is in the dairy industry in areas of Western Europe. In this system, calves are born in spring, then reared indoors until summer, when they are put onto pasture previously grazed by autumn-born, and therefore relatively naive stock. The ingestion of over-wintered L3 by these autumn-born animals has increased pasture contamination, and the second generation of L3 is now on pasture and available for ingestion by the younger cohort of animals.

The epizootiology of *Nematodirus* spp. has evolved to take advantage of the presence of young naive stock. While these parasites are relatively pathogenic, immunity develops quickly and clinical disease is limited to young animals in early spring. The paradigm around *Nematodirus* spp. is that eggs deposited onto pasture may persist undeveloped until the next season, when they embryonate and rapidly develop to L3, to be ingested by susceptible stock. However, it is equally likely that L3 are available all year round (Sutherland and Leathwick, unpublished observations) but are unable to establish or fully develop in older animals.

Insufficient age-related immunity

Effective immunity to most of the GIN species develops in ruminants by 4–7 months of age and may develop even in the absence of parasitism (Armour, 1980). The aetiology of age-related immunity is poorly understood and is highly variable between parasite species.

Insufficient age-related immunity appears to be primarily important with *O. ostertagi* in cattle, and a number of studies report clinical disease in adult cattle following exposure of (previously unexposed) stock to parasite challenge.

The introduction of infected stock to a clean environment

The profile of GIN species found in the major livestock producing regions of the world is remarkably similar. There are certainly differences in the relative abundance of species, influenced primarily by the suitability of particular macro- and microclimates, but in general, most important species of parasites tend to be present to some degree. This is hardly surprising, as movement of infected stock on a global scale occurred before the introduction of effective broad-spectrum anthelmintics. So, while the horse may have bolted with respect to most GIN species, there are always exceptions to any rule. An example is the absence of the pathogenic cattle parasite *H. placei* from New Zealand, which one assumes has been plain luck, as the prevailing conditions would certainly be favourable for its survival and development.

Epidemiology of cattle parasites

There is less of a PPRI in cattle than in sheep, and therefore a lower contribution on terms of eggs passed onto pasture to subsequently infect young stock; spring-born calves will therefore acquire most of their parasite challenge from over-wintered L3 (Brunsdon, 1980). While a few L3 are available for ingestion in spring and early summer, numbers rise rapidly in mid-summer (Michel *et al.*, 1970) and present a significant threat to animal health (Brunsdon, 1980). Indeed, it has been estimated that early in the grazing season, the number of larvae of *O. ostertagi* ingested per host per day is only 0.0001 (repeated in Smith & Grenfell, 1985).

An obvious factor in the epidemiology of cattle parasites is the practice of housing of animals over winter in some regions. This will significantly affect the pattern of L3 availability on pasture in comparison to areas such as New Zealand and Australia, where cattle are maintained on pasture all year.

Population biology in the parasitic phase

A detailed knowledge of the population dynamics of individual parasite species in their preferred host has the potential to provide critical information which could be utilised in control strategies. However, despite the enormous cumulative cost of GIN to the livestock industries worldwide, remarkably little work has been carried out into the population biology of the parasites. It could be argued that there are good reasons for this; the major constraint in these types of studies is cost, with serial necropsies of animals necessary at regular intervals. Given the inherent variability in parasitism between even closely related animals, prohibitively large numbers of animals may be required to provide robust and relevant information. A range of other factors may also influence parasite population biology and need to be taken into account when designing experiments. These include the plane of nutrition, while the commonly observed effects of indoor housing vs. maintenance in the field on host–parasite biology should be considered. For studies on population biology of GIN to be relevant, experiments should be designed to, as much as is practically possible, reflect the pattern and size of exposure grazing ruminants would encounter on farm. This requires parasite L3 to be administered often, in what is commonly referred to as a trickle-infection or trickle-challenge regime, rather than as a single large dose. Neither should overly large numbers of L3 be administered, as the host response may well diverge from that which occurs in a 'normal' on-farm situation.

The impact of the host immune system is a major factor in parasite population biology; the various components of immunity (whether protective or not) are discussed more fully in Chapter 12. The current chapter will, therefore, be limited to a description of the impact of immunity on population dynamics.

All the factors mentioned above make precise measurements of parasite population dynamics difficult. Despite this, a number of elegant studies have been performed which have significantly contributed to our knowledge base.

As with many other aspects of GIN biology and control, some of the greatest contributions were made some decades ago.

Sheep parasites

As expected, given the costs involved in studies of parasite population biology in the host, significantly more research has been conducted in sheep than in cattle.

Studies of the population biology of GIN in sheep have focussed mainly on the three most economically important species, i.e. *H. contortus* and *T. circumcincta* in the abomasum and *T. colubriformis* in the small intestine.

H. contortus

With *H. contortus* infections in young lambs grazed on pasture, the size of the resulting adult worm is directly related to the number of larvae ingested. However, the rate of accumulation of the adult worm burden slows and no further increase in numbers occurs by approximately 3 weeks of exposure to parasites. As the accumulation of adults decreases, however, the number of arrested L4 increases (Courtney *et al.*, 1983). Courtney *et al.* (1983) concluded that these data were consistent with at least two mechanisms of population regulation. In the first, a rapid turnover of adult worms occurs and in the second, adult worms accumulate until a threshold is reached and incoming larvae become arrested (Dineen *et al.*, 1965).

The parasitic phase of the *H. contortus* life cycle was reconstructed using a mathematical model (Smith, 1988). In this model, parasite death was assumed to be attributable to at least three processes: (1) failure of L3 to exsheath following ingestion, (2) failure to become established via immune exclusion, and (3) mortality of L4 and adult worms. Smith (1988) proposed that the proportion of worms able to establish follows a declining sigmoidal function of the duration of infection during continual exposure to L3. As the number of L3 able to establish decreases, the death rate of L4 and adult worms increases, this time as a linear function related to exposure to L3.

T. circumcincta

The population biology of *T. circumcincta* is very similar to that of *H. contortus*. In a single infection with varying numbers of *T. circumcincta* (3,000, 10,000 or 33,000 L3), worm count data indicated a plateau phase during which the numbers of adult worms present remained stable. This period was followed by a 'loss phase' in which worms were expelled. However, the duration of this plateau phase decreased as inoculation size increased (Hong *et al.*, 1986). It was noted by the authors that approximately 50% of L3 established regardless of inoculum size and absolute numbers of adults. At the higher inoculum rate, arrested larvae began to develop, with data for worm lengths displaying a bimodal distribution. As this was a single infection, however, the proportion of those larvae found to be arrested decreased over the next 5 weeks, as they resumed development. These larvae never reached the same length as the cohort which developed through to adults first. This hypothesis was supported by the observation that vulval development was inhibited – this reduced flap development has been associated with host immunity; given the fact that worms relatively increased exposure to conditions in the host prior to the completion of the life cycle, it seems reasonable to assume that the hypothesis is correct.

The authors also proposed that an increase in the size of the inoculum results in similar population biology as observed in more immune hosts, and further state that this is not due to a 'crowding' effect but is due to increased arrested development.

The same authors undertook a subsequent experiment which extended this work to measurements of the population biology of *T. circumcincta* in animals that were given different numbers of L3, but this time as a 'trickle' infection (Hong *et al.*, 1987). Groups of 18-week old lambs were given either 250, 500 or 1,000 L3 daily and then cohorts of animals were killed at days 30, 60, 110 and 140. As with the single infections, this study demonstrated that the size of the adult worm burden was positively correlated with the infection rate and that the rate of loss of adult worms was related to the size of the resident population. This was proposed to be the primary mechanism of population regulation.

A more recent study included monthly counts of adult *T. circumcincta* in lambs challenged three times weekly from weaning as part of the experimental design (Sutherland and Leathwick, unpublished). The results demonstrate the initial peak of worm burdens followed by a sharp decline as protective immunity develops and are shown in Figure 3.2.

However, as with the authors' previous study, this effect became clear at the highest inoculum dose, at which worm numbers were lower than would be expected, implying a shorter worm life expectancy at higher rates of challenge. The peak rates of infection in the experiment, based on FEC and worm

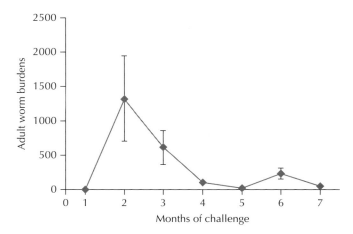

Figure 3.2 Worm counts from lambs challenged three times weekly with 2000 L3 of *T. circumcincta* (Sutherland, Brown and Leathwick, unpublished).

count, were also reached earlier at day 30 for the highest rate of challenge, but were observed to be at day 60 for the lower two dose rates.

Mathematical modelling of the population biology of *T. circumcincta* has been attempted on a number of occasions (Callinan & Arundel, 1982; Paton & Gettinby, 1983; Paton *et al.*, 1984; Smith, 1988). A comparison of how well these models fitted experimental data determined that none in fact did so completely (Smith, 1989). Neither of the two discrete-time models (Paton & Gettinby, 1983; Paton *et al.*, 1984) was able to mimic the rise and fall in parasite numbers observed in trickle-infection experiments (Hong *et al.*, 1987), presumably because both models proposed that parasite mortality was constant with a constant infection rate. Conversely, two continuous-time models (Callinan & Arundel, 1982; Smith, 1988) can mimic trickle-infection experiments as they utilise parasite mortality as a function of the infection rate and duration of infection. Where these models fall down is that neither accurately takes into account between-animal variability in infection rate and are therefore less than ideal for predicting field intensity of parasitism (Smith, 1989).

T. colubriformis

The population biology of *T. colubriformis* is very different from the previous two species discussed. In general, *T. colubriformis* L3 are ingested, develop and then accumulate as adults in the small intestine. The size of the adult worm burden is determined by the infection rate and the age of the host, with the highest numbers of adults recovered from young animals given a high challenge (Dobson, 1990). As the immune response to challenge with *T. colubriformis* develops, the establishment and development of L3 is reduced (Courtney *et al.*, 1983; Dobson *et al.*, 1990; Waller *et al.*, 1981), although there is evidence of parasites becoming arrested at the exsheathed L3 stage (Barnes & Dobson, 1993; Eysker, 1978). This is followed by a period of 4–8 weeks during which worm burdens remain stable, implying that adult *T. colubriformis* have a relatively long lifespan (Courtney *et al.*, 1983). The adult worms are then expelled and the host displays a high level of immunity to subsequent re-infection (Dobson *et al.*, 1990, 1992; Eysker, 1987; Waller *et al.*, 1981).

Cattle parasites

Compared to small ruminant research, primarily in sheep, there has been relatively little work performed on the population dynamics of GIN in cattle, almost certainly due to the inherent cost constraints. That said, however, it is somewhat paradoxical that a number of ground-breaking studies in the area were conducted on cattle parasites – most notably those on *O. ostertagi* by Michel and co-workers.

Having performed worm counts over several months of infection with *O. ostertagi* L3, a pattern of infection was observed in which worm burdens accumulated over the first 2–3 months of infection, declined and then rose again before a second, sustained decline by 9–10 months of age (Michel, 1963, 1969; Michel *et al.*, 1970).

Michel noted that regardless of the number of L3 administered to calves, the pattern of egg output in faeces, including the size of the peak of egg production, was remarkably similar (Michel, 1967, 1969). The same study demonstrated this to be the case even when the numbers of adult worms present were different. Administration of immunosuppressant removed this effect, and infections with larger numbers of adult worms then produced correspondingly larger quantities of eggs (Michel, 1967, 1969). The obvious implication was that the immune response of the host was somehow regulating egg production. Michel further demonstrated that groups of immunosuppressed animals infected with differing numbers of L3 produced similar quantities of eggs, suggesting that the effect of immunosuppression was on this regulatory process and not on the worms themselves. The observation that egg output from calves infected with *O. ostertagi* was effectively independent of worm burden resulted in Michel developing two important hypotheses. The first was that pasture contamination from infected calves is not determined by the level of worm burden, while the second stated that worm burdens of calves could not be determined by measuring egg output (Michel, 1967).

Research on the dynamics of *O. ostertagi* infections in calves has also demonstrated strong density-dependent effects on the establishment and persistence of infection. Thus, as the infection rate increases, the proportion of L3 developing through to adults reduces (Michel *et al.*, 1970). Within the framework of this density dependence, however, the number of adult worms present is related to the size of larval challenge. Furthermore, as the numbers of adult worms present increase, so too does the death rate of those worms (Anderson & Michel, 1977), which was estimated as between 20–50 days under continuous challenge with L3 (Michel *et al.*, 1970). As a result, the size of the resident worm burden at any time reflects the number of L3 ingested 2–3 weeks previously. Like *T. circumcincta* in sheep, therefore, the dynamics of *O. ostertagi* in cattle is characterised by a continuous turnover of the established population which is strongly driven by larval challenge.

Arrested development of *O. ostertagi* is a source of some concern, as resumed development can result in significant pathology in animals with no observable egg counts. The numbers of parasites becoming inhibited at the L4 stage, approximately 3–4 days following ingestion, increase with the duration of infection (Michel, 1963). This inhibition has been shown to be due to the development of an immune response to infection (Michel *et al.*, 1970, 1979), although there may also be a significant impact of environmental effects on the free-living stages prior to ingestion (Armour & Bruce, 1974; Armour *et al.*, 1969).

References

ANDERSEN, F. L., LEVINE, N. D. & BOATMAN, P. A. (1970). Survival of third-stage *Trichostrongylus colubriformis* larvae on pasture. *Journal of Parasitology*, **56**, 209–232.

ANDERSON, N. (1971). Ostertagiasis in beef cattle. *Victorian Veterinary Proceedings*, **30**, 36–38.

ANDERSON, R. M. & MICHEL, J. F. (1977). Density-dependent survival in populations of *Ostertagia ostertagi*. *International Journal for Parasitology*, **7**, 321–329.

ARMOUR, J. (1980). The epidemiology of helminth disease in farm animals. *Veterinary Parasitology*, **6**, 7–46.

ARMOUR, J. & BRUCE, R. G. (1974). Inhibited development in *Ostertagia ostertagi* infections, a diapause phenomenon in a nematode. *Parasitology*, **69**, 161–174.

ARMOUR, J. & DUNCAN, M. (1987). Arrested larval development in cattle nematodes. *Parasitology Today*, **3**, 171–176.

ARMOUR, J., JENNINGS, F. W. & URQUHART, G. M. (1969). Inhibition of *Ostertagia ostertagi* at the early fourth larval stage. II. The influence of environment on host or parasite. *Research in Veterinary Science*, **10**, 238–244.

BARNES, E. H. & DOBSON, R. J. (1993). Persistence of acquired immunity to *Trichostrongylus colubriformis* in sheep after termination of infection. *International Journal for Parasitology*, **23**, 1019–1026.

BAZELY, D. R. (1990). Rules and cues used by sheep foraging in monocultures. *Behavioural Mechanisms of Food Selection*, 343–367.

BLITZ, N. M. & GIBBS, H. C. (1972). Studies on the arrested development of *Haemonchus contortus* in sheep – I. The induction of arrested development. *International Journal for Parasitology*, **2**, 5–12.

BORGSTEEDE, F. H. M. (1977). The epidemiology of gastro-intestinal helminth infections in young cattle in The Netherlands. Ph.D. Thesis, University of Utrecht.

BRUNSDON, R. V. (1964). The seasonal variations in the nematode egg counts of sheep: A comparison of the spring rise phenomenon in breeding and unmated ewes. *New Zealand Veterinary Journal*, **12**, 75–80.

BRUNSDON, R. V. (1980). Principles of helminth control. *Veterinary Parasitology*, **6**, 185–215.

CALLINAN, A. P. L. (1978). The ecology of the free-living stages of *Ostertagia circumcincta*. *International Journal for Parasitology*, **8**, 233–237.

CALLINAN, A. P. L. (1979). The ecology of the free-living stages of *Trichostrongylus vitrinus*. *International Journal for Parasitology*, **9**, 133–136.

CALLINAN, A. P. L. & WESTCOTT, J. M. (1986). Vertical distribution of trichostrongylid larvae on herbage and in soil. *International Journal for Parasitology*, **16**, 241–244.

CALLINAN, A. P. L. & ARUNDEL, J. H. (1982). Population dynamics of the parasitic stages of *Ostertagia* spp. in sheep. *International Journal for Parasitology*, **12**, 531–535.

CAMERON, C. D. T. & GIBBS, H. C. (1966). Effects of stocking density and flock management on internal parasitism in lambs. *Canadian Journal of Animal Science*, **46**, 121–124.

CONNAN, R. M. (1974). Arrested development in *Chabertia ovina*. *Research in Veterinary Science*, **16**, 240–243.

COOPER, J., GORDON, I. J. & PIKE, A. W. (2000). Strategies for the avoidance of faeces by grazing sheep. *Applied Animal Behaviour Science*, **69**, 15–33.

COURTNEY, C. H., PARKER, C. F., MCCLURE, K. E. & HERD, R. P. (1983). Population dynamics of *Haemonchus contortus* and *Trichostrongylus* spp. in sheep. *International Journal for Parasitology*, **13**, 557–560.

COYNE, M. J., SMITH, G. & JOHNSTONE, C. (1991). Fecundity of gastrointestinal trichostrongylid nematodes of sheep in the field. *American Journal of Veterinary Research*, **52**, 1182–1188.

CROFTON, H. D. (1954). The vertical migration of infective larvae of strongyloid nematodes. *Journal of Helminthology*, **28**, 35–52.

CROFTON, H. D. (1958). Nematode parasite populations in sheep on lowland farms. V. Further observations on the post-parturient rise and a discussion of its significance. *Parasitology*, **48**, 251–260.

DINEEN, J. K., DONALD, A. D., WAGLAND, B. M. & OFFNER, J. (1965). The dynamics of the host:parasite relationship. III. The response of sheep to primary infection with *Haemonchus contortus*. *Parasitology*, **55**, 515–525.

DOBSON, R. J., BARNES, E. H. & WINDON, R. G. (1992). Population dynamics of *Trichostrongylus colubriformis* and *Ostertagia circumcincta* in single and concurrent infections. *International Journal for Parasitology*, **22**, 997–1004.

DOBSON, R. J., DONALD, A. D., BARNES, E. H. & WALLER, P. J. (1990). Population dynamics of *Trichostrongylus colubriformis* in sheep: Model to predict to the worm pupulation over time as a function of infection rate and host age. *International Journal for Parasitology*, **20**, 365–373.

DONALD, A. D. (1964). Nematode parasite populations in cattle in Fiji: A humid tropical environment. *Parasitology*, **54**, 273–287.

DONALD, A. D. (1968). Ecology of the free-living stages of nematode parasites of sheep. *Australian Veterinary Journal*, **44**, 139–144.

DONALD, A. D., MORLEY, F. H. W. & WALLER, P. J. (1982). Effects of reproduction, genotype and anthelmintic treatment of ewes on *Ostertagia* spp. populations. *International Journal for Parasitology*, **12**, 403–411.

EYSKER, M. (1978). Inhibition of the development of *Trichostrongylus* spp. as third stage larvae in sheep. *Veterinary Parasitology*, **4**, 29–33.

EYSKER, M. (1987). Regulation of *Trichostrongylus vitrinus* and *T. colubriformis* populations in naturally infected sheep in The Netherlands. *Research in Veterinary Science*, **42**, 267–271.

EYSKER, M. (1993). The role of inhibited development in the epidemiology of *Ostertagia* infections. *Veterinary Parasitology*, **46**, 259–269.

GIBSON, M. (1981). The effect of constant and changing temperatures on the development rates of the eggs and larvae of *Ostertagia ostertagi*. *Journal of Thermal Biology*, **6**, 389–394.

GIBSON, T. E. & EVERETT, G. (1972). The ecology of the free-living stages of *Ostertagia circumcincta*. *Parasitology*, **64**, 451–460.

GORDON, H. M. (1948). The epidemiology of parasitic diseases, with special reference to studies with nematode parasites of sheep. *Australian Veterinary Journal*, **24**, 17–45.

GORDON, H. M. (1973). Epidemiology and control of gastrointestinal nematodoses of ruminants. *Advances in Veterinary Science and Comparative Medicine*, **17**, 395–437.

GRUNER, L. & SAUVE, C. (1982). The distribution of trichostrongyle infective larvae on pasture and grazing behaviour in calves. *Veterinary Parasitology*, **11**, 203–213.

GULLAND, F. M. D. (1992). The role of nematode parasites in Soay sheep (*Ovis aries L.*) mortality during a population crash. *Parasitology*, **105**, 493–503.

HERLICH, H. & MERKAL, R. S. (1963). Serological and immunological responses of calves to infection with *Trichostrongylus axei*. *J Parasitol*, **49**, 623–627.

HOBERG, E. P. (2005). Coevolution and biogeography among nematodirinae (Nematoda: Trichostrongylina) Lagomorpha and Artiodactyla (Mammalia): Exploring determinants of history and structure for the northern fauna across the Holarctic. *Journal of Parasitology*, **91**, 358–369.

HONG, C., MICHEL, J. F. & LANCASTER, M. B. (1986). Populations of *Ostertagia circumcincta* in lambs following a single infection. *International Journal for Parasitology*, **16**, 63–67.

HONG, C., MICHEL, J. F. & LANCASTER, M. B. (1987). Observations on the dynamics of worm burdens in lambs infected daily with *Ostertagia circumcincta*. *International Journal for Parasitology*, **17**, 951–956.

HSU, C. K. & LEVINE, N. D. (1977). Degree-day concept in development of infective larvae of *Haemonchus contortus* and *Trichostrongylus colubriformis* under constant and cyclic conditions. *American Journal of Veterinary Research*, **38**, 1115–1119.

HUTCHINGS, M. R., KYRIAZAKIS, I., ANDERSON, D. H., GORDON, I. J. & COOP, R. L. (1998). Behavioural strategies used by parasitized and non-parasitized sheep to avoid ingestion of gastro-intestinal nematodes associated with faeces. *Animal Science*, **67**, 97–106.

HUTCHINGS, M. R., KYRIAZAKIS, I., PAPACHRISTOU, T. G., GORDON, I. J. & JACKSON, F. (2000). The herbivores' dilemma: Trade-offs between nutrition and parasitism in foraging decisions. *Oecologia*, **124**, 242–251.

JASMER, D. P., WESCOTT, R. B. & CRANE, J. W. (1986). Influence of cold temperatures upon development and survival of eggs of Washington isolates of *Haemonchus contortus* and *Ostertagia circumcincta*. *Proceedings of the Helminthological Society of Washington*, **53**, 244–247.

JEWELL, P. A. (1995). Soay sheep. *St Kilda; the Continuing Story of the Islands*, 73–93.

JØRGENSEN, L. T., LEATHWICK, D. M., CHARLESTON, W. A. G., GODFREY, P. L., VLASSOFF, A. & SUTHERLAND, I. A. (1998). Variation between hosts in the developmental success of the free-living stages of trichostrongyle infections of sheep. *International Journal for Parasitology*, **28**, 1347–1352.

KELLY, J. D. & LINEEN, J. K. (1973). The suppression of rejection of *Nippostrongylus brasiliensis* in Lewis strain rats treated with ovine prolactin: The site of the immunological defect. *Immunology*, **24**, 551–558.

LANGROVA, I. & JANKOVSKA, I. (2004). Arrested development of *Trichostrongylus colubriformis* in experimentally infected rabbits. Effect of decreasing photoperiod, low temperature and desiccation. *Helminthologia*, **41**, 85–90.

LANGROVA, I., MAKOVCOVA, K., VADLEJCH, J., JANKOVSKA, I., PETRTYL, M., FECHTNER, J., KEIL, P., LYTVYNETS, A. & BORKOVCOVA, M. (2008). Arrested development of sheep strongyles: Onset and resumption under field conditions of Central Europe. *Parasitology Research*, **103**, 387–392.

LE JAMBRE, L. F. & RATCLIFFE, L. H. (1971). Seasonal change in a balanced polymorphism in a *Haemonchus contortus* population. *Parasitology*, **62**, 151–155.

LEATHWICK, D. M., GODFREY, P. L., MILLER, C. M. & VLASSOFF, A. (1999). Temperature, resistance status and host effects on the development of nematode eggs. *New Zealand Journal of Zoology*, **26**, 76.

LEVINE, N. D. (1963). Weather, climate and the bionomics of ruminant nematode larvae. *Advances in Veterinary Science*, **8**, 215–261.

MARSH, R. & CAMPLING, R. C. (1970). Fouling of pastures by dung. *Herbage Abstracts*, **40**, 123–130.

MCKENNA, P. B. (1998). The effect of previous cold storage on the subsequent recovery of infective third stage nematode larvae from sheep faeces. *Veterinary Parasitology*, **80**, 167–172.

MICHEL, J. F. (1963). The phenomena of host resistance and the course of infection of *Ostertagia ostertagi* in calves. *Parasitology*, **53**, 63–84.

MICHEL, J. F. (1967). Regulation of egg output of populations of *Ostertagia ostertagi*. *Nature*, **215**, 1001–1002.

MICHEL, J. F. (1969). The epidemiology of some nematode infections in calves. *Veterinary Record*, **85**, 323–326.

MICHEL, J. F., LANCASTER, M. B. & HONG, C. (1970). Field observations on the epidemiology of parasitic gastro-enteritis in calves. *Research in Veterinary Science*, **11**, 255–259.

MICHEL, J. F., LANCASTER, M. B. & HONG, C. (1974). Studies on arrested development of *Ostertagia ostertagi* and *Cooperia oncophora*. *Journal of Comparative Pathology*, **84**, 539–554.

MICHEL, J. F., LANCASTER, M. B. & HONG, C. (1975). Arrested development of *Ostertagia ostertagi* and *Cooperia oncophora*. Effect of temperature at the free living third stage. *Journal of Comparative Pathology*, **85**, 133–138.

MICHEL, J. F., LANCASTER, M. B. & HONG, C. (1979). The effect of age, acquired resistance, pregnancy and lactation on some reactions of cattle to infection with *Ostertagia ostertagi*. *Parasitology*, **79**, 157–168.

MORLEY, F. H. W. & DONALD, A. D. (1980). Farm management and systems of helminth control. *Veterinary Parasitology*, **6**, 105–134.

O'CONNOR, L. J., WALKDEN-BROWN, S. W. & KAHN, L. P. (2006). Ecology of the free-living stages of major trichostrongylid parasites of sheep. *Veterinary Parasitology*, **142**, 1–15.

O'SULLIVAN, B. M. & DONALD, A. D. (1970). A field study of nematode parasite populations in lactating ewes. *Parasitology*, **61**, 301–315.

PANDEY, V. S. (1972). Effect of temperature on development of the free-living stages of Ostertagia ostertagi. *Journal of Parasitology*, **58**, 1037–1041.

PATON, G. & GETTINBY, G. (1983). The control of a parasitic nematode population in sheep represented by a discrete time network with stochastic inputs. *Proceedings – Royal Irish Academy, Section B*, **83 B**, 267–280.

PATON, G., THOMAS, R. J. & WALLER, P. J. (1984). A prediction model for parasitic gastro-enteritis in lambs. *International Journal for Parasitology*, **14**, 439–445.

REES, G. (1950). Observation on the vertical migrations of the third stage larvae of *Haemonchus contortus* (Rud.) on experimental plots of *Lolium perenne* S24, in relation to meteorological and micrometeorological factors. *Parasitology*, **40**, 127–143.

ROGERS, W. P. (1940). The effects of environmental conditions on the accessibility of third-stage trichostrongyle larvae to grazing animals. *Parasitology*, **32**, 209–233.

ROSE, J. H. & SMALL, A. J. (1984). Observations on the bionomics of the free-living stages of *Trichostrongylus vitrinus*. *Journal of Helminthology*, **58**, 49–58.

ROSSANIGO, C. E. & GRUNER, L. (1995). Moisture and temperature requirements in faeces for the development of free-living stages of gastrointestinal nematodes of sheep, cattle and deer. *Journal of Helminthology*, **69**, 357–362.

SAKWA, D. P., WALKDEN-BROWN, S. W., DOBSON, R. J., KAHN, L. P., LEA, J. M. & BAILLIE, N. D. (2003). Pasture microclimate can influence early development of *Haemonchus contortus* in sheep faecal pellets in a cool temperate climate. *Proceedings of the Australian Sheep Veterinary Society*, 33–40.

SALISBURY, J. R. & ARUNDEL, J. H. (1970). Peri-parturient deposition of nematode eggs by ewes and residual pasture contamination as sources of infection for lambs. *Australian Veterinary Journal*, **46**, 523–529.

SARGISON, N. D., WILSON, D. J., BARTLEY, D. J., PENNY, C. D. & JACKSON, F. (2007). Haemonchosis and teladorsagiosis in a Scottish sheep flock putatively associated with the overwintering of hypobiotic fourth stage larvae. *Veterinary Parasitology*, **147**, 326–331.

SCIACCA, J., KETSCHEK, A., FORBES, W. M., BOSTON, R., GUERRERO, J., ASHTON, F. T., GAMBLE, H. R. & SCHAD, G. A. (2002). Vertical migration by the infective larvae of three species of parasitic nematodes: Is the behaviour really a response to gravity? *Parasitology*, **125**, 553–560.

SILANGWA, S. M. & TODD, A. C. (1964). Vertical migration of Trichostrongylid larvae on grasses. *Journal of Parasitology*, **50**, 278–285.

SMEAL, M. G., ROBINSON, G. G. & FRASER, G. C. (1980). Seasonal availability of nematode larvae on pastures grazed by cattle in New South Wales. *Australian Veterinary Journal*, **56**, 74–79.

SMITH, G. (1988). The population biology of the parasitic stages of *Haemonchus contortus*. *Parasitology*, **96**, 105–115.

SMITH, G. (1989). Population biology of the parasitic phase of *Ostertagia circumcincta*. *International Journal for Parasitology*, **19**, 385–393.

SMITH, G. & GRENFELL, B. T. (1985). The population biology of *Ostertagia ostertagi*. *Parasitology Today*, **1**, 76–81.

TETLEY, J. H. (1941). The epidemiology of low-plane nematode infection in sheep in Manawatu District, New Zealand. *Cornell Veterinarian*, **31**, 243–265.

TETLEY, J. H. (1949). Rhythms in nematode parasitism of sheep. *Bulletin 96*.

TETLEY, J. H. (1959). The availability of the infective stages of nematode parasites to sheep in early spring. *Journal of Helminthology*, **33**, 289–292.

TODD, K. S., JR, LEVINE, N. D. & BOATMAN, P. A. (1976). Effect of temperature on survival of free-living stages of *Haemonchus contortus*. *American Journal of Veterinary Research*, **37**, 991–992.

VAN DIJK, J. & MORGAN, E. R. (2008). The influence of temperature on the development, hatching and survival of *Nematodirus battus* larvae. *Parasitology*, **135**, 269–283.

VLASSOFF, A. (1973). Seasonal incidence of infective trichostrongyle larvae on pasture grazed by lambs. *New Zealand Journal of Experimental Agriculture*, **1**, 293–301.

VLASSOFF, A. (1976). Seasonal incidence of infective trichostrongyle larvae on pasture: The contribution of the ewe and the role of the residual pasture infestation as sources of infection to the lamb. *New Zealand Journal of Experimental Agriculture*, **4**, 281–284.

VLASSOFF, A. (1982). Biology and population dynamics of the free-living stages of gastrointestinal nematodes of sheep. *Control of Internal Parasites in Sheep*, 11–20.

VLASSOFF, A., LEATHWICK, D. M. & HEATH, A. C. G. (2001). The epidemiology of nematode infections of sheep. *New Zealand Veterinary Journal*, **49**, 213–221.

WALLER, P. J., DONALD, A. D. & DOBSON, R. J. (1981). Arrested development of intestinal *Trichostrongylus* spp. in grazing sheep and seasonal changes in the relative abundance of *T. colubriformis* and *T. vitrinus*. *Research in Veterinary Science*, **30**, 213–216.

WALLER, P. J. & THOMAS, R. J. (1983). Arrested development of *Nematodirus* species in grazing lambs. *Research in Veterinary Science*, **34**, 357–361.

WATKINS, A. R. J. & FERNANDO, M. A. (1984). Arrested development of the rabbit stomach worm *Obeliscoides cuniculi*: Manipulation of the ability to arrest through processes of selection. *International Journal for Parasitology*, **14**, 559–570.

WILLIAMS, J. C. & BILKOVICH, F. R. (1971). Development and survival of infective larvae of the cattle nematode, *Ostertagia ostertagi*. *Journal of Parasitology*, **57**, 327–338.

WILLIAMS, J. C. & KNOX, J. W. (1976). Effect of nematode parasite infection on the performance of stocker cattle at high stocking rates on coastal Bermuda grass pastures. *American Journal of Veterinary Research*, **37**, 453–463.

YAZWINSKI, T. A. & GIBBS, H. C. (1975). Survey of helminth infections in Maine dairy cattle. *American Journal of Veterinary Research*, **36**, 1677–1682.

4 The principles of gastrointestinal nematode control

The previous chapter on the epidemiology, or epizootiology, of gastrointestinal nematode (GIN) parasites infecting grazing livestock introduced some of the basic biological principles which make these parasites difficult to eradicate. Persistence of the infective L3 on pasture and/or in infected host animals and the relatively rapid utilisation of favourable climatic conditions by the parasites, often when susceptible young stock are present, mean that in the 21st century, GIN parasites are still considered to be of the highest economic importance in sheep- and cattle-producing regions of the world (McLeod, 1995; Nieuwhof & Bishop, 2005; Perry et al., 2002).

Adequate control of GIN is required not only to ensure acceptable levels of animal health and welfare but to enable the intensification of pastoral agriculture. While this is necessary to ensure profitability in most cases, the increase in grazing pressure and associated larval challenge can also feed back into increased problems with parasitism. It seems the pastoral industries have created their own Red Queen scenario in which we are running as fast as we can to remain in the same place (Karieva, 1999). The continued development and application of sustainable worm control strategies remains as vital now as ever before.

While there are countless variations in worm control strategies across the world's pastoral industries, almost all have relied for decades on at least one of the two basic tactics – the application of anthelmintic drenches or grazing management practices.

Control of parasites with anthelmintic drenches

Since the development of the benzimidazoles in the 1960s, the control of GIN in grazing ruminants has relied on the regular or strategic application of broad-spectrum anthelmintic drenches. While there are numerous other strategies which may influence the effectiveness of GIN control within an integrated parasite management framework, the majority of the industry, on a global basis, continues to place a heavy reliance on the effectiveness of drenches (Vlassoff *et al.*, 2001). Vlassoff *et al.* (2001) also note that in New Zealand at least, while the number of drench treatments given has remained stable in recent years, the introduction and adoption of persistent drenches suggests that exposure of GIN to drenches throughout the season has actually increased.

Drench programmes

The value of strategic drench control programmes became apparent as a result of epidemiological observations which demonstrated the seasonal pattern of pasture contamination with L3 (Gordon, 1948). This led to the development of strategic control programmes designed to prevent the build-up of this contamination, thus preventing productivity losses which would certainly occur if larval challenge was allowed to continue unchecked (Brunsdon, 1966; Gordon, 1948). Obviously, given the effect of climate on the seasonal pattern of contamination, strategic control programmes will vary in timing and number of drenches between regions (Reinecke, 1980). However, the general aim to reduce contamination remains the same.

This practice of preventive strategic drenching became synonymous with the provision of 'safe pasture' (this will be discussed in relation to its impact on anthelmintic resistance in Chapters 7 and 8). In addition to the strategic use of anthelmintics, the movement of stock onto pasture with low (or zero) numbers of L3, as a means of providing 'safe pasture', is a vital part of integrated worm control programmes.

Some researchers have recommended that 'safe pasture' can be provided by the tactical use of anthelmintics, and that the use of such 'tactical drench treatments' negates the need to move stock to less-contaminated pasture. This is based on the principle of treating animals at times of the year in which larval development on pasture is at its lowest. This results in reduced re-infection of treated stock and ensures that a high proportion of the parasite population on a property are subjected to drug treatment (Southcott *et al.*, 1976). In Victoria, Australia, it was demonstrated that only two anthelmintic treatments, in an area characterised by a long dry period over the summer months, was sufficient to provide safe pasture for lambs in autumn and winter (Anderson, 1972, 1973). The first treatment is administered in early summer, at the beginning of the dry period, with the second given in mid-summer. These tactical treatments were shown to reduce pasture contamination by 90% and were claimed to be economically preferable to strategic drenching programmes which used more and regular drenching (Anderson *et al.*, 1976). Tactical drenching to provide safe pasture has also been used for GIN control in cattle. A study in England demonstrated that four fortnightly treatments of young calves, after the animals were turned out in spring, enabled them to graze pastures, which would otherwise have been heavily contaminated (Potts *et al.*, 1974). These treatments were estimated to reduce pasture contamination by 97% and resulted in a weight gain of 135.7% compared to calves grazing contaminated pastures (Potts *et al.*, 1974). In New Zealand, set stocking of calves in highly intensive systems with regular application of drenches to reduce the effects of parasitism is a common practice, and has almost certainly been a major contributor to the severity of anthelmintic resistance in the cattle of that country (Chapter 6).

With the benefit of hindsight, it has become obvious that developing and applying drenching programmes which increase the proportion of the population exposed to treatment will result in an increased selective advantage for resistant parasites. In this situation, not only is there a higher likelihood of resistant, but not susceptible, adult worms surviving, but few L3 are available on pasture to replace or dilute resistant survivors. These issues are discussed more fully in subsequent chapters.

Strategic drenching programmes

As stated above, the basic principle underpinning strategic drenching programmes is the reduction in the number of larvae contaminating pasture (Brunsdon, 1980). Obviously, the pattern and intensity of contamination with the various GIN species of grazing livestock will change significantly with factors such as climate and the type of farming system.

In temperate countries such as New Zealand, parasite epidemiology is characterised by relatively high over-wintering of L3, with a relatively lower contribution from adult stock during lactation. In this situation, lambs begin to produce eggs early in the season, meaning worm numbers on pasture and in susceptible hosts can increase markedly by autumn (Brunsdon, 1980). This has led to the development of 5- or 6-drench preventive worm control programmes for lambs, beginning in spring and continuing on a monthly basis through summer and autumn (Vlassoff & Brunsdon, 1981). The early drenches of this programme are not designed to cure any clinical disease in young lambs *per se*, but rather to knock back the first generation of parasites infecting the naïve stock, with the intention of substantially reducing future pasture contamination. This preventive programme is often supplemented by treatments to adult stock, as well as additional treatments of young stock, either based on signs of infection or in years in which the climatic conditions are deemed to be especially favourable for parasite development and survival (Beckett, 1993; Bisset *et al.*, 1986; Brunsdon *et al.*, 1983; Familton, 1991; Milligan, 1982). In addition to preventive drenching in lambs, treatment of adult stock pre-lambing has been recommended by some researchers as a means of reducing pasture contamination over the period of lactation, with the aim of limiting the numbers of L3 available to naïve stock (Beckett, 1993; Familton, 1991).

In some geographic regions, such as the northern parts of Europe or in more arid areas of Australia and South Africa, the climate is less conducive to over-wintering, and eggs produced by adult stock during the PPRI represent the major source of contamination for young animals (Boag & Thomas, 1971a, b; Heath & Michel, 1969; Reinecke, 1980). In this situation, the generation produced by the young stock results in a moderately sized second wave of pasture contamination in the autumn (Boag & Thomas, 1971a), and treatment regimes should be designed with this in mind.

Comparing the various strategic drench systems which have been developed for use across Australia illustrates perfectly how a one-size fits all approach to parasite control is not recommended. The country is so large that it has major sheep- and cattle-producing regions in a number of distinct climatic zones, with associated differences in parasite epizootiology; these have encouraged the development of targeted regional control programmes.

Recommendations for worm control in Australia have continued to evolve since the introduction of broad-spectrum anthelmintics. The 1970s saw such practices as the deliberate use of low doses of levamisole to prevent outbreaks of Haemonchosis (Waller, 2006), while many properties adopted an increasing frequency of drenches each year to maintain productivity and control. Eventually, with the realisation that resistance was becoming a serious issue for sheep farmers, strategic drench programmes were developed which aimed to minimise the frequency of drenching, in the belief that selection for resistance would also decrease (see Chapter 7). By the mid-1990s, for example, it was recommended for all sheep producing areas of the country that lambs should be drenched at weaning and moved to safe pasture, followed by a further two drenches at 8-week intervals (Barger, 1997).

Unfortunately, it has become obvious that this blanket recommendation had not in fact slowed the development of resistance, and a number of different strategic drenching programmes have now been developed, which largely reflect the ability of L3 to develop and survive on pasture in each of the various climatic zones (Barger, 1993; Waller *et al.*, 1995). These can be divided into five basic models.

Summer drenching: winter rainfall regions of temperate zones

The summer drenching programme (Drenchplan) is used most commonly from south-east South Australia, east to Tasmania and across to southern Western Australia. This programme is designed to utilise hot dry conditions in summer to limit pasture infectivity following summer drenching. For reasons related to the development and survival of L3 on pasture, the programme is relatively less successful in cooler Tasmania than in the other areas. The first drench is administered in early summer as pasture is becoming dry, with a subsequent drench for young stock 2–3 months later if required (based on egg counts). Various other interventions may be required depending on area, climate and age of lambing. With regards to the latter factor, lambing out of season, while potentially profitable, can cause problems if stock are faced with unusually high levels of parasite challenge at times of stress such as during lactation.

A major challenge in this drench programme is the possibility of outbreaks of *Haemonchus contortus*, which can occur before egg counts become obvious. In periods of high risk, whether this is based on climate or experience of local conditions, treatments with a persistent anthelmintic are advisable.

Summer drenching: winter rainfall regions in Mediterranean zones

This programme has been developed in recent years as a modification to the summer drenching programme described above to suit the climatic conditions – principally hot dry summers – common in the Mediterranean regions of Western Australia (Besier, 2001). In these conditions, survival of L3 over summer is negligible; during this period, a high proportion of the total worm population is present in the hosts, and therefore most of the population becomes subject to treatment. Following on from this is the likelihood that these worms provide the majority of subsequent parasite populations. The likelihood of developing resistance, which will be greater as the proportion of the population treated increases, has led to the development of a more complex, but hopefully more sustainable drenching programme (Besier, 2001).

In the spring or early summer, a drench is given to weaner lambs – this is timed to coincide with a move to safe pasture or a climate-driven reduction in pasture contamination. At the same time, a drench should be administered to adult sheep on a needs basis, normally based on faecal egg counts. Any further treatments of either lambs or adult stock should be administered only when egg counts signal potential impacts on productivity or pasture contamination. It is recognised that in this area, the problem of resistance has increased to the point at which additional drenches may be required to minimise pasture contamination and productivity losses solely due to the presence of sufficient numbers of resistant parasites (Besier, 2001).

Summer rainfall: agricultural regions

In the 1980s, the 'Wormkill' programme was developed for application in areas of south-east Australia in which *H. contortus*, and to a lesser extent *Trichostrongylus* spp., were the major cause of productivity losses. The essence of Wormkill was to minimise pasture contamination with *H. contortus* for extended periods through the strategic use of the narrow-spectrum anthelmintic closantel (Barger *et al.*, 1991), with the addition of broad-spectrum drenches to control *Trichostrongylus* spp. (Dash, 1986). In the Wormkill programme, assuming resistance has not become a major problem, closantel is administered in spring to all animals to prevent any pasture contamination from hypobiotic larvae; this is followed by additional closantel treatments in early summer, mid-summer and autumn. Broad-spectrum anthelmintics are also administered to lambs and weaners at these times.

In recent years, the problem of closantel resistance has lessened the effectiveness of this drug (Rolfe *et al.*, 1990), and it has been replaced where necessary by other anthelmintics, including persistent products such as moxidectin (Abbott *et al.*, 1995) or controlled-release capsules releasing ivermectin (Allerton *et al.*, 1998). Additional treatments can be administered as required, based on egg counts, although routine drenches may be given regardless at weaning.

Low rainfall cereal zones

In any area in which the intensity of animal production is low, such as primarily arable areas, worm control is less problematic, particularly due to prevailing low levels of pasture contamination. In these areas, a weaning drench may be administered to lambs, although this may not be necessary if egg counts are sufficiently low. Adult sheep may be drenched if necessary, but only based on egg counts. Although pasture contamination and therefore worm burdens are normally low, favourable climatic conditions such as rainfall – can quickly lead to a build-up of larvae on pasture, particularly in areas where *H. contortus* is present.

Low rainfall pastoral zones

Due to low stocking density of animals in semi-arid or arid conditions, pasture contamination throughout most of the year is minimal, and adequate worm control is possible with few drenches. However, due to the same extensive nature of the enterprises, management options are reduced as farmers rarely handle stock. When climatic conditions are favourable, there may still be significant losses following a rapid increase in pasture contamination.

Principles of worm control in cattle

While most of the preceding section has described a number of alternate strategies for the control of parasitism of small ruminants, the general principles of reducing pasture contamination apply equally to cattle. There is some variability in areas in which cattle are housed over winter, as this practice undoubtedly alters the pattern of larval availability compared to regions in which animals graze pasture year round (Michel, 1969). Furthermore, the widespread practice of administering persistent treatments as injectable or pour-on formulations may influence the frequency of treatment within strategic drenching programmes.

Control of GIN by grazing management

In addition to the application of a drench, moving treated stock onto relatively uncontaminated pasture – so-called 'clean' or 'safe' pasture – can significantly reduce the severity of parasitism in weaned lambs (Brunsdon, 1980). A study in Australia (Donald, 1974) demonstrated the use of drench and move to clean pasture and suggested that a single drench was sufficient to control parasitism over the entire grazing season. It was noted, however, that the provision of truly 'safe' pastures in areas where animals are grazed all year round is unusual (Donald & Waller, 1973), and the provision of such 'safe' pastures would require the treatment of adult animals over autumn and winter.

The economic benefits of drench and move were illustrated by Brunsdon (1980), who measured a 6.3 kg advantage from a single drench to lambs at weaning when it was followed by a move to 'safe' pasture. In contrast, drenching the lambs and leaving them on the 'dirty' paddocks resulted in a weight advantage of only 0.8 kg. As a general rule, therefore, it appears that reducing the intensity of pasture contamination underpins the control of GIN or at least plays a key role in reducing production losses from livestock.

In addition to a basic programme of drenching and moving stock to pastures which have remained free of animals for a significant enough period for larval numbers to decline, there are numerous other management practices which can be introduced to minimise the ingestion of L3 by a susceptible host animal-without recourse to (or used in conjunction with) anthelmintic treatment. Most of these practices are more or less applicable depending on the prevailing climate, farm-type and farming practices. The most widespread practice is to utilise grazing animals which are less susceptible to the particular larval contamination assumed to be present. This may involve mixed or alternate grazing with different host species or with different stock classes.

Alternate/mixed grazing with different host species or stock classes

Grazing systems which utilise both sheep and cattle are based primarily on the premise that most of the GIN of each of the host species is either poorly or completely non-adapted to the alternate species (Amarante *et al.*, 1997; Borgsteede, 1981; Roberts, 1942). As ingested L3 are destroyed during passage through the gastrointestinal tract in an unsuitable host, each species should therefore act as a net remover of larval challenge for the other in a mixed or alternate grazing system.

The value of this approach has been investigated on a number of occasions. Grazing sheep and cattle together so that the animal equivalence was 70, 50, 40 or 30% (sheep to cattle), resulted in a progressive decrease in the worm burdens in the sheep of GIN species normally associated with that host species, such as *Teladorsagia circumcincta* and *Nematodirus spathiger*, but a corresponding increase in the numbers of parasites normally associated with cattle, such as *Cooperia oncophora* and *Trichostrongylus axei* (Arundel & Hamilton, 1975). Due to the observed low worm burdens in all treatments in this study, no conclusions could be drawn concerning the impact of mixed grazing on animal productivity. Similar results were obtained in another study which quantified the impact of alternate grazing on worm burdens, although on this occasion grazing with sheep reduced burdens of *Ostertagia ostertagi* and *T. axei* in calves, but had no effect on *C. oncophora* (Barger & Southcott, 1975). A subsequent extension to this study determined that worm burdens of most GIN could be reduced in either of the host species when the period of alternate grazing was sufficiently long – reductions were observed using 12-week, but not 6-week periods (Southcott & Barger, 1975).

While there is a large degree of host specificity within the GIN of sheep and cattle, it is obvious from the research reviewed above that it is by no means absolute, with some species able to establish in either host. Examples of this are *T. axei* (which is found in a number of host species, including horses), *H. contortus* and *Cooperia* spp. (Borgsteede, 1981; Roberts, 1942). For this reason, any mixed-species grazing system should not be regarded as a foolproof method for parasite control by itself, but as part of an integrated control package. This was demonstrated in a 4-year alternate grazing trial alternating sheep and cattle in which reduced parasite burdens in the cattle were observed in the first 2 years of the study, but thereafter no benefit was apparent (Bairden *et al.*, 1995).

The value of mixed or alternate grazing systems which use different stock classes of the same species has also been investigated. Here, the rationale is similar to that of mixed-species grazing, as in most cases older animals have developed an effective immune response to parasite challenge and therefore also act as net removers of pasture contamination (Charleston, 1986). A recent study in New Zealand, which was primarily designed to determine the impact of alternate grazing with lambs and ewes on the development of resistance, also demonstrated significant productivity benefits for the lambs (Leathwick *et al.*, 2008).

In contrast to the use of adult stock of the same species, there is little evidence of any productivity benefit through the application of alternate-species grazing strategies. However, this is not true of mixed grazing systems using cattle and sheep which simultaneously graze the same pasture. Here, however, the evidence suggests that differences in sward structure and pasture utilisation resulting from differences in diet selection was the key to improved productivity, as opposed to a reduction in parasitism *per se* (Abaye *et al.*, 1994, 1997; Jordan *et al.*, 1988).

It is evident that using unsuitable hosts in a grazing management system, whether they be an alternate species or immune individuals, can be an important tool in an integrated control programme for GIN control. However, as almost every chapter in this book will reveal, the reality, and the practicality of its application on-farm, is more complex than it first appears.

Even where parasites may not establish patent infections, they may still have a negative impact on productivity. For example, while the cattle parasite *O. ostertagi* did not reach patency in experimental infections in sheep, the challenged animals mounted an immune response which, although less pronounced than in animals challenged with the closely-related *T. circumcincta*, would almost certainly have imposed a cost in terms of productivity. It should be noted, however, that the same study also demonstrated that exposure of sheep to challenge with *O. ostertagi* conferred a degree of immunity to subsequent challenge with *T. circumcincta* (Sutherland *et al.*, 1999).

As a result of these observations, it is proposed that mixed/alternate grazing can be a useful management strategy, but care must be taken that the 'resistant' animals are in fact able to withstand larval challenge. Thus, sheep/cattle grazing or young/adult grazing is for the most part of value. However, given the similarity in GIN species profiles, mixed grazing between sheep and goats does not provide a similar benefit. Indeed, given the track record of the development of anthelmintic resistance in goats, and the subsequent transfer of the resistant worms to sheep, this particular version of mixed grazing is considered unwise.

Resistance to treatment

The inevitable outcome of sustained worm control, regardless of the treatment protocol, is the eventual development of resistance to the applied treatment (Smith *et al.*, 1999). If allowed to become serious enough, drench resistance will become a major threat to the sustainability of worm control worldwide. The subsequent chapters are devoted to reviewing the status of resistance, the mechanisms used by the worms, the influence of the various drench types and finally the major risk factors for resistance and how to minimise the selective advantage for resistant worms.

Before dealing with these various facets of resistance, it is necessary to highlight the possible impacts of worm control on parasite epidemiology, and the potential advantage this can confer to those worms capable of surviving treatment.

The major principles of worm control are to minimise the exposure of stock to parasite challenge and then to remove worm burdens which may cause productivity losses. It could be considered rather obvious that sustained treatment results in selective advantage; however, there are certain factors which deserve special consideration when designing sustainable worm control programmes.

Firstly, when the **proportion** of resistant worms in the population is low, then any measure which reduces the size of the population will favour those with resistant genes (see Chapter 7). Also, any practice which reduces the extent of pasture contamination, whether through drenching or the use of particular grazing management practices, is likely to confer a selective advantage for resistant worms. An excellent example of how drenching programmes and grazing management can combine to produce resistance is the practice of drench and move to clean pasture. In this situation, all parasites in the host are subject to drug treatment; then, following a move to 'clean' pasture, only those resistant survivors have the opportunity to provide progeny to future generations (Figure 4.1).

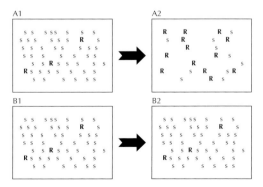

Figure 4.1 A1 to A2 depicts the effect of drench and move to 'safe' or 'clean' pasture, although the assumption has been made that a limited number of susceptible genotypes (s) are present to reduce the proportion of resistant (R) genotypes. B1 to B2 depicts the consequence of drenching and moving onto 'dirty' pasture.

Furthermore, following drench and move, there are no susceptible L3 on pasture which can be ingested to dilute or replace the resistant drench survivors. A similar effect can be seen when farmers attempt to use drench to provide 'clean' pasture through intense chemotherapy or in arid areas in which the development and survival of the free-living stages of parasites is low. An initially surprising observation from a large-scale survey of anthelmintic resistance in New Zealand was that those farms which utilised mixed grazing of sheep and cattle tended to have a higher prevalence of drench-resistant parasites. The obvious explanation for this is that the net removal of L3 from pasture by the unsuitable hosts had a relatively greater effect on the population of susceptible L3 available to the suitable host animals.

Each of these scenarios reduces the overall contribution of susceptible parasites to the parasite population and confers a selective advantage to those worms able to survive anthelmintic treatment.

References

ABAYE, A. O., ALLEN, V. G. & FONTENOT, J. P. (1994). Influence of grazing cattle and sheep together and separately on animal performance and forage quality. *Journal of Animal Science*, **72**, 1013–1022.

ABAYE, A. O., ALLEN, V. G. & FONTENOT, J. P. (1997). Grazing sheep and cattle together or separately: Effect on soils and plants. *Agronomy Journal*, **89**, 380–386.

ABBOTT, K. A., COBB, R. M. & HOLM GLASS, M. (1995). Duration of the persistent activity of moxidectin against *Haemonchus contortus* in sheep. *Australian Veterinary Journal*, **72**, 408–410.

ALLERTON, G. R., GOGOLEWSKI, R. P., RUGG, D., PLUE, R. E., BARRICK, R. A. & EAGLESON J. S. (1998). Field trials evaluating ivermectin controlled-release capsules for weaner sheep and for breeding ewes. *Australian Veterinary Journal*, **76**, 39–43.

AMARANTE, A. F. T., BAGNOLA, J., AMARANTE, M. R. V. & BARBOSA, M. A. (1997). Host specificity of sheep and cattle nematodes in São Paulo state, Brazil. *Veterinary Parasitology*, **73**, 89–104.

ANDERSON, N. (1972). Trichostrongylid infections of sheep in a winter rainfall region. I. Epizootiological studies in the western district of Victoria, 1966–67. *Australian Journal of Agricultural Research*, **23**, 1113–1129.

ANDERSON, N. (1973). Trichostrongylid infections of sheep in a winter rainfall region. II. Epizootiological studies in the western district of Victoria, 1967–68. *Australian Journal of Agricultural Research*, **24**, 599–611.

ANDERSON, N., MORRIS, R. S. & McTAGGART, I. K. (1976). An economic analysis of two schemes for the anthelmintic control of helminthiasis in weaned lambs. *Australian Veterinary Journal*, **52**, 174–180.

ARUNDEL, J. H. & HAMILTON, D. (1975). The effect of mixed grazing of sheep and cattle on worm burdens in lambs. *Australian Veterinary Journal*, **51**, 436–439.

BAIRDEN, K., ARMOUR, J. & DUNCAN, J. L. (1995). A 4-year study on the effectiveness of alternate grazing of cattle and sheep in the control of bovine parasitic gastroenteritis. *Veterinary Parasitology*, **60**, 119–132.

BARGER, I. (1997). Control by management. *Veterinary Parasitology*, **72**, 493–506.

BARGER, I. A. (1993). Control of gastrointestinal nematodes in Australia in the 21st century. *Veterinary Parasitology*, **46**, 23–32.

BARGER, I. A., HALL, E. & DASH, K. M. (1991). Local eradication of *Haemonchus contortus* using closantel. *Australian Veterinary Journal*, **68**, 347–348.

BARGER, I. A. & SOUTHCOTT, W. H. (1975). Control of nematode parasites by grazing management. I. Decontamination of cattle pastures by grazing with sheep. *International Journal for Parasitology*, **5**, 39–44.

BECKETT, F. W. (1993). An evaluation of a modified preventive drenching programme on commercial sheep farms. *New Zealand Veterinary Journal*, **41**, 116–122.

BESIER, R. B. (2001). Re-thinking the summer drenching program. *Journal of Agriculture of Western Australia*, **42**, 6–9.

BISSET, S. A., BRUNSDON, R. V., HEATH, A. C. G., VLASSOFF, A. & MASON, P. C. (1986). Guide to livestock parasite control. *New Zealand Farmer*, **107**, 5–22.

BOAG, B. & THOMAS, R. J. (1971a). Epidemiological studies on gastro-intestinal nematode parasites of sheep. I. Infection patterns on clean and autumn contaminated pasture. *Research in Veterinary Science*, **12**, 132–139.

BOAG, B. T. & THOMAS, R. J. (1971b). Epidemiological studies on gastro-intestinal nematode parasites of sheep. The control of infection in lambs on clean pasture. *Research in Veterinary Science*, **14**, 11–20.

BORGSTEEDE, F. H. M. (1981). Experimental cross-infections with gastrointestinal nematodes of sheep and cattle. *Zeitschrift fur Parasitenkunde Parasitology Research*, **65**, 1–10.

BRUNSDON, R. V. (1966). Further studies of the effect of infestation by nematodes of the family Trichostrongylidae in sheep: An evaluation of a strategic drenching programme. *New Zealand Veterinary Journal*, **14**, 71–83.

BRUNSDON, R. V. (1980). Principles of helminth control. *Veterinary Parasitology*, **6**, 185–215.

BRUNSDON, R. V., KISSLING, R. & HOSKING, B. C. (1983). A survey of anthelmintic usage for sheep: A time for change? *New Zealand Veterinary Journal*, **31**, 24–29.

CHARLESTON, W. A. G. (1986). Parasites. In *Sheep Production. 2. Feeding, Growth and Health* (eds McCutcheon, S. N., McDonald, M. F. & Wickham, G. A.), New Zealand Institute of Agricultural Science and Ray Richards Publisher, Auckland, NZ, pp. 204–243.

DASH, K. M. (1986). Control of helminthosis in lambs by strategic treatment with closantel and broad-spectrum anthelmintics. *Australian Veterinary Journal*, **63**, 4–7.

DONALD, A. D. (1974). Some recent advances in the epidemiology and control of helminth infection in sheep. *Proceedings of the Australian Society for Animal Production*, **10**, 148–155.

DONALD, A. D. & WALLER, P. J. (1973). Gastro-intestinal nematode parasite populations in ewes and lambs and the origin and time course of infective larval availability in pastures. *International Journal for Parasitology*, **3**, 219–233.

FAMILTON, A. S. (1991). Re-examination of gastrointestinal parasite control – The contribution of the ewe. *Proceedings of the 21st Seminar of the Sheep and Beef Cattle Society of the New Zealand Veterinary Association*, **21**, 25–35.

GORDON, H. M. (1948). The epidemiology of parasitic diseases, with special reference to studies with nematode parasites of sheep. *The Australian Veterinary Journal*, **24**, 17–45.

HEATH, G. B. & MICHEL, J. F. (1969). A contribution to the epidemiology of parasitic gastro-enteritis in lambs. *Veterinary Record*, **85**, 305–308.

JORDAN, H. E., PHILLIPS, W. A., MORRISON, R. D., DOYLE, J. J. & MCKENZIE, K. (1988). A 3-year study of continuous mixed grazing of cattle and sheep: Parasitism of offspring. *International Journal for Parasitology*, **18**, 779–784.

KARIEVA, P. (1999). Coevolutionary arms races: Is victory possible? *Proceedings of the National Academy of Sciences USA*, **96**, 8–10.

LEATHWICK, D. M., MILLER, C. M., ATKINSON, D. S., HAACK, N. A., WAGHORN, T. S. & OLIVER, A. M. (2008). Managing anthelmintic resistance: Untreated adult ewes as a source of unselected parasites, and their role in reducing parasite populations. *New Zealand Veterinary Journal*, **56**, 184–195.

MCLEOD, R. S. (1995). Costs of major parasites to the Australian livestock industries. *International Journal for Parasitology*, **25**, 1363–1367.

MICHEL, J. F. (1969). The epidemiology of some nematode infections in calves. *Veterinary Record*, **85**, 323–326.

MILLIGAN, K. (1982). Drenching adult sheep: Is it worth while? *New Zealand Journal of Agriculture*, **144**, 18.

NIEUWHOF, G. J. & BISHOP, S. C. (2005). Costs of the major endemic diseases of sheep in Great Britain and the potential benefits of reduction in disease impact. *Animal Science*, **81**, 23–29.

PERRY, B. D., RANDOLPH, T. F., MCDERMOTT, J. J., SONES, K. R. & THORNTON, P. K. (2002). *Investing in Animal Health Research to Alleviate Poverty*. International Livestock Research Institute (ILRI), Nairobi, Kenya.

POTTS, K. M., JONES, R. M. & CORNWELL, R. L. (1974). Control of bovine parasitic gastro-enteritis by reduction of pasture larval levels. *Proceedings of the 3rd International Congress for Parasitology*, Munich, 747–748.

REINECKE, R. K. (1980). Chemotherapy in the control of helminthosis. *Veterinary Parasitology*, **6**, 255–292.

ROBERTS, F. H. S. (1942). The host specificity of sheep and cattle helminths, with particular reference to the use of cattle in cleansing sheep pastures. *Australian Veterinary Journal*, **18**, 19–27.

ROLFE, P. F., BORAY, J. C., FITZGIBBON, C., PARSONS, G., KEMSLEY, P. & SANGSTER, N. (1990). Closantel resistance in *Haemonchus contortus* from sheep. *Australian Veterinary Journal*, **67**, 29–31.

SMITH, G., GRENFELL, B. T., ISHAM, V. & CORNELL, S. (1999). Anthelmintic resistance revisited: Under-dosing, chemoprophylactic strategies, and mating probabilities. *International Journal for Parasitology*, **29**, 77–91.

SOUTHCOTT, W., MAJOR, G. & BARGER, I. (1976). Seasonal pasture contamination and availability of nematodes for grazing sheep. *Australian Journal of Agricultural Research*, **27**, 277–286.

SOUTHCOTT, W. H. & BARGER, I. A. (1975). Control of nematode parasites by grazing management. II. Decontamination of sheep and cattle pastures by varying periods of grazing with the alternate host. *International Journal for Parasitology*, **5**, 45–48.

SUTHERLAND, I. A., BROWN, A. E., GREEN, R. S., MIILER, C. M. & LEATHWICK, D. M. (1999). The immune response of sheep to larval challenge with *Ostertagia circumcincta* and *O. ostertagi*. *Veterinary Parasitology*, **84**, 125–135.

VLASSOFF, A. & BRUNSDON, R. V. (1981). Control of gastro-intestinal nematodes: Advantages of a preventive anthelmintic drenching programme for lambs on pasture. *New Zealand Journal of Experimental Agriculture*, **9**, 221–225.

VLASSOFF, A., LEATHWICK, D. M. & HEATH, A. C. G. (2001). The epidemiology of nematode infections of sheep. *The New Zealand Veterinary Journal*, **49**, 213–221.

WALLER, P. J. (2006). From discovery to development: Current industry perspectives for the development of novel methods of helminth control in livestock. *Veterinary Parasitology*, **139**, 1–14.

WALLER, P. J., DASH, K. M., BARGER, I. A., LE JAMBRE, L. F. & PLANT, J. (1995). Anthelmintic resistance in nematode parasites of sheep: Learning from the Australian experience. *Veterinary Record*, **136**, 411–413.

5 Anthelmintics

'Most anthelmintics will cure a parasitic disease, or will at least reduce the effects of the infestation, but few will reduce the worm burden to a level at which the risks of re-infestation are negligible. The very high efficiency of phenothiazine against both the mature and immature worms, and its effects on egg production and on the development of the eggs and larvae in faeces, give it a true preventive effect. Some theoretical examples will illustrate these points. It was found (Gordon, unpublished) that the mixture of copper sulphate and nicotine sulphate, commonly used against Trichostrongylus spp. in sheep, had a mean efficiency of 57 per cent., whereas phenothiazine had a mean efficiency of 80 per cent. Suppose that two sheep harbour 20,000 Trichostrongylus spp. each. Following treatment with the copper sulphate-nicotine sulphate mixture, the residual worm burden will be 8,600, whereas the residual worm burden following the use of phenothiazine will be 4,000. If half of the residual worms are females and each female produces 200 eggs per day (Gordon, unpublished), the total daily egg output for the first sheep will be 860,000 and for the second 400,000. If a second treatment is carried out, the residual worm burden becomes 3,700 and 800, and the daily egg output becomes 370,000 and 80,000 respectively.'

The quote above is from an address to the Australian Veterinary Association in 1947, which was reproduced a year later in the *Australian Veterinary Journal* (Gordon, 1948). The enthusiasm of the author for phenothiazine is understandable; in the 1930s, he had assessed the efficacy of such treatments as sodium arsenite, tetrachloroethylene, carbon tetrachloride and combinations of sodium arsenite/copper sulphate, copper sulphate/carbon bisulphide and copper sulphate/nicotine sulphate (Gordon, 1935). [It is also interesting to note that phenothiazine and related compounds have an alternative application as tranquilisers (Kurland *et al.*, 1961), which raises questions regarding its full impact on treated livestock.]

While some of the treatments assessed were relatively effective, it is inconceivable that such concoctions would have any place in modern agricultural practice. Indeed, the quote from Gordon is reproduced here to illustrate the extent to which the introduction of modern anthelmintics has revolutionised the control of gastrointestinal nematodes (GIN) in grazing ruminants. This chapter briefly describes what constitutes an anthelmintic, then describes the currently available anthelmintic families as well as some compounds which may become available in the near future.

What are anthelmintics?

Anthelmintics are drugs which are effective in removing existing burdens or which prevent establishment of ingested L3. Despite the impact of helminths in veterinary medicine, there have been very few successful, broad-spectrum anthelmintic families discovered and commercialised for use in grazing livestock in the last 50 years. This has been a source of considerable concern as productivity, and therefore profitability, of the livestock sectors are reliant on a small number of effective treatments.

The primary reason behind this lack of success in developing novel active families appears to be economic. The size of the drench market in grazing livestock is much smaller than that of companion animals or humans. Together with increasing costs of development and increasingly stringent regulatory requirements, there has been little appetite for developing new anthelmintics within the major pharmaceutical companies.

There has been another potential factor in the lack of drug discovery in recent years; for many years, the success of ivermectin and related compounds appeared to make the development of any other compounds unnecessary. Almost paradoxically, however, it has been the increasing failure of these (and previous) drugs as the prevalence of resistance to treatment has increased that may finally make pharmaceutical companies reconsider the potential commercial benefits of anthelmintic discovery.

How effective does an anthelmintic have to be?

As a representative example of what is required for any compound to claim anthelmintic efficacy, the following passage is quoted from New Zealand Food Safety Authority guidelines: http://www.nzfsa.govt.nz/acvm/publications/standards-guidelines/anthelminticfinal.pdf

'Claims made for a genus, rather than a species, in a dose confirmation trial are not acceptable as there are known differences between species in some genera with some anthelmintics.

Each of six animals in each respective treatment group should be infected with each stage and species of parasite for which a claim is to be made. If this cannot be established antemortem, it will be assumed for the treatment group if all control animals are infected.

Efficacy claims must be in line with WAAVP recommendations that such claims should be expressed as a percentage against each separate genus/species as:

- *highly effective (>98%);*
- *effective (90–98%);*
- *moderately effective (80–89%); or*
- *insufficiently active or inactive (<80%).*

Such claims can be made only for the species and stage of infection for which this reduction is achieved.'

Realistically, any new anthelmintic released commercially would be required to display at least 95% efficacy against all of the major GIN species to be accepted by the industry. It is also obvious that different active families should utilise a different mode of action on nematodes. This not only provides a point of difference for marketing purposes, but also the opportunity for a new (or existing) anthelmintic to effectively kill parasites which are resistant to another family. When developing a new anthelmintic, it has now become necessary that any candidate compound is able to remove worm burdens of parasites which are known to be resistant to at least the three major existing active families.

Which species does an anthelmintic against GIN need to remove?

There is little variability in the range of target species for anthelmintics in either the sheep or cattle sectors worldwide, although the relative importance of particular species may vary with factors such as climate. There is also some cross-infection between species associated with either sheep or cattle. The major species of nematodes known to be effectively removed by anthelmintics are listed below by host species and by organ as follows:

Sheep GIN

Abomasum: *Haemonchus contortus, Teladorsagia (Ostertagia) circumcincta, Trichostrongylus axei.*

Small intestine: *Trichostrongylus colubriformis, T. vitrinus, Cooperia curticei, C. oncophora, C. punctata, Nematodirus spathiger, N. filicollis, N. battus, Bunostomum trigonocephalum, Strongyloides papillosus.*

Large intestine: *Chabertia ovina, Trichuris ovis, Oesophagostomum columbianum, Oe. venulosum.*

Cattle GIN

Abomasum: *Ostertagia ostertagi, O. leptospicularis, T. axei, H. placei, H. contortus.*

Small intestine: *B. phlebotomum, C. oncophora, C. punctata, C. spatulata, C. pectinata, C. surnabada, S. papillosus.*

Large intestine: *C. ovina, O. radiatum, T. ovis.*

Description, efficacy, profile and mode of action of anthelmintic families

1. Benzimidazoles such as thiabendazole and albendazole

'Sir,
   We wish to report the discovery of a new class of anthelmintic agents possessing a broad spectrum of activity for gastrointestinal parasites of domestic animals. Some of the compounds are among the most potent chemotherapeutic agents known, complete larvacidal activity being manifest in vitro at 10^{-5} γ/ml.'
Brown et al. (1961)

Description

Following on from the quote reproduced at the beginning of this chapter, the discovery of thiabendazole, and subsequently other benzimidazole and pro-benzimidazole drugs, heralded the era of effective and affordable broad-spectrum control of GIN in grazing livestock. The original member of the class, the synthetic molecule thiabendazole, was originally used as a fungicide. All of the other members of the benzimidazole class of compounds are derivatives of the same chemical family.

Efficacy

Brown *et al.* (1961), first demonstrated the efficacy of thiabendazole against a range of GIN. Quoting again from the *Nature* paper which reported the drug's discovery, *'In sheep, for example, thiabendazole in a single oral dose of 50 mg./kg. of body weight removed more than 95% of the worms belonging to ten genera of gastrointestinal parasites (Trichostrongylus, Cooperia, Nematodirus, Ostertagia, Haemonchus, Oesophagostomum, Bunostomum, Strongyloides, Chabertia, Trichuris). In addition to removing the adult parasites, thiabendazole inhibits production of eggs and interferes with development of larval forms.'*

Subsequent studies also demonstrated excellent efficacy of thiabendazole against the inhibited forms of *T. circumcincta* (Armour *et al.*, 1975) and *H. contortus* (McKenna, 1974).

The initial member of the family was soon followed by other, more effective, benzimidazoles such as mebendazole (Kelly *et al.*, 1975), fenbendazole (Eslami & Anwar, 1976) and albendazole (Borgsteede, 1979; Theodorides *et al.*, 1976).

The pro-benzimidazole drugs, such as thiophanate and netobimin, are also highly effective against GIN (Eichler, 1973; Richards *et al.*, 1987).

Profile

The original member of the family, thiabendazole (Figure 5.1), reaches a maximum plasma concentration by 5 hours post-oral administration in sheep and is then rapidly excreted over the next 48–72 hours (Tocco *et al.*, 1964). Subsequent benzimidazoles, presumably because of reduced solubility (Bogan & Armour, 1986), have a slower dissolution rate and absorption into the circulation. For example, maximum concentrations of fenbendazole and oxfendazole are reached between 24 and 36 hours post-oral administration in sheep (Marriner & Bogan, 1981a, b) and cattle (Ngomyuo *et al.*, 1984). The benzimidazoles associate strongly with particulate matter in the rumen, which may be important in extending the period during which the drugs may be absorbed (Hennessy, 1997).

Mode of Action

Originally thought to act by inhibiting the enzyme fumarate reductase (Prichard, 1970), the mode of action of the benzimidazoles has since been characterised as binding to, and interfering with, the polymerisation of nematode beta-tubulin, resulting in the inhibition of microtubule polymerisation. As these microtubules are necessary for the transport of secretory granules and enzyme secretion within the cytoplasm, cell death eventually occurs (Kohler, 2001).

2. Imidazothiazoles/tetrahydropyrimidines – including levamisole and morantel tartrate

Description

These two families of compounds are routinely considered together as they share a common mode of action (Sanchez Bruni *et al.*, 2006). The initial member of this active class was the aminothiazol derivative tetramisole, which was observed to have anthelmintic activity against three nematode species in chickens (Thienpont *et al.*, 1966). Tetramisole was subsequently found to be a racemic mixture of 50% L- and D-isomers. When the D-isomer was demonstrated to have little anthelmintic activity, the L-isomer was developed and commercialised as levamisole (Figure 5.2). The removal of the D-isomer was particularly helpful as

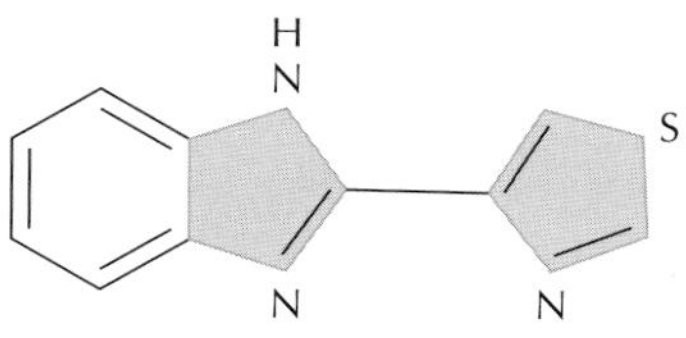

Figure 5.1   Chemical structure of thiabendazole.

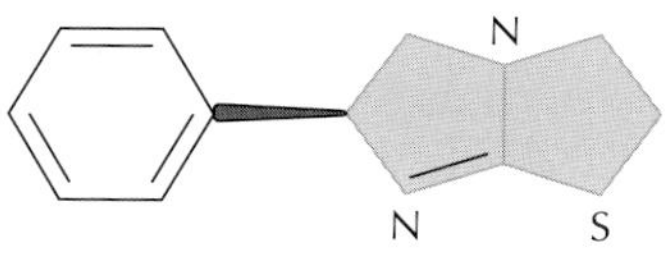

Figure 5.2   Chemical structure of levamisole.

both L and D had equal toxicity in the mammalian host (Sanchez Bruni *et al.*, 2006).

The tetrahydropyrimidine, morantel tartrate, is the methyl analogue of pyrantel tartrate (Bogan & Armour, 1986) and has been consistently used in cattle in the northern hemisphere. It is noted that, unlike the benzimidazoles and most of the MLs, both levamisole and morantel tartrate can be toxic at high doses (Bogan & Armour, 1986).

Efficacy

Levamisole was found to be effective against GIN in both sheep (Kates *et al.*, 1971; Turton, 1974) and cattle at an oral dose rate of 7.5 mg/kg (Leland *et al.*, 1971; Turton, 1969), although the efficacy against *O. ostertagi* in cattle is relatively low against all stages (Williams *et al.*, 1991). By contrast, the drug does have good efficacy against the inhibited larvae of *T. circumcincta* in sheep (Reid *et al.*, 1976). Morantel tartrate, administered as a bolus to cattle, has good efficacy against most, but not all, of the major GIN of cattle; efficacy is particularly poor against *O. ostertagi* (87%) and *T. axei* (96%). In nine controlled experimental trials conducted across Europe efficacy determined by worm counts against field-derived mixed infections averaged 79% (Jones & Bliss, 1983).

Profile

At an oral dose of 7.5 mg/kg in sheep, levamisole reached peak plasma concentrations of 3.1 µg/ml when given subcutaneously, but only 0.7 and 0.8 µg/ml when given via the oral and intra-ruminal routes respectively (Bogan *et al.*, 1982). Peak concentrations were reached in plasma by 1 hour following subcutaneous administration and after approximately 6 hours by the other two routes. Regardless of the route of administration, drug concentrations in plasma had declined to be almost undetectable after 24 hours (Bogan *et al.*, 1982).

Mode of action

These anthelmintics have been characterised as nicotinic agonists, acting selectively at synaptic and extra-synaptic nicotinic acetylcholine receptors. This results in spastic paralysis of the worms, leading to expulsion from the host (Martin, 1997). In the large nematode *Ascaris suum*, patch clamping was used to demonstrate that these anthelmintics increase membrane conductance by opening cation–ion channels permeable to Na^+ and K^+ (Evans & Martin, 1993; Robertson & Martin, 1993).

3. The avermectin and milbemycin macrocyclic lactones (MLs)

Description

The commercial release of ivermectin as an oral drench for livestock (Chabala *et al.*, 1980) heralded a new era of worm control (Chabala *et al.*, 1980).

Effective against a wider range of parasites than existing families, including arthropods (Lancaster *et al.*, 1982; Meleney *et al.*, 1982), and at a lower dose rate, the product quickly became the dominant anthelmintic for both sheep and cattle.

The avermectins are a group of closely related complex MLs and are fermentation products of the actinomycete bacterial species *Streptomyces avermitilis*.

Originally found in a soil sample from a Japanese golf course, the avermectins were established to have anthelmintic activity during routine screening in a nematode–mouse model (*Nematospiroides dubius*). The avermectins have a macrocyclic backbone with a disaccharide substituent at C13. Ivermectin is a semi-synthetic derivative of the naturally occurring avermectins (Figure 5.3), comprising around 80% 22, 23-dihydroavermectin B_{1a} and around 20% B_{1b}. Abamectin is the natural precursor to ivermectin and has a double bond at the C22–23 position. Other avermectins of note for the control of GIN are doramectin (25-cyclohexyl-avermectin B_1) and eprinomectin (90:10 mix of 4″-epi-acetylamino-4″-deoxyavermectin B_{1a} and B_{1b}).

While similar to the avermectins, the milbemycin compound moxidectin is a fermentation product of a different bacterial species, *S. cyanogriseus noncyanogenus*. Unlike the avermectins, moxidectin has an unsaturated C-25 chain.

Each of the MLs is strongly lipophilic, which is assumed to account for improved distribution throughout the body of treated subjects.

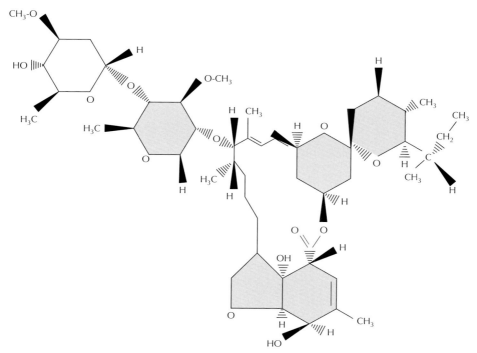

Figure 5.3   Chemical structure of 22,23-dihydroavermectin B_{1a}.

Efficacy

At an oral dose rate of 0.2 mg/kg, ivermectin was highly effective against all of the important GIN species in both sheep (Wescott & LeaMaster, 1982; Yazwinski *et al.*, 1983) and cattle (Egerton *et al.*, 1981) and was also effective against inhibited larval stages (Williams *et al.*, 1981).

Abamectin, used orally at 0.2 mg/kg, was also shown to be highly effective against all species and stages of GIN in sheep (Alka *et al.*, 2004) and cattle (Heinze-Mutz *et al.*, 1993; Williams *et al.*, 1992). Furthermore, studies have demonstrated the ability of abamectin to remove burdens of worms which are resistant to ivermectin (Alka *et al.*, 2004; Sutherland *et al.*, 2002).

Doramectin, administered subcutaneously to cattle, was effective against GIN (Goudie *et al.*, 1993; Jones *et al.*, 1993; Mehlhorn *et al.*, 1993), while an injectable formulation for sheep was also effective (Sisodia *et al.*, 1996). Cattle treated with doramectin are protected from reinfection with susceptible parasites for around 20 days post-administration (Vercruysse *et al.*, 1993).

Eprinomectin for cattle, given at a dose rate of 0.1 ml/kg, was highly effective against GIN (Gogolewski *et al.*, 1997c; Shoop *et al.*, 1996). Eprinomectin is also effective against GIN in sheep (Cringoli *et al.*, 2003), although it is rarely used.

Moxidectin has been described as the most potent of the MLs, and by logical extension, the most potent of all available anthelmintics against all of the major GIN species in sheep and cattle, although it is less effective against some arthropods than ivermectin (Gill & Lacey, 1998; Kieran, 1994; McKellar & Benchaoui, 1996; Shoop *et al.*, 1995; Sutherland *et al.*, 1999). Moxidectin, given to sheep as an oral drench at a dose rate of 0.2 mg/kg, can confer protection against reinfection with susceptible parasites for up to 21 days post-treatment (Barnes *et al.*, 2001; Sutherland *et al.*, 1997). An extended period of protection in some GIN species was observed in cattle treated with a 10% injectable formulation of moxidectin (Geurden *et al.*, 2004).

Profile

There is significant variability in the pharmacokinetic profiles of the commercially available MLs. Ivermectin, administered as an oral drench to sheep and cattle, reaches a peak in plasma within 1 day and has a half-life of approximately 2.7 days (Fink & Porras, 1989). Administration of ivermectin by other routes, e.g. subcutaneously, topical or as a controlled-release bolus, significantly lengthens both the time-to-peak plasma concentration and the half-life (Alvinerie *et al.*, 1999; Lifschitz *et al.*, 1999).

There is little information available on the profile of abamectin, although when given as an oral drench, it is presumed to be roughly similar to ivermectin (Sutherland *et al.*, 2002).

Doramectin, regardless of the route of administration, has a significantly longer half-life than ivermectin, which is presumed to result from the lipophilic cyclohexyl moiety (Lanusse *et al.*, 1997). Similarly, eprinomectin has an extended half-life, as well as having little if any partitioning into milk, which is presumed to result from substitutions at the 4″ position (Lanusse *et al.*, 1997; Shoop & Soll, 2002).

Moxidectin, given as an oral drench, rapidly attains peak plasma concentrations (as does ivermectin), but this is then followed by a relatively longer half-life (Afzal *et al.*, 1994). Again, this is presumed to result from the high level of lipophilicity of the compound (Alvinerie *et al.*, 1996).

As with the benzimidazoles, the MLs associate strongly with particulate matter in the rumen, which may be important in extending the period during which the drugs may be absorbed (Hennessy, 1997).

Mode of action

The MLs were originally postulated to act on invertebrates by inducing the release of the neurotransmitter GABA, which then interferes with neuronal transmission. More recently, however, this has been amended, and the drugs have been shown to potentiate the effects of GABA in the worms. The mode of action, meanwhile, has been more clearly defined as a receptor-mediated potentiation of glutamate-gated chloride channels (GluCl), which results in a number of phenotypic effects such as an inability to move, feed and oviposit (Prichard, 2001). Products of the genes avr-15, avr-14 and GLC-1 have been postulated to respond to ivermectin exposure; avr-15 is expressed in pharyngeal muscle, while the others are expressed in extrapharyngeal neurons (Dent *et al.*, 1997, 2000).

4. Emodepside

Description

While the cyclic octadepsipeptide, emodepside, is currently marketed only for use as an anthelmintic in cats, it is included here as an example of the ability of pharmaceutical companies to discover a new active family (Scherkenbeck *et al.*, 2002). Derived from PF1022A, a secondary metabolite of the fungus *Mycelia sterilia* (Miyadoh *et al.*, 2000), emodepside is made up of four N-methyl-L-leucins, two D-lactic acids and two D-phenyllic acids to which has been added a morpholine at each D-phenyllic acid (Sasaki *et al.*, 1992).

Efficacy

Emodepside was determined to have a high efficacy against a range of nematode species and life-cycle stages in both small (Akyol *et al.*, 1993) (Terada *et al.*, 1993) and large animals (Von Samson-Himmelstjerna *et al.*, 2005). Populations of *H. contortus* in sheep, which were known to be resistant to benzimidazole, levamisole and ivermectin, and a population of *C. oncophora* in cattle with resistance to ivermectin, were all effectively removed by treatment with emodepside (and, incidentally, PF1022A) (Von Samson-Himmelstjerna *et al.*, 2005).

Profile

No information is available in the literature.

Mode of action

PF1022A was initially demonstrated to inhibit motility of *Angiostrongylus cantonensis in vitro* (Terada, 1992). The activity was partially reversed using gabergic antagonists, and completely reversed using N-methylcytisine, and by the addition of Ca^{2+} (Terada, 1992). Terada (1992) concluded therefore that the anthelmintic activity came via stimulation of the GABAergic mechanism while also inhibiting cholinergic activity. However, later studies have concluded that this new class of anthelmintic acts via an interaction with a presynaptic latrophilin-like receptor. Activation of Gqα protein and phospholipase-Cβ then induces mobilisation of diacylglycerol which in turn induces expression of the proteins UNC-13 and synaptobrevin. This pathway ultimately results in the release of an as yet undefined transmitter or modulator which inhibits pharyngeal pumping and somatic function (Amliwala *et al.*, 2004; Harder *et al.*, 2003).

5. Paraherquamide

Description

Paraherquamide is an oxindole alkaloid metabolite derived from the fungal species *Penicillium paraherqui* and *P. charlesii* (Yamazaki *et al.*, 1981). In recent years, there has been renewed interest in this class of anthelmintic, following the modification of paraherquamide to 2-desoxoparaherquamide A, which is claimed to be as active as its predecessor but with more of an improved safety profile (Lee *et al.*, 2002). At the time of writing, however, no treatment for grazing livestock is commercially available.

Efficacy

Paraherquamide is safe and effective (>95% efficacy) against most of the major GIN species in calves at a dose rate between 1.0 and 4.0 mg/kg. An exception iwas *C. punctata*, with even the highest dose of 4.0 mg/kg reducing worm numbers by only 89% (Shoop *et al.*, 1992). In sheep, paraherquamide was also effective against most species of GIN, but in this case, the dose-limiting species was *Oe. columbianum* in which a dose of 2 mg/kg removed only 79% of the adult worms (Shoop *et al.*, 1990).

Profile

No information is available in the literature.

Mode of action

Paraherquamide exerts its effect by activating the blockage of cholinergic neuromuscular transmission, causing flaccid paralysis (Robertson *et al.*, 2002; Zinser *et al.*, 2002). The activity of paraherquamide against levamisole-resistant *Oe. dentatum*, however, suggests that the mode of action is different between the two drugs (Martin *et al.*, 2003).

6. The organophosphates, including naphthalophos and trichlorphon

Description

These drugs were originally designed as insecticides and were subsequently found to have some anthelmintic activity against GIN in ruminants (Gibson, 1960, 1961). Naphthalophos was used in Australia to control *H. contortus* between the 1960s and 1980s, then was re-released in 1993 in response to the problem of anthelmintic resistance (Kotze *et al.*, 1999). The organophosphates (OPs) have a restricted utility in ruminants due to low efficacy against some species and risks of toxicity (Brander, 1991).

Efficacy

The OPs are highly effective against *H. contortus*, including inhibited larval stages (Le Jambre & Barger, 1979), but are less effective against other GIN species, removing around 70–90% of adult worms (Kotze *et al.*, 1999).

Profile

Unlike their predecessors, the organochlorines (e.g. DDT, dieldrin), the organophosphate anthelmintics are rapidly absorbed and metabolised; peak plasma levels are attained within 2 hours (for dichlorvos), with levels becoming undetectable by 8 hours post-administration (Brander, 1991).

Mode of action

The OPs act, as they do in insects (and humans and grazing ruminants), by inhibiting the worms' acetylcholinesterase activity, leading to an accumulation of acetylcholine which interferes with neuronal transmission and results in paralysis (Aiello, 1998; Martin *et al.*, 1997).

7. The salicylanilide, closantel

Description

A substituted salicylanilide, closantel (CL) binds strongly to plasma proteins (Rothwell *et al.*, 2000).

Efficacy

The narrow-spectrum anthelmintic closantel, while highly active against trematodes, has a limited activity against GIN. A notable exception, however, is the haematophagous *H. contortus*, and other species which reside in the bile duct or have a site of predilection distal to the bile duct (e.g. *Oesophagostomum* spp.) (Hall *et al.*, 1980). This spectrum of activity is obviously related to the albumin-binding characteristics of the drug.

Profile

Closantel reaches peak plasma concentrations post-oral administration between 8 and 48 hours, then has a long half-life of 2–3 weeks, possibly due to strong binding to serum albumin (Lanusse & Prichard, 1993; Michiels *et al.*, 1987; Mohammed-Ali & Bogan, 1987; Rothwell *et al.*, 2000), and can therefore confer protection against infection with susceptible parasites for several weeks post-administration (Rana *et al.*, 2001).

Mode of action

The mode of action of closantel was originally described as via an uncoupling of the oxidative phosphorylation pathway in both nematode and mammalian mitochondria (Kane *et al.*, 1980), while the drug also appears to affect ion and fluid homoeostasis across cell membranes (Rothwell, 1996). *In vivo*, however, strong albumin binding prevents this occurring to the host, enabling its use as an anthelmintic. The probable explanation for the relatively superior efficacy against *H. contortus* is ingestion of sufficient blood containing the drug, while uncoupling of the drug–albumin complex in bile may explain the relatively greater efficacy against large intestinal GIN species (Mohammed-Ali & Bogan, 1987).

8. The acetonitrile derivatives – monepantel

> '*Here we report the discovery of the amino-acetonitrile derivatives (AADs) as a new chemical class of synthetic anthelmintics and describe the development of drug candidates that are efficacious against various species of livestock-pathogenic nematodes.*'
>
> *Kaminsky et al. (2008a)*

Description

The AADs are low molecular weight pre-biotic compounds produced by alkylation of phenols with chloroacetone, Strecker reaction and alkylation of the amine with aroyl chlorides (Ducray *et al.*, 2008; Kaminsky *et al.*, 2008a). Over 600 AADs were tested for anthelmintic efficacy and one, monepantel (Figure 5.4), was chosen as an anthelmintic development candidate (Kaminsky *et al.*, 2008b). As an interesting aside, a literature

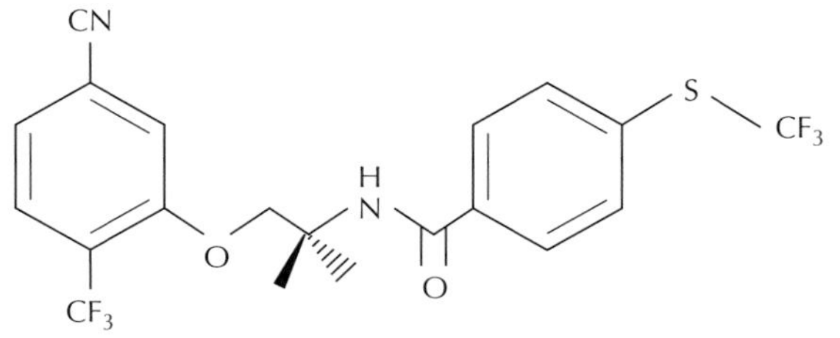

Figure 5.4   Chemical structure of monepantel.

search for amino-acetonitrile compounds revealed that the compounds are found in the interstellar medium (Wirstrom, 2007), although it is presumed that the developers of monepantel had a more readily available supply of material.

At the time of writing, monepantel is not commercially available, although there are suggestions that the regulatory process is well advanced and that the first new anthelmintic family since 1981 will be available soon.

Efficacy

Monepantel was effective against a wide range of GIN species in both sheep and cattle at dosages of 2.5 and 5 mg/kg. No activity was observed against any arthropod species tested (Kaminsky *et al.*, 2008b).

Profile

Pharmacokinetic data has been published for several of the AADs, but not monepantel. Available information (Kaminsky *et al.*, 2008a) demonstrates that the compounds are rapidly absorbed into plasma following oral administration of 20 mg/kg. This is followed by the rapid decline of plasma levels within 2 days, then a subsequent, relatively long half-life in plasma of 215 hours.

Mode of action

Studies in *Caenorhabditis elegans* mutants and a resistant line of *H. contortus* point to the mode of action of monepantel as nicotinic agonism but mediated via a unique nicotinic acetylcholinesterase receptor (Kaminsky *et al.*, 2008a).

Combination of anthelmintic treatments

Combining two or more anthelmintic families into one product can extend the spectrum of activity or result in improved efficacy. Extending the spectrum of activity is usually relevant in areas where tapeworm or fluke is perceived to be production or health issues and which are not controlled by the active family used to target the GIN. Improved efficacy, on the other hand, should only become relevant when worms resistant to one or more of the constituent families are present. The relationship between combinations and resistance is discussed in the following chapter.

Modifying the delivery of anthelmintics

As with combination therapy, a major driver for modifying the route of delivery of anthelmintics is either ease of use or an attempt to increase persistence as a method of overcoming resistance; this latter relationship is discussed more fully in the following chapter.

Parenteral administration

This term covers both pour-on and injectable formulations of anthelmintics.

While pour-on treatments for cattle containing either benzimidazole or levamisole have been developed and are in use, parenteral administration has been largely dominated by the MLs (Hennessy, 1997). This is mostly due to issues around dose size and solubility of the earlier classes (Dorn & Federmann, 1976), which were overcome with the development of the MLs. With a few exceptions, such as the introduction of injectable and pour-on moxidectin and doramectin for use in sheep, parenteral administration has been used most often in cattle. This is partly because of the ease of administration of pour-ons in large animals and partly because of the relative impenetrability of sheep wool (Hennessy, 1997). It seems incredible, now that the industry has become accustomed to the ease of use of pour-on formulations, that they were preceded by a system of intra-ruminal injection of drench for cattle, in an attempt to get enough active into the animal without the need for head restraint (Borgsteede & Reid, 1982).

Controlled release of anthelmintics

The first controlled release devices for use in grazing ruminants was the Paratect bolus, developed in the early 1980s by Pfizer, and were for use only in cattle. The devices stayed in the rumen through gravity, much of which was conferred by the heavy metal spike around which the drug was packed. Needless to say, these products were met with some consternation in the rendering plants of abattoirs. The boluses, which released 150 mg of morantel tartrate/day over a 90-day period, were designed to make the control of parasitism easier compared to orally dosing or injecting adult cattle with drenches. These boluses were highly effective against resident and incoming GIN (Armour *et al.*, 1981). The use of persistent treatments to provide 'safe pasture' had begun.

The initial impetus behind the development of sustained-release devices for anthelmintics in sheep came from an investigation into why members of the benzimidazole family had different efficacies and pharmacokinetic profiles (Prichard *et al.*, 1978). Given that the modes of action of the individual drugs were the same, the obvious conclusion to explain the difference in efficacy was the variability in pharmacokinetic profile. Empirical evidence determined that repeated administration of thiabendazole significantly increased efficacy against arrested *O. ostertagi* larvae in cattle, and the conclusion was made that increasing the duration of exposure to toxic levels of the drug improved the efficacy (Prichard *et al.*, 1978).

The next logical step was to incorporate a benzimidazole anthelmintic into a sustained-release device or bolus (Laby, 1978). This device is administered orally and then alters shape to be retained in the rumen. The original experiments used a bolus releasing oxfendazole at 0.5 mg/kg per day (compared to the oral dose of 5.0 mg/kg) and demonstrated the removal of *T. circumcincta* from treated sheep within 4 days of administration, while pasture contamination with worm eggs was reduced below the limit of detection for at least 86 days by the sequential use of two capsules, each with a pay-out of 40 days (Anderson *et al.*, 1980). Albendazole replaced oxfendazole in what became the first commercially available controlled-release capsule for sheep. These boluses releases approximately 0.5 mg/kg/day of albendazole for 100 days (Sutherland *et al.*, 2000).

In 1995, the use of a compressed ivermectin tablet for control of parasitism was reported (Gogolewski *et al.*, 1995) and was soon followed by the incorporation of ivermectin tablets into a controlled-release bolus. This bolus releases 0.8 mg/kg/day for 100 days and was highly effective against GIN (Gogolewski *et al.*, 1997a, b).

More recent developments, utilising the same base technology, include a bolus releasing sequential doses of albendazole and ivermectin (Extender Max, www.merial.com), and, in New Zealand, another bolus releasing a combination of albendazole and abamectin for 100 days (Leathwick, personal communication).

Injectable formulations

The ML compounds, moxidectin and doramectin, when given as injectable treatments, are inherently persistent. However, recent products containing both these compounds have increased the period of drug release still further.

Bioavailability

The mechanism/s by which most nematodes and anthelmintics interact in the gastrointestinal tract remain unclear. While it may be obvious for *H. contortus*, it is less so for species of mucous browsers. Do they have to physically ingest anthelmintic partitioned from blood or which has flowed unabsorbed down the gastrointestinal tract? Or are the drugs absorbed across the cuticle of the worm?

References

AFZAL, J., STOUT, S. J., DACUNHA, A. R. & MILLER, P. (1994). Moxidectin: Absorption, tissue distribution, excretion, and biotransformation of 14C-labeled moxidectin in sheep. *Journal of Agricultural and Food Chemistry*, **42**, 1767–1773.

AIELLO, S. E. (1998). The Merck Veterinary Manual, Merck & Co., USA.

AKYOL, C. V., KINO, H. & TERADA, M. (1993). Effects of PF1022A, a newly developed gabergic anthelmintic, on adult stage of *Angiostrongylus cantonensis* in rats. *Japanese Journal of Parasitology*, **42**, 220–226.

ALKA, GOPAL, R. M., SANDHU, K. S. & SIDHU, P. K. (2004). Efficacy of abamectin against ivermectin-resistant strain of *Trichostrongylus colubriformis* in sheep. *Veterinary Parasitology*, **121**, 277–283.

ALVINERIE, M., SUTRA, J. F., GALTIER, P., LIFSCHITZ, A., VIRKEL, G., SALLOVITZ, J. & LANUSSE, C. (1999). Persistence of ivermectin in plasma and faeces following administration of a sustained-release bolus to cattle. *Research in Veterinary Science*, **66**, 57–61.

ALVINERIE, M., SUTRA, J. F., LANUSSE, C. & GALTIER, P. (1996). Plasma profile study of moxidectin in a cow and its suckling calf. *Veterinary Research*, **27**, 545–549.

AMLIWALA, K., BULL, K., WILLSON, J., HARDER, A., HOLDEN-DYE, L. & WALKER, R. J. (2004). Emodepside, a cyclo-octadepsipeptide anthelmintic with a novel mode of action. *Drugs of the Future*, **29**, 1015–1024.

ANDERSON, N., LABY, R. H., PRICHARD, R. K. & HENNESSY, D. (1980). Controlled release of anthelmintic drugs: A new concept for prevention of helminthosis in sheep. *Research in Veterinary Science*, **29**, 333–341.

ARMOUR, J., BAIRDEN, K. & DUNCAN, J. L. (1981). Studies on the control of bovine ostertagiasis using a morantel sustained release bolus. *Veterinary Record*, **108**, 532–535.

ARMOUR, J., BAIRDEN, K. & REID, J. F. S. (1975). Effectiveness of thiabendazole against inhibited larvae of sheep *Ostertagia* spp. *Veterinary Record*, **96**, 131–132.

BARNES, E. H., DOBSON, R. J., STEIN, P. A., LE JAMBRE, L. F. & LENANE, I. J. (2001). Selection of different genotype larvae and adult worms for anthelmintic resistance by persistent and short-acting avermectin/milbemycins. *International Journal for Parasitology*, **31**, 720–727.

BOGAN, J. A. & ARMOUR, J. (1986). Anthelmintics for ruminants. *Parasitology - Quo Vadit*, 483–491.

BOGAN, J. A., MARRINER, S. E. & GALBRAITH, E. A. (1982). Pharmacokinetics of levamisole in sheep. *Research in Veterinary Science*, **32**, 124–126.

BORGSTEEDE, F. H. (1979). The activity of albendazole against adult and larval gastrointestinal nematodes in naturally infected calves in The Netherlands. *Tijdschrift voor diergeneeskunde*, **104**, 181–188.

BORGSTEEDE, F. H. M. & REID, J. F. (1982). Oxfendazole efficacy in calves: A comparison of oral and intraruminal routes of administration. *Veterinary Quarterly*, **4**, 139–141.

BRANDER, G. C., PUGH, D. M., BYWATER, R. J. & JENKINS, W. L. (1991). *Veterinary Applied Pharmacology & Therapeutics*, Bailliere Tindall, London.

BROWN, H. D., MATZUK, A. R., ILVES, I. R. *et al.* (1961). Antiparasitic drugs. IV. 2-(4-thiazolyl)-benzimidazole, a new anthelmintic [5]. *Journal of the American Chemical Society*, **83**, 1764–1765.

CHABALA, J. C., MROZIK, H., TOLMAN, R. L. *et al.* (1980). Ivermectin, a new broad-spectrum antiparasitic agent. *Journal of Medicinal Chemistry*, **23**, 1134–1136.

CRINGOLI, G., RINALDI, L., VENEZIANO, V. & CAPELLI, G. (2003). Efficacy of eprinomectin pour-on against gastrointestinal nematode infections in sheep. *Veterinary Parasitology*, **112**, 203–209.

DENT, J. A., DAVIS, M. W. & AVERY, L. (1997). avr-15 encodes a chloride channel subunit that mediates inhibitory glutamatergic neurotransmission and ivermectin sensitivity in *Caenorhabditis elegans*. *EMBO Journal*, **16**, 5867–5879.

DENT, J. A., SMITH, M. M., VASSILATIS, D. K. & AVERY, L. (2000). The genetics of ivermectin resistance in *Caenorhabditis elegans*. *Proceedings of the National Academy of Sciences of the United States of America*, **97**, 2674–2679.

DORN, H. & FEDERMANN, M. (1976). Citarin-l spot on a new form of administration of an established anthelmintic. *Veterinary Medicine Reviews*, **1**, 5–16.

DUCRAY, P., GAUVRY, N., PAUTRAT, F. *et al.* (2008). Discovery of amino-acetonitrile derivatives, a new class of synthetic anthelmintic compounds. *Bioorganic and Medicinal Chemistry Letters*, **18**, 2935–2938.

EGERTON, J. R., EARY, C. H. & SUHAYDA, D. (1981). The anthelmintic efficacy of ivermectin in experimentally infected cattle. *Veterinary Parasitology*, **8**, 59–70.

EICHLER, D. A. (1973). The anthelmintic activity of thiophanate in sheep and cattle. *British Veterinary Journal*, **129**, 533–543.

ESLAMI, A. H. & ANWAR, M. (1976). Anthelmintic efficiency of fenbendazole on ovine gastrointestinal nematodes. *Veterinary Record*, **99**, 214–215.

EVANS, A. M. & MARTIN, R. J. (1993). On the block by morantel of nicotinic acetylcholine channels isolated from *Ascaris suum*: Rate constants for multi-ion block estimated by maximum likelihood. *Journal of Physiology*, **467**, 254.

FINK, D. W. & PORRAS, A. G. (1989). Pharmacokinetics of ivermectin in animals and humans. *Ivermectin and Abamectin*, 113–130, Campbell, W.C. (ed), Springer-Verlag.

GEURDEN, T., CLAEREBOUT, E., DEROOVER, E. & VERCRUYSSE, J. (2004). Evaluation of the chemoprophylactic efficacy of 10% long acting injectable moxidectin against gastrointestinal nematode infections in calves in Belgium. *Veterinary Parasitology*, **120**, 331–338.

GIBSON, T. E. (1960). Controlled tests with four new anthelmintic substances against *Trichostrongylus axei* in sheep. *Veterinary Record*, **72**, 343–344.

GIBSON, T. E. (1961). Controlled tests with three organic phosphorus compounds as anthelmintics against *Haemonchus contortus* in sheep. *Veterinary Record*, **73**, 230–231.

GILL, J. H. & LACEY, E. (1998). Avermectin/milbemycin resistance in trichostrongyloid nematodes. *International Journal for Parasitology*, **28**, 863–877.

GOGOLEWSKI, R. P., ALLERTON, G. R., LANGHOLFF, W. K., CRAMER, L. G. & EAGLESON, J. S. (1995). An ivermectin tablet for sheep: Efficacy against gastro-intestinal nematodes and a bioavailability comparison with a liquid ivermectin formulation. *Veterinary Parasitology*, **60**, 297–302.

GOGOLEWSKI, R. P., ALLERTON, G. R., RUGG, D., KAWHIA, D., BARRICK, R. A. & EAGLESON, J. S. (1997a). Demonstration of the sustained anthelmintic efficacy of a controlled-release capsule formulation of ivermectin in weaner lambs under field conditions in New Zealand. *New Zealand Veterinary Journal*, **45**, 158–161.

GOGOLEWSKI, R. P., RUGG, D., ALLERTON, G. R., KAWHIA, D., BARRICK, R. A. AND EAGLESON, J. S. (1997b). Demonstration of the sustained anthelmintic activity of a controlled-release capsule formulation of ivermectin in ewes under field conditions in New Zealand. *New Zealand Veterinary Journal*, **45**, 163–166.

GOGOLEWSKI, R. P., SLACEK, B., FAMILTON, A. S. *et al.* (1997c). Efficacy of a topical formulation of eprinomectin against endoparasites of cattle in New Zealand. *New Zealand Veterinary Journal*, **45**, 1–3.

GORDON, H. M. (1935). Efficiency of certain drugs against *Haemonchus contortus*. *The Australian Veterinary Journal*, **35**, 109–113.

GORDON, H. M. (1948). The epidemiology of parasitic diseases, with special reference to studies with nematode parasites of sheep. *The Australian Veterinary Journal*, **24**, 7–45.

GOUDIE, A. C., EVANS, N. A., GRATION, K. A. F. *et al.* (1993). Doramectin – A potent novel endectocide. *Veterinary Parasitology*, **49**, 5–15.

HALL, C. A., MCDONELL, P. A. & GRAHAM, J. M. (1980). Anthelmintic activity of closantel against benzimidazole resistant strains of *Haemonchus contortus* and *Trichostrongylus colubriformis* in sheep. *The Australian Veterinary Journal*, **56**, 461–462.

HARDER, A., SCHMITT-WREDE, H. P., KRÜCKEN, J. *et al.* (2003). Cyclooctadepsipeptides – An anthelmintically active class of compounds exhibiting a novel mode of action. *International Journal of Antimicrobial Agents*, **22**, 318–331.

HEINZE-MUTZ, E. M., PITT, S. R., BAIRDEN, K., BAGGOTT, D. G., ARMOUR, J., BARTH, D. & CRAMER, L. G. (1993). Efficacy of abamectin against nematodes in cattle. *Veterinary Record*, **132**, 35–37.

HENNESSY, D. R. (1997). Modifying the formulation or delivery mechanism to increase the activity of anthelmintic compounds. *Veterinary Parasitology*, **72**, 367–390.

JONES, R. M. & BLISS, D. H. (1983). An economic and efficacy comparison between morantel (when administered from an intraruminal bolus) and conventional anthelmintic treatment in grazing cattle. *Veterinary Parasitology*, **12**, 297–306.

JONES, R. M., LOGAN, N. B., WEATHERLEY, A. J., LITTLE, A. S. & SMOTHERS, C. D. (1993). Activity of doramectin against nematode endoparasites of cattle. *Veterinary Parasitology*, **49**, 27–37.

KAMINSKY, R., DUCRAY, P., JUNG, M. *et al.* (2008a). A new class of anthelmintics effective against drug-resistant nematodes. *Nature*, **452**, 176–180.

KAMINSKY, R., GAUVRY, N., SCHORDERET WEBER, S. *et al.* (2008b). Identification of the amino-acetonitrile derivative monepantel (AAD 1566) as a new anthelmintic drug development candidate. *Parasitology Research*, **103**, 931–939.

KANE, H. J., BEHM, C. A. & BRYANT, C. (1980). Metabolic studies on the new fasciolicidal drug, closantel. *Molecular and Biochemical Parasitology*, **1**, 347–355.

KATES, K. C., COLGLAZIER, M. L., ENZIE, F. D., LINDAHL, I. L. & SAMUELSON, G. (1971). Comparative activity of thiabendazole, levamisole, and parbendazole against natural infections of helminths in sheep. *Journal of Parasitology*, **57**, 356–362.

KELLY, J. D., CHEVIS, R. A. F. & WHITLOCK, H. V. (1975). The anthelmintic efficacy of mebendazole against adult *Fasciola hepatica* and a concurrent mixed nematode infection in sheep. *New Zealand Veterinary Journal*, **23**, 81–84.

KIERAN, P. J. (1994). Moxidectin against ivermectin-resistant nematodes – A global view. *Australian Veterinary Journal*, **71**, 18–20.

KOHLER, P. (2001). The biochemical basis of anthelmintic action and resistance. *International Journal for Parasitology*, **31**, 336–345.

KOTZE, A. C., STEIN, P. A. & DOBSON, R. J. (1999). Investigation of intestinal nematode responses to naphthalophos and pyrantel using a larval development assay. *International Journal for Parasitology*, **29**, 1093–1099.

KURLAND, A. A., HANLON, T. E., TATOM, M. H. & SIMOPOULOS, A. L. (1961). Comparative studies of the phenothiazine tranquilizers: Methodological and logistical considerations. *Journal of Nervous and Mental Disease*, **132**, 61–74.

LABY, R. H. (1978). Australian Patent Application No. 35908/78.

LANCASTER, J. L., JR, SIMCO, J. S. & KILGORE, R. L. (1982). Systematic efficacy of ivermectin MK-933 against the lone star tick. *Journal of Economic Entomology*, **75**, 242–244.

LANUSSE, C., LIFSCHITZ, A., VIRKEL, G. *et al.* (1997). Comparative plasma disposition kinetics of ivermectin, moxidectin and doramectin in cattle. *Journal of Veterinary Pharmacology and Therapeutics*, **20**, 91–99.

LANUSSE, C. E. & PRICHARD, R. K. (1993). Relationship between pharmacological properties and clinical efficacy of ruminant anthelmintics. *Veterinary Parasitology*, **49**, 123–158.

LE JAMBRE, L. F. & BARGER, I. A. (1979). Efficiency of rafoxanide and naphthalophos against inhibited *Haemonchus contortus*. *Australian Veterinary Journal*, **55**, 346–347.

LEE, B. H., CLOTHIER, M. F., DUTTON, F. E. *et al.* (2002). Marcfortine and paraherquamide class of anthelmintics: Discovery of PNU-141962. *Current Topics in Medicinal Chemistry*, **2**, 779–793.

LELAND, S. E., JR, CALEY, H. K. & RIDLEY, R. K. (1971). Efficacy of levamisole (l-tetramisole) and thiabendazole in reduction of helminth egg counts in cattle. *Journal of the American Veterinary Medical Association*, **158**, 1373–1375.

LIFSCHITZ, A., VIRKEL, G., PIS, A. *et al.* (1999). Ivermectin disposition kinetics after subcutaneous and intramuscular administration of an oil-based formulation to cattle. *Veterinary Parasitology*, **86**, 203–215.

MARRINER, S. E. & BOGAN, J. A. (1981a). Pharmacokinetics of fenbendazole in sheep. *American Journal of Veterinary Research*, **42**, 1146–1148.

MARRINER, S. E. & BOGAN, J. A. (1981b). Pharmacokinetics of oxfendazole in sheep. *American Journal of Veterinary Research*, **42**, 1143–1145.

MARTIN, R. J. (1997). Modes of action of anthelmintic drugs. *Veterinary Journal*, **154**, 11–34.

MARTIN, R. J., BAI, G., CLARK, C. L. & ROBERTSON, A. P. (2003). Methyridine (2-[2-methoxyethyl]-pyridine) and levamisole activate different ACh receptor subtypes in nematode parasites: A new lead for levamisole-resistance. *British Journal of Pharmacology*, **140**, 1068–1076.

MARTIN, R. J., ROBERTSON, A. P. & BJORN, H. (1997). Target sites of anthelmintics. *Parasitology*, **114** (Suppl), S111–S124.

MCKELLAR, Q. A. & BENCHAOUI, H. A. (1996). Avermectins and milbemycins. *Journal of Veterinary Pharmacology and Therapeutics*, **19**, 331–351.

MCKENNA, P. B. (1974). The anthelmintic efficacy of thiabendazole and levamisole against inhibited *Haemonchus contortus* larvae in sheep. *New Zealand Veterinary Journal*, **22**, 163–166.

MEHLHORN, H., JONES, H. L., WEATHERLEY, A. J. & SCHUMACHER, B. (1993). Doramectin, a new avermectin highly efficacious against gastrointestinal nematodes and lungworms of cattle and pigs: Two studies carried out under field conditions in Germany. *Parasitology Research*, **79**, 603–607.

MELENEY, W. P., WRIGHT, F. C. & GUILLOT, F. S. (1982). Residual protection against cattle scabies afforded by ivermectin. *American Journal of Veterinary Research*, **43**, 1767–1769.

MICHIELS, M., MEULDERMANS, W. & HEYKANTS, J. (1987). The metabolism and fate of closantel (flukiver) in sheep and cattle. *Drug Metabolism Reviews*, **18**, 235–251.

MIYADOH, S., KAWASAKI, H., AOYAGI, K., YAGUCHI, T., OKADA, T. & SUGIYAMA, J. (2000). Taxonomic position of the fungus producing the anthelmintic PF1022 based on the 18S rRNA gene base sequence. *Nippon Kingakukai Kaiho*, **41**, 183–188.

MOHAMMED-ALI, N. A. & BOGAN, J. A. (1987). The pharmacodynamics of the flukicidal salicylanilides, rafoxanide, closantel and oxyclosanide. *Journal of Veterinary Pharmacology and Therapeutics*, **10**, 127–133.

NGOMYUO, A. J., MARRINER, S. E. & BOGAN, J. A. (1984). The pharmacokinetics of fenbendazole and oxfendazole in cattle. *Veterinary Research Communications*, **8**, 187–193.

PRICHARD, R. K. (1970). Mode of action of the anthelminthic thiabendazole in *Haemonchus contortus*. *Nature*, **228**, 684–685.

PRICHARD, R. K. (2001). Genetic variability following selection of *Haemonchus contortus* with anthelmintics. *Trends in Parasitology*, **17**, 445–453.

PRICHARD, R. K., HENNESSY, D. R. & STEEL, J. W. (1978). Prolonged administration: A new concept for increasing the spectrum and effectiveness of anthelmintics. *Veterinary Parasitology*, **4**, 309–315.

RANA, K. K., SINGH, S. & CHAUDHRI, S. S. (2001). Therapeutic and persistent efficacy of ivermectin, moxidectin and closantel against fenbendazole resistant *Haemonchus contortus* in sheep. *Indian Journal of Animal Sciences*, **71**, 1107–1110.

REID, J. F. S., DUNCAN, J. L. & BAIRDEN, K. (1976). Efficacy of levamisole against inhibited larvae of *Ostertagia* spp. in sheep. *Veterinary Record*, **98**, 426–427.

RICHARDS, L. S., ZIMMERMAN, G. L., HOBERG, E. P., SCHONS, D. J. & DAWLEY, S. W. (1987). The anthelmintic efficacy of netobimin against naturally acquired gastrointestinal nematodes in sheep. *Veterinary Parasitology*, **26**, 87–94.

ROBERTSON, A. P., CLARK, C. L., BURNS, T. A. *et al.* (2002). Paraherquamide and 2-deoxy-paraherquamide distinguish cholinergic receptor subtypes in Ascaris muscle. *Journal of Pharmacology and Experimental Therapeutics*, **302**, 853–860.

ROBERTSON, S. J. & MARTIN, R. J. (1993). Levamisole-activated single-channel currents from muscle of the nematode parasite *Ascaris suum*. *British Journal of Pharmacology*, **108**, 170–178.

ROTHWELL, J. T., LACEY, E. & SANGSTER, N. C. (2000). The binding of closantel to ovine serum albumin, and homogenate fractions of *Haemonchus contortus*. *International Journal for Parasitology*, **30**, 769–775.

ROTHWELL, J. T. & SANGSTER, N.C. (1996). The effects of closantel treatment on the ultrastructure of *Haemonchus contortus*. *International Journal for Parasitology*, **26**, 49–57.

SANCHEZ BRUNI, S. F., JONES, D. G. & MCKELLAR, Q. A. (2006). Pharmacological approaches towards rationalizing the use of endoparasitic drugs in small animals. *Journal of Veterinary Pharmacology and Therapeutics*, **29**, 443–457.

SASAKI, T., TAKAGI, M., YAGUCHI, T., MIYADOH, S., OKADA, T. & KOYAMA, M. (1992). A new anthelmintic cyclodepsipeptide, PF1022A. *Journal of Antibiotics*, **45**, 692–697.

SCHERKENBECK, J., JESCHKE, P. & HARDER, A. (2002). PF1022A and related cyclodepsipeptides – a novel class of anthelmintics. *Current Topics in Medicinal Chemistry*, **2**, 759–777.

SHOOP, W. & SOLL, M. (2002). Ivermectin, abamectin and eprinomectin. *Macrocyclic Lactones in Antiparasitic Therapy*, 1–29, CABI Publishing, New York.

SHOOP, W. L., EGERTON, J. R., EARY, C. H. *et al.* (1996). Eprinomectin: A novel avermectin for use as a topical endectocide for cattle. *International Journal for Parasitology*, **26**, 1237–1242.

SHOOP, W. L., EGERTON, J. R., EARY, C. H. & SUHAYDA, D. (1990). Anthelmintic activity of paraherquamide in sheep. *Journal of Parasitology*, **76**, 349–351.

SHOOP, W. L., MICHAEL, B. F., HAINES, H. W. & EARY, C. H. (1992). Anthelmintic activity of paraherquamide in calves. *Veterinary Parasitology*, **43**, 259–263.

SHOOP, W. L., MROZIK, H. & FISHER, M. H. (1995). Structure and activity of avermectins and milbemycins in animal health. *Veterinary Parasitology*, **59**, 139–156.

SISODIA, S. L., PATHAK, K. M. L. & KAPOOR, M. (1996). Anthelmintic efficacy of doramectin against naturally occurring gastrointestinal nematodes of sheep. *Indian Veterinary Journal*, **73**, 1167–1171.

SUTHERLAND, I. A., BROWN, A. E. & LEATHWICK, D. M. (2000). Selection for drug-resistant nematodes during and following extended exposure to anthelmintic. *Parasitology*, **121**, 217–226.

SUTHERLAND, I. A., LEATHWICK, D. M. & BROWN, A. E. (1999). Moxidectin: Persistence and efficacy against drug-resistant *Ostertagia circumcincta*. *Journal of Veterinary Pharmacology and Therapeutics*, **22**, 2–5.

SUTHERLAND, I. A., LEATHWICK, D. M., BROWN, A. E. & MILLER, C. M. (1997). Prophylactic efficacy of persistent anthelmintics against challenge with drug-resistant and susceptible *Ostertagia circumcincta*. *Veterinary Record*, **141**, 120–123.

SUTHERLAND, I. A., LEATHWICK, D. M., MOEN, I. C. & BISSET, S. A. (2002). Resistance to therapeutic treatment with macrocyclic lactone anthelmintics in *Ostertagia circumcincta*. *Veterinary Parasitology*, **109**, 91–99.

TERADA, M. (1992). Neuropharmacological mechanism of action of PF1022A, an antinematode anthelmintic with a new structure of cyclic depsipeptide, on *Angiostrongylus cantonensis* and isolated frog rectus. *Japanese Journal of Parasitology*, **41**, 108–117.

TERADA, M., ISHIH, A., TUNGTRONGCHITR, A., SANO, M. & SHOMURA, T. (1993). Effects of PF1022A on developing larvae of *Angiostrongylus costaricensis* in mice, with special reference to route, dose and formulation. *Japanese Journal of Parasitology*, **42**, 199–210.

THEODORIDES, V. J., NAWALINSKI, T. & CHANG, J. (1976). Efficacy of albendazole against *Haemonchus*, *Nematodirus*, *Dictyocaulus* and *Moniezia* of sheep. *American Journal of Veterinary Research*, **37**, 1515–1516.

THIENPONT, D., VANPARIJS, O. F. J., RAEYMAEKERS, A. H. M. *et al.* (1966). Tetramisole (R 8299), a new, potent broad spectrum anthelmintic. *Nature*, **209**, 1084–1086.

TOCCO, D. J., BUHS, R. P., BROWN, H. D. *et al.* (1964). The metabolic fate of thiabendazole in sheep. *Journal of Medicinal Chemistry*, **7**, 399–405.

TURTON, J. A. (1969). Anthelmintic action of levamisole injection in cattle. *Veterinary Record*, **85**, 264–265.

TURTON, J. A. (1974). Controlled trials to determine the anthelmintic efficacy of levamisole against *Ostertagia circumcincta* and *Trichostrongylus colubriformis* in lambs. *Research in Veterinary Science*, **16**, 152–155.

VERCRUYSSE, J., DORNY, P., HONG, C. *et al.* (1993). Efficacy of doramectin in the prevention of gastrointestinal nematode infections in grazing cattle. *Veterinary Parasitology*, **49**, 51–59.

VON SAMSON-HIMMELSTJERNA, G., HARDER, A., SANGSTER, N. C. & COLES, G. C. (2005). Efficacy of two cyclooctadepsipeptides, PF1022A and emodepside, against anthelmintic-resistant nematodes in sheep and cattle. *Parasitology*, **130**, 343–347.

WESCOTT, R. B. & LEAMASTER, B. R. (1982). Efficacy of ivermectin against naturally acquired and experimentally induced nematode infections in sheep. *American Journal of Veterinary Research*, **43**, 531–533.

WILLIAMS, J. C., KNOX, J. W., BAUMANN, B. A., SNIDER, T. G., KIMBALL, M. G. & HOERNER, T. J. (1981). Efficacy of ivermectin against inhibited larvae of *Ostertagia ostertagi*. *American Journal of Veterinary Research*, **42**, 2077–2080.

WILLIAMS, J. C., KNOX, J. W., MARBURY, K. S., SWALLEY, R. A. & EDDI, C. S. (1991). Efficacy of levamisole against *Ostertagia ostertagi* in Louisiana cattle during maturation of inhibited larvae (September) and during minimal inhibition (December/January). *Veterinary Parasitology*, **40**, 73–85.

WILLIAMS, J. C., LOYACANO, A. F., NAULT, C., RAMSEY, R. T. & PLUE, R. E. (1992). Efficacy of abamectin against natural infections of gastrointestinal nematodes and lungworm of cattle with special emphasis on inhibited, early fourth stage larvae of *Ostertagia ostertagi*. *Veterinary Parasitology*, **41**, 77–84.

WIRSTROM, E. S., BERGMAN, P., HJALMARSON, A & NUMMELIN, A. (2007). A search for pre-biotic molecules in hot cores. *Astronomy and Astrophysics*, **473**, 177–180.

YAMAZAKI, M., OKUYAMA, E., KOBAYASHI, M. & INOUE, H. (1981). The structure of paraherquamide, a toxic metabolite from *Penicillium paraherquei*. *Tetrahedron Letters*, **22**, 135–136.

YAZWINSKI, T. A., GREENWAY, T. & PRESSON, B. L. (1983). Antiparasitic efficacy of ivermectin in naturally parasitized sheep. *American Journal of Veterinary Research*, **44**, 2186–2187.

ZINSER, E. W., WOLF, M. L., ALEXANDER-BOWMAN, S. J. *et al.* (2002). Anthelmintic paraherquamides are cholinergic antagonists in gastrointestinal nematodes and mammals. *Journal of Veterinary Pharmacology and Therapeutics*, **25**, 241–250.

6 Anthelmintic resistance

What is anthelmintic resistance?

'Resistance is present when there is a greater frequency of individuals within a population able to tolerate doses of compound than in a normal population of the same species and is heritable.'

Prichard et al. (1980)

The development of resistance to what became widely-used anthelmintic treatments, particularly following the introduction of the benzimidazoles, was of course inevitable. As stated in a review of anthelmintic resistance (Wolstenholme *et al.*, 2004), 'biological reality reasserts itself'. Historical attempts to eliminate any organism with high fecundity and an ability to reassemble its genotype through, e.g. sexual reproduction, presents a litany of failure ranging from the malaria parasite *Plasmodium falciparum* (and its definitive host, the anopheline mosquito), rabbits and multiple-resistant bacteria in 21st century hospitals.

One of the most heartening developments in veterinary parasitology over the past few years has been the realisation by most of the major pharmaceutical companies (whether driven by profit or not is irrelevant) that their products should be used as responsibly and sustainably as possible. Meanwhile, everyone with a vested interest in livestock production, from farmers to veterinarians and scientists, should proceed in the knowledge that resistance will always occur to any anthelmintic product, whether it is an existing product or belongs to a completely new action family.

Most of the information in this chapter has been presented before in a number of excellent and thorough reviews – particularly regarding the prevalence of resistance (Craig, 1993; Jabbar *et al.*, 2006; Jackson & Coop, 2000; Kaplan, 2004; Prichard, 1994; Waller, 1987). What follows is therefore a general overview of the evolution of the global resistance problem.

Evolution of anthelmintic resistance

Within 3 years of the publication of the discovery of thiabendazole in 1961, a report appeared in the literature of variability in the effectiveness of the drug against *H. contortus* (Conway, 1964) and against mixed infections in sheep (Drudge *et al.*, 1964). Reports of resistance to various members of the benzimidazole family in *H. contortus*, *T. circumcincta* and *T. colubriformis* then began to appear in the 1970s and 1980s in a variety of geographically distinct countries (Britt & Oakley, 1986; Cawthorne & Whitehead, 1983; Green *et al.*, 1981; Hall *et al.*, 1979; Hotson *et al.*, 1970; Kerboeuf & Hubert, 1985; Kettle *et al.*, 1982; Theodorides *et al.*, 1970).

The problem of benzimidazole resistance appeared to be most serious in the *H. contortus* endemic region of Australia (Waller & Prichard, 1985). While this was tentatively linked to the high use of anthelmintic use in the region, another possible reason was that the relatively greater pathogenicity of this parasite resulted in a greater focus than on other parasites in the same or other regions (Waller, 1987, 1994). *This is an excellent example of one of the maxims of drug resistance in any biological system – there is no such thing as resistance until an effort is made to detect it.*

Levamisole resistance was first reported in laboratory-maintained strains in Australia (Le Jambre *et al.*, 1976, 1977, 1978), with the first case of resistance in the field observed in 1981, also in Australia (Green *et al.*, 1981). Paradoxically, this was reported in *H. contortus*, a species against which levamisole continues to perform remarkably well.

Seven years after the release of ivermectin in 1981, a laboratory-selected population of *H. contortus* was reported (Egerton *et al.*, 1988). This was quickly followed by reports of resistance in the same parasite from the field (Echevarria & Trindade, 1989; Van Wyk & Malan, 1988).

Resistance to moxidectin first appeared in a population of *T. circumcincta* in goats in New Zealand (Leathwick, 1995), then in *Cooperia* spp. in cattle in the same country (Vermunt *et al.*, 1996). Resistance to moxidectin was later described in *H. contortus* in sheep in the field (Love *et al.*, 2003) and more recently in *T. colubriformis* infecting goats in the USA (Kaplan *et al.*, 2007).

Worldwide occurrence of anthelmintic resistance

It is notable that anthelmintic resistance, regardless of which active family is involved, has tended to appear earlier and become more widespread in southern hemisphere countries. Most of the first reports of resistance in sheep in the field were from either Australia (Hall *et al.*, 1979), New Zealand (Kettle *et al.*, 1982; Vlassoff & Kettle, 1980), South Africa (Van Wyk & Malan, 1988) or South America (Echevarria & Trindade, 1989). There are now farms in South Africa and Australia in which the resistance problem in sheep has become so bad that farming is no longer possible.

The incidence of resistance in cattle remains lower than in sheep, for reasons which remain unclear, although populations of *O. ostertagi* resistant to fenbendazole (Borgsteede, 1986) and morantel tartrate (Borgsteede, 1988) were reported from Europe. Once again, however, resistance appears to be more widespread in the southern hemisphere, with reports indicating the problem to be particularly severe in South America (Mejia *et al.*, 2003) and New Zealand, where a recent report demonstrated that over 90% of farms surveyed had detectable resistance, almost always to ivermectin in *Cooperia* spp. (Waghorn *et al.*, 2006). It seems, therefore, that while resistance has been recorded more often around the world in sheep than has been the case in cattle, there is no underlying reason preventing the development of resistance in cattle parasites. One possibility for the relative imbalance in the severity of resistance between sheep and cattle is the transfer of parasite populations from goats to sheep. As a result of differences in the pharmacokinetic profile of anthelmintics in goats (Bogan, 1987), browsing animals which have presumably evolved ways to quickly detoxify plant secondary metabolites (PSM), the effective dose of drugs is significantly higher than in sheep. It is noticeable that resistance in goats occurs more quickly, in more parasite species and against more anthelmintic classes than it does in sheep. Furthermore, the majority of gastrointestinal nematode (GIN) species of sheep readily utilise goats as an alternative host.

Resistance to one or more active families by one or more species

Worms can be readily controlled on farms despite the development of resistance to one, or even two of the commercially available action families, if the farmer knows the resistance status and switches to an alternative and effective anthelmintic.

Thus, even on farms with serious levels of e.g. benzimidazole and levamisole resistance, changing to an ML should ensure effective control. However, this will almost certainly result in a relatively high selection pressure for worms to become resistant to the third active family (Besier & Love, 2003).

The first recorded case of resistance to more than one action family occurred in goats in Victoria, Australia, where a population of *T. colubriformis* survived treatment with concurrent doses of a benzimidazole and levamisole (Barton *et al.*, 1985). This was quickly followed by populations of the same species with recorded resistance to the same drugs on two sheep properties in New South Wales, Australia (Dash, 1986). In 1991–1992, a survey of 881 sheep farms in Australia demonstrated that 85% of the properties had populations of GIN which were resistant to benzimidazoles, 65% had worms resistant to levamisole and 34% were resistant to benzimidazole–levamisole combination products (Overend *et al.*, 1994). While it was not proven at the time, there was a suggestion that multiple species of GIN may have developed resistance.

Following the development of resistance to the most recently introduced class of anthelmintics, the MLs, observations of triple resistance in one or more GIN species have steadily increased in sheep (and goats) in Australasia (Besier & Love, 2003; Sutherland *et al.*, 2008; Wrigley *et al.*, 2006), Africa

(Van Wyk *et al.*, 1999), South America (Nari *et al.*, 1996; Waller *et al.*, 1996) and Asia (Chandrawathani *et al.*, 2003, 2004).

The situation in cattle remains less severe than in small ruminants; resistance is most often confined to the MLs in *Cooperia* spp., although multiple resistance of *Cooperia* spp. to MLs and benzimidazoles was found on 74% of farms surveyed in New Zealand (Waghorn *et al.*, 2006), while ML and benzimidazole *C. oncophora*, and benzimidazole-resistant *C. punctata, O. ostertagi* and *H. placei* have been recorded in South America (Mejia *et al.*, 2003).

Impact of resistance on productivity

One of the problems scientists and veterinarians face when discussing anthelmintic resistance with farmers is that very little impact is observed until the problem has become severe (Pomroy, 2006). However, it has been observed that productivity parameters change in relative proportion to the effectiveness of the treatment (Besier, 1996). Besier and Love (2003) measured the impact of resistance in the summer rainfall region of Western Australia, where resistance had become a serious problem for producers, and estimated that drenches which were 65% effective against resident worm burdens, resulted in lambs producing 10% less wool than those given a fully effective treatment. When treatment was 85% effective, wool production fell by just 2%. The lost value of using a 65% or 85% effective drench was estimated as AU$6.60 and $2.45, respectively. Should the situation progress as it has in recent years, the likely economic impact of anthelmintic resistance on the Australian economy is estimated to reach $700 million by 2010. In New Zealand, a small reduction of 3 kg between lambs treated with either an effective or an ineffective drench was observed, although it was noted that the groups were grazed together (Macchi *et al.*, 2001).

Mechanisms of resistance

Benzimidazole resistance is associated with alterations to β-tubulin genes, the result of which is to prevent the drugs binding to their intended target (Lacey & Gill, 1994). The first described change was the substitution of a tyrosine for a phenylalanine at amino acid 200 of isotype 1 β-tubulin (Elard *et al.*, 1996; Kwa *et al.*, 1994), although resistant populations of worms have been observed to retain the phenylalanine at amino acid 200, but instead have the mutation at position 167 (Prichard, 2001). In the cattle nematode *C. oncophora*, benzimidazole resistance was associated with the amino acid 200 substitution (Winterrowd *et al.*, 2003).

Early studies using mutants of the free-living nematode *Caenorhabditis elegans* (Lewis *et al.*, 1980) demonstrated an association between resistance to levamisole with the loss of some of the worms' acetylcholine receptors, and that the levamisole resistance genes *lev-1, unc-29* and *unc-38* encoded subunits of acetylcholine-gated cation channels, which included levamisole (and morantel) binding sites (Fleming *et al.*, 1997). Among GIN parasites, *Oe. dentatum* has several cholinergic channels which vary in their response to levamisole exposure (Martin *et al.*, 1997) while *H. contortus* has a number of levamisole-binding sites on their cholinergic receptor subunits which vary in their affinity for the drug, with the low-affinity receptors being associated with resistance (Sangster *et al.*, 1998). These studies suggest that resistance to levamisole and morantel is complex and involves multiple genes. Further work is required to provide a definitive explanation of the mechanisms of resistance to these anthelmintics.

Elucidating the mechanism of resistance to the MLs has proved to be extremely complex. The drugs act on multiple targets, including locomotion, feeding and reproduction, although the relative importance of these may vary between parasite species (Wolstenholme *et al.*, 2004) and may even vary within populations of one species (Gill & Lacey, 1998). This has led to suggestions that multiple genes are involved in ML resistance (Prichard, 2001; Wolstenholme *et al.*, 2004). It is certainly the case that multiple mutations are necessary for high levels of resistance to be expressed in *C. elegans* (Dent *et al.*, 2000). An increase in the relative proportion of low-affinity L-glutamate binding sites has been observed in resistant populations of both *H. contortus* (Hejmadi *et al.*, 2000) and *T. circumcincta* (Paiement *et al.*, 1999), while other studies have observed an effect of polymorphisms in a GluCl channel from *C. oncophora* on reducing sensitivity to ivermectin in *Xenopus* oocysts (Njue *et al.*, 2004). Alterations in nematode amphids – the receptors responsible for environmental sensing – have also been observed to differ in association with ML resistance (Freeman *et al.*, 2003), although it is unclear how this results in reduced sensitivity to treatment. Another amino acid-gated ion channel, HG1, may also be selected for in ML-resistant worms (Prichard, 2001).

More recently, evidence suggested that ML resistance was associated with mutations in one or more P-glycoprotein genes, with a resulting increase in drug efflux. An ML-resistant mutant of *C. elegans*, developed through step-wise exposure to increasing levels of ivermectin, was demonstrated to express a multiple resistance phenotype, having side resistance to moxidectin and also to the unrelated anthelmintics levamisole and pyrantel, but not albendazole (James & Davey, 2009). The resistance was associated with multi-drug resistance proteins (MDRP) and P-glycoproteins and was reversed following administration of MDRP inhibitors. An important distinction was made between low- and high-level resistances. In the former, resistance was associated with increased expression of the proteins mrp-1, pgp-1 and decreased glutathione, while high-level resistance was associated with increased expression of P-glycoproteins (James & Davey, 2009). Interestingly, recent evidence suggests that ML resistance tends to be more multigenic in cattle nematodes than in field-derived resistant sheep parasites (Geldhof *et al.*, 2008). It is possible that, given the observation of multigenic resistance in parasites selected in the laboratory following exposure to low drug concentrations that a similar scenario has occurred in cattle due to sustained use of pour-on and injectable drench formulations.

Resistance to the most recently developed anthelmintic, the AAD monepantel, was investigated in three populations of *H. contortus* in which the resistance was selected by *in vitro* selection. In all three populations, the resistant parasites lacked at least part of a gene the research group named *H. contortus des-2* homologue, due to its similarity to the *des-2* gene in *C. elegans* (Kaminsky *et al.*, 2008). However, a *C. elegans* mutant lacking *des-2* did not express a resistant phenotype. Yet another gene, acr-23, was at least partly missing in all of the *H. contortus* populations and in a resistant *C. elegans* mutant, implying this may be at least one conserved mechanisms of monepantel resistance (Kaminsky *et al.*, 2008).

How does resistance develop?

Simplistically put, observable resistance will develop when individual worms are able to survive drug treatment, then pass on their resistant genes to subsequent generations; assuming no positive effects of the resistant mutations other than the ability to survive treatment, these subsequent generations also need to be subjected to drug selection. Ultimately, there are sufficient numbers of resistant worms to successfully breed with each other. There are a number of factors which influence how likely and how quickly this process can occur: (a) presence of resistance genes in the treated population, (b) drug efficacy is insufficient to remove worms with resistance genes, (c) selection for resistance is correlated with the proportion of the population exposed to treatment, (d) susceptible worms are unable to establish and to dilute or replace resistance genes and (e) resistant worms establish and multiply in naïve hosts.

There are two obvious routes via which GIN become resistant to anthelmintics. First, drug treatment selects for those individuals in a population with a necessary mutation. Certainly the extremely high genetic variability of GIN suggests this to be a reasonable theory; this would include the situation in which resistant individuals were already present before an anthelmintic was developed and also where mutations occur subsequent to drug development. Alternatively, resistance could develop by selecting those individuals which are resistant to sub-optimal drug exposure i.e. by under-dosing. There is good evidence available to suggest that both of these routes have resulted in the selection of resistant populations of GIN. Furthermore, evidence suggests that selection via these routes results in two distinct types of resistance.

Selection of resistance to 'full-dose' therapy in the field generally produces worms with monogenic resistance, whereby a single mutation is involved, often conferring a 'high' level of resistance. Conversely, selection of resistant worms by exposure to low levels of drug in the laboratory often results in worms with polygenic resistance, either involving more than one gene conferring resistance against a single drug or more than one gene conferring resistance to more than one drug. It is noted that observations of ML resistance mechanisms in *Cooperia* spp. from cattle appear to involve polygenic resistance; this may have arisen due to the regular use of topical applications such as pour-on and injectable formulations leading to effective under-dosing. Other indirect evidence for the likelihood of under-dosing selecting for resistance is the number of resistant populations which have arisen in goats.

Anthelmintics have markedly different pharmacokinetic profiles in these animals compared to the situation in sheep, which may significantly reduce the peak of exposure to treatment.

It should be noted, however, that actually determining what quantum of *in vivo* drug exposure will provide significant selection advantages to worms in the early stages of developing resistance is impossible.

Inheritance of resistance

The mechanisms by which resistance is inherited will significantly influence the ability of resistant genes to survive and spread through worm populations. Simplistically, a heterozygote-resistant worm in which the resistance is inherited as a dominant trait may survive treatment, which would effectively remove a heterozygote-resistant worm in which the resistance is inherited as a recessive trait. Assume that a worm population within a host consists of a mixture of 90% fully susceptible worms, 9% heterozygote-resistant worms and 1% homozygous-resistant ones. Further assume that a treatment removes all of the susceptible worms but none of the homozygous-resistant worms. Depending on whether the resistance is inherited as a dominant or recessive trait, either 10% or 1% of the resident worms may survive treatment and go on to produce progeny with resistant genes.

The actual situation in resistant GIN is of course much more complex, particularly with polygenic resistance. Furthermore, there can be significant variability in the inheritance of resistance to the same anthelmintic between the various GIN species.

Benzimidazole resistance inherited in *T. colubriformis* is incompletely recessive and is maternally influenced. However, in *H. contortus*, resistance is inherited through more than one gene, was semi-dominant and autosomal, and has further been described as multigenic, autosomal but recessive. Subsequent studies established that resistance was inherited similarly between these two species. At least two loci are involved in the inheritance of high levels of benzimidazole resistance.

Resistance to levamisole in *H. contortus* is inherited as a recessive autosomal trait, while the resistance in *T. colubriformis* is inherited via a single sex-linked gene. Nematodes have an XX (female) and XO (male) system of sex determination, and sex-linked recessive traits are therefore recessive in females but dominant in males.

Interestingly, following *in vitro* treatment of *H. contortus* to benzimidazole or levamisole, no evidence was found to suggest sex linkage in either inheritance. As stated above, this may reflect differences in the methods of selection of resistant isolates between field/monogenic and laboratory/polygenic.

Resistance to ivermectin in *H. contortus* is inherited as a completely dominant trait (Dobson *et al.*, 1996; Le Jambre *et al.*, 2000), while in *T. circumcincta*, ivermectin resistance is inherited as a dominant trait (Sutherland *et al.*, 2002) but was effectively incompletely recessive to moxidectin (Sutherland *et al.*, 2002). However, a subsequent study demonstrated that the resistance was dominant during the period of declining drug activity, which is responsible for the persistent efficacy of moxidectin (Sutherland *et al.*, 2003). Interestingly, the same study established that resistance was partially dominant/recessive under treatment with controlled-release capsules releasing ivermectin. In *T. colubriformis*, ivermectin resistance is inherited as an incompletely dominant/recessive trait which appears to be multigenic (Gill & Lacey, 1998; Gopal *et al.*, 2001).

No information is available on the inheritance of resistance to any of the important GIN in cattle.

Detection of resistance

Faecal egg count reduction test

The gold standard method of determining the resistance status of a parasite population, or all parasite species/populations on a property, is the faecal egg count reduction test (FECRT). In the FECRT, animals are allocated to groups of 10 based on pre-treatment FEC, with one group of 10 for each anthelmintic treatment tested and a further untreated control group. In many regions, this requires the use of 40 animals, given there are three active families available. In some regions where combinations containing benzimidazoles and levamisole have been administered to sheep for long periods, a further group may be included to test for resistance to the dual combination. In addition to sampling for FEC, a bulked faecal sample should be cultured for larval differentiation to species or (at least) genus. The appropriate treatments should be calculated for individual liveweight, then administered by syringe for accuracy. Thereafter, 7–14 days later, each individual is sampled for FEC, while bulk samples of faeces are cultured for larval differentiation. A full FECRT is understandably expensive and takes a significant length of time before farmers are presented with the results of their resistance profile. Accurate larval differentiation also demands a high degree of skill.

Care must be taken when conducting an FECRT to delay sampling animals until at least 7–20 days post-treatment; some drench products, particularly the MLs, can cause a temporary suppression on egg production from resistant female survivors (Sutherland *et al.*, 1999), and there is a danger of a misdiagnosis should samples be taken too early.

Any species for which the reduction in egg count is less than 95% is then considered to be resistant. This unfortunately highlights two major deficiencies of the FECRT and of resistance testing in general. The first of these concerns seasonal variability in nematode populations, e.g., in New Zealand, *T. circumcincta*, the parasite of most concern in surveys of ML resistance is more prevalent in early summer. Resistance testing at other times of the year, even if egg counts may be higher, may not detect resistant populations of this species. The second caveat inherent in the FECRT is the use of the 95% threshold for reduction in FEC. While this may have some practical benefit in simplifying outputs, it most certainly does not present a firm line in the sand in which a 95% reduction means no resistance is present or is likely to become a problem on any given property. There are a number of situations in which an example 96% reduction in FEC in an FECRT (or where treatment removes 96% of resident worms) may provide dangerously misleading conclusions. For example, the use of a persistent treatment which is 96% effective is likely to confer a strong advantage to resistant worms, while the presence of large numbers of eggs of a susceptible population may effectively mask the presence of resistant worms belonging to another species. Clearly, a faster, accurate method of resistance monitoring would be welcomed by the industry.

Egg hatch assay

Developed for use with the benzimidazole anthelmintics (Le Jambre, 1976), the egg hatch test is not suitable for use with the other action families currently on the market. This is unfortunate, as the assay is simple to operate and results are obtained by a maximum of 30 hours after collection of faeces.

Larval development assay

This assay can be performed either in a liquid medium or in liquid over an agar matrix containing the drug under investigation. Eggs are extracted from faeces and added to wells of a 96-well microtitre plate in a medium containing lyophilised *Escherichia coli*, yeast extract and the fungicide Amphotericin B. Plates are incubated at 25°C for 7 days, then the numbers of L3 are counted. This test is relatively simple, easy to set up and robust and enables the identification of L3 to species or genus on its conclusion. The lipophilicity of the MLs means attaining a clear discriminating dose is difficult in the Larval development assay (LDA).

Larval migration inhibition assay

L3s are extracted from cultured faeces and placed in the upper side of a chamber divided in half by a mesh. Different concentrations of the drug under investigation are then added to the medium with the larvae. Given the normal swimming behaviour of trichostrongylid L3, the worms will eventually migrate through the mesh into the lower chamber. This migration will be inhibited should the L3 be paralysed or inhibited by exposure to drug. Obviously, resistant L3 will be better able to migrate than those susceptible to the applied drug. This assay is simple to operate and relatively rapid. It also enables identification of L3 to species/genus.

Molecular markers for anthelmintic resistance

Given that anthelmintic resistance has a genetic basis, it should be feasible to reliably identify DNA markers which could be utilised in detecting resistance alleles. However, this has not been, and will not be, a straightforward process.

Our understanding of the mechanisms of resistance to many drugs remains imprecise, which adds difficulty to associating biological events with potential DNA markers. Furthermore, GIN are astoundingly variable at the genetic level, which adds a further layer of complexity.

It is also of some concern that detecting resistance in a parasite population is in itself inherently complex: sheep and cattle harbour several species of worms, which also have to be identified in the assay procedure, and any one of these species will be susceptible or resistant to one or more of several anthelmintic families.

At the time of writing, markers are available for benzimidazole resistance only (a phenylalanine to tyrosine mutation at residue 200 of the isotype 1 β-tubulin gene) (Prichard *et al.*, 2007), although there are promising signs that markers for levamisole/morantel tartrate resistance are close, with a recent study reporting on the discovery of numerous transcript-derived fragments of *H. contortus* which were absent from two levamisole-susceptible populations but present in two levamisole-resistant populations (Neveu *et al.*, 2007).

Identifying markers for ML resistance has proved extremely difficult thus far, as multiple mechanisms may be involved across various populations of various species (Prichard *et al.*, 2007).

Future options for detecting resistance

The ability to easily and quickly detect eggs and/or larvae of different parasite species in a post-drench faecal sample would be significantly faster, cheaper and possibly more accurate than the existing FECRT. Attempts to develop such a test have utilised reagents such as lectins (Colditz *et al.*, 2002) but with little obvious success so far.

References

BARTON, N. J., TRAINOR, B. L., URIE, J. S., ATKINS, J. W., PYMAN, M. F. & WOLSTENCROFT, I. R. (1985). Anthelmintic resistance in nematode parasites of goats. *Australian Veterinary Journal*, **62**, 224–227.

BESIER, R. B. (1996). Ivermectin resistant *Ostertagia* in Western Australia. *Proceedings of Sheep Sessions, Second Pan-Pacific Veterinary Conference*, Sydney, 195–207.

BESIER, R. B. & LOVE, S. C. J. (2003). Anthelmintic resistance in sheep nematodes in Australia: The need for new approaches. *Australian Journal of Experimental Agriculture*, **43**, 1383–1391.

BOGAN, J., BENOIT, E. & DELATOUR, P. (1987). Pharmacokinetics of oxfendazole in goats: A comparison with sheep. *Journal of Veterinary Pharmacology and Therapeutics*, **10**, 305–309.

BORGSTEEDE, F. H. M. (1986). Resistance of *Cooperia curticei* against fenbendazole. *Research in Veterinary Science*, **41**, 423–424.

BORGSTEEDE, F. H. M. (1988). The difference between two strains of *Ostertagia ostertagi* in resistance to morantel tartrate. *International Journal for Parasitology*, **18**, 499–502.

BRITT, D. P. & OAKLEY, G. A. (1986). Anthelmintic evaluation of a thiabenda-zole-resistant strain of *Ostertagia circumcincta* recovered from sheep in England. *Veterinary Parasitology*, **19**, 95–101.

CAWTHORNE, R. J. G. & WHITEHEAD, J. D. (1983). Isolation of benzimidazole resistant strains of *Ostertagia circumcincta* from British sheep. *Veterinary Record*, **112**, 274–277.

CHANDRAWATHANI, P., WALLER, P. J., ADNAN, M. & HOGLUND, J. (2003). Evolution of high-level, multiple anthelmintic resistance on a sheep farm in Malaysia. *Tropical Animal Health and Production*, **35**, 17–25.

CHANDRAWATHANI, P., YUSOFF, N., WAN, L. C., HAM, A. & WALLER, P. J. (2004). Total anthelmintic failure to control nematode parasites of small rumi-nants on government breeding farms in Sabah, East Malaysia. *Veterinary Research Communications*, **28**, 479–489.

COLDITZ, I. G., LE JAMBRE, L. F. & HOSSE, R. (2002). Use of lectin bind-ing characteristics to identify gastrointestinal parasite eggs in faeces. *Veterinary Parasitology*, **105**, 219–227.

CONWAY, D. P. (1964). Variance in the effectiveness of thiabendazole against *Haemonchus contortus* in sheep. *American Journal of Veterinary Research*, **25**, 106–107.

CRAIG, T. M. (1993). Anthelmintic resistance. *Veterinary Parasitology*, **46**, 121–131.

DASH, K. M. (1986). Multiple anthelmintic resistance in *Trichostrongylus colubri-formis*. *Australian Veterinary Journal*, **63**, 45–47.

DENT, J. A., SMITH, M. M., VASSILATIS, D. K. & AVERY, L. (2000). The genet-ics of ivermectin resistance in *Caenorhabditis elegans*. *Proceedings of the National Academy of Sciences of the United States of America*, **97**, 2674–2679.

DOBSON, R. J., LE JAMBRE, L. & GILL, J. H. (1996). Management of anthelmintic resistance: Inheritance of resistance and selection with persistent drugs. *International Journal for Parasitology*, **26**, 993–1000.

DRUDGE, J. H., SZANTO, J., WYANT, Z. N. & ELAM, G. (1964). Field studies on parasite control in sheep: Comparison of thiabendazole, ruelene, and phenothi-azine. *American Journal of Veterinary Research*, **25**, 1512–1518.

ECHEVARRIA, F. A. M. & TRINDADE, G. N. P. (1989). Anthelminthic resistance by *Haemonchus contortus* to ivermectin in Brazil: A preliminary report. *Veterinary Record*, **124**, 147–148.

EGERTON, J. R., SUHAYDA, D. & EARY, C. H. (1988). Laboratory selection of *Haemonchus contortus* for resistance to ivermectin. *Journal of Parasitology*, **74**, 614–617.

ELARD, L., COMES, A. M. & HUMBERT, J. F. (1996). Sequences of b-tubulin cDNA from benzimidazole-susceptible and -resistant strains of *Teladorsagia cir-cumcincta*, a nematode parasite of small ruminants. *Molecular and Biochemical Parasitology*, **79**, 249–253.

FLEMING, J. T., SQUIRE, M. D., BARNES, T. M. *et al.* (1997). *Caenorhabditis ele-gans* levamisole resistance genes lev-1, unc-29, and unc-38 encode functional nico-tinic acetylcholine receptor subunits. *Journal of Neuroscience*, **17**, 5843–5857.

FREEMAN, A. S., NGHIEM, C., LI, J. *et al.* (2003). Amphidial structure of ivermec-tin-resistant and susceptible laboratory and field strains of *Haemonchus contortus*. *Veterinary Parasitology*, **110**, 217–226.

GELDHOF, P., VAN ZEVEREN, A., EL-ABDELLATI, A., DE GRAEF, A., CLAEREBOUT, E., & VERCUYSSE, J. (2008). Molecular mechanisms of mac-rocyclic lactone resistance in the cattle parasites *Ostertagia ostertagi* and *Cooperia oncophora*. *Proceedings of the Australian Society for Parasitology Annual Meeting*, Glenelg, Adelaide, Australia.

GILL, J. H. & LACEY, E. (1998). Avermectin/milbemycin resistance in trichostrongy-loid nematodes. *International Journal for Parasitology*, **28**, 863–877.

GOPAL, R. M., POMROY, W. E., WEST, D. M. & GARRICK, D. J. (2001). Inheritance of ivermectin resistance in a field isolate of *Trichostrongylus colubriformis*. *New Zealand Veterinary Journal*, **28**, 229–230.

GREEN, P. E., FORSYTH, B. A., ROWAN, K. J. & PAYNE, G. (1981). The isola-tion of a field strain of *Haemonchus contortus* in Queensland showing multiple anthelmintic resistance. *Australian Veterinary Journal*, **57**, 79–84.

HALL, C. A., CAMPBELL, N. J. & CARROLL, S. N. (1979). Resistance of thia-bendazole in a field population of *Ostertagia circumcincta* from sheep. *Australian Veterinary Journal*, **55**, 229–231.

HEJMADI, M. V., JAGANNATHAN, S., DELANY, N. S. *et al.* (2000). L-Glutamate binding sites of parasitic nematodes an association with ivermectin resistance? *Parasitology*, **120**, 535–545.

HOTSON, I. K., CAMPBELL, N. J. & SMEAL, M. G. (1970). Anthelmintic resistance in *Trichostrongylus colubriformis*. *Australian Veterinary Journal*, **46**, 356–360.

JABBAR, A., IQBAL, Z., KERBOEUF, D. *et al.* (2006). Anthelmintic resistance: The state of play revisited. *Life Sciences*, **79**, 2413–2431.

JACKSON, F. & COOP, R. L. (2000). The development of anthelmintic resistance in sheep nematodes. *Parasitology*, **120**, 95–107.

JAMES, C. E. AND DAVEY, M. W. (2009). Increased expression of ABC trans-port proteins is associated with ivermectin resistance in the model nematode *Caenorhabditis elegans*. *International Journal for Parasitology*, **39**, 213–220.

KAMINSKY, R., DUCRAY, P., JUNG, M. *et al.* (2008). A new class of anthelmintics effective against drug-resistant nematodes. *Nature*, **452**, 176–180.

KAPLAN, R. M. (2004). Drug resistance in nematodes of veterinary importance: A status report. *Trends in Parasitology*, **20**, 477–481.

KAPLAN, R. M., VIDYASHANKAR, A. N., HOWELL, S. B., NEISS, J. M., WILLIAMSON, L. H. & TERRILL, T. H. (2007). A novel approach for combin-ing the use of *in vitro* and *in vivo* data to measure and detect emerging moxid-ectin resistance in gastrointestinal nematodes of goats. *International Journal for Parasitology*, **37**, 795–804.

KERBOEUF, D. & HUBERT, J. (1985). Benzimidazole resistance in field strains of nematodes from goats in France. *Veterinary Record*, **116**, 133–133.

KETTLE, P. R., VLASSOFF, A., AYLING, J. M., MCMURTY, L. W., SMITH, S. J. & WATSON, A. J. (1982). A survey of nematode control measures used by sheep farmers and anthelmintic resistance on these farms. Part 2. South Island excluding the Nelson region. *New Zealand Veterinary Journal*, **30**, 79–81.

KWA, M. S. G., VEENSTRA, J. G. & ROOS, M. H. (1994). Benzimidazole resistance in *Haemonchus contortus* is correlated with a conserved mutation at amino acid 200 in b-tubulin isotype 1. *Molecular and Biochemical Parasitology*, **63**, 299–303.

LACEY, E. & GILL, J. H. (1994). Biochemistry of benzimidazole resistance. *Acta Tropica*, **56**, 245–262.

LE JAMBRE, L. F. (1976). Egg hatch as an *in vitro* assay of thiabendazole resistance in nematodes. *Veterinary Parasitology*, **2**, 385–391.

LE JAMBRE, L. F., GILL, J. H., LENANE, I. J. & BAKER, P. (2000). Inheritance of avermectin resistance in *Haemonchus contortus*. *International Journal for Parasitology*, **30**, 105–111.

LE JAMBRE, L. F., SOUTHCOTT, W. H. & DASH, K. M. (1976). Resistance of selected lines of *Haemonchus contortus* to thiabendazole, morantel tartrate and levamisole. *International Journal for Parasitology*, **6**, 217–222.

LE JAMBRE, L. F., SOUTHCOTT, W. H. & DASH, K. M. (1977). Resistance of selected lines of *Ostertagia circumcincta* to thiabendazole, morantel tartrate and levamisole. *International Journal for Parasitology*, 7, 473–479.

LE JAMBRE, L. F., SOUTHCOTT, W. H. & DASH, K. M. (1978). Development of simultaneous resistance in *Ostertagia circumcincta* to thiabendazole, morantel tartrate and levamisole. *International Journal for Parasitology*, 8, 443–447.

LEATHWICK, D. M. (1995). A case of moxidectin failing to control ivermectin resistant *Ostertagia* species in goats. *Veterinary Record*, 136, 443–444.

LEWIS, J. A., WU, C. H., LEVINE, J. H. & BERG, H. (1980). Levamisole-resistant mutants of the nematode *Caenorhabditis elegans* appear to lack pharmacological acetylcholine receptors. *Neuroscience*, 5, 967–989.

LOVE, S. C. J., NEILSON, F. J. A., BIDDLE, A. J. & MCKINNON, R. (2003). Moxidectin-resistant *Haemonchus contortus* in sheep in northern New South Wales. *Australian Veterinary Journal*, 81, 359–360.

MACCHI, C., POMROY, W. E., MORRIS, R. S., PFEIFFER, D. U. & WEST, D. M. (2001). Consequences of anthelmintic resistance on live-weight gain of lambs on commercial sheep farms. *New Zealand Veterinary Journal*, 49, 48–53.

MARTIN, R. J., ROBERTSON, A. P., BJORN, H. & SANGSTER, N. C. (1997). Heterogeneous levamisole receptors: A single-channel study of nicotinic acetylcholine receptors from *Oesophagostomum dentatum*. *European Journal of Pharmacology*, 322, 249–257.

MEJIA, M. E., FERNANDEZ IGARTUA, B. M., SCHMIDT, E. E. & CABARET, J. (2003). Multispecies and multiple anthelmintic resistance on cattle nematodes in a farm in Argentina: The beginning of high resistance? *Veterinary Research*, 34, 461–467.

NARI, A., SALLES, J., GIL, A., WALLER, P. J. & HANSEN, J. W. (1996). The prevalence of anthelmintic resistance in nematode parasites of sheep in Southern Latin America: Uruguay. *Veterinary Parasitology*, 62, 213–222.

NEVEU, C., CHARVET, C., FAUVIN, A., CORTET, J., CASTAGNONE-SERENO, P. & CABARET, J. (2007). Identification of levamisole resistance markers in the parasitic nematode *Haemonchus contortus* using a cDNA-AFLP approach. *Parasitology*, 134, 1105–1110.

NJUE, A. I., HAYASHI, J., KINNE, L., FENG, X. P. & PRICHARD, R. K. (2004). Mutations in the extracellular domains of glutamate-gated chloride channel a3 and b subunits from ivermectin-resistant *Cooperia oncophora* affect agonist sensitivity. *Journal of Neurochemistry*, 89, 1137–1147.

OVEREND, D. J., PHILLIPS, M. L., POULTON, A. L. & FOSTER, C. E. (1994). Anthelmintic resistance in Australian sheep nematode populations. *Australian Veterinary Journal*, 71, 117–121.

PAIEMENT, J. P., PRICHARD, R. K. & RIBEIRO, P. (1999). *Haemonchus contortus*: Characterization of a glutamate binding site in unselected and ivermectin-selected larvae and adults. *Experimental Parasitology*, 92, 32–39.

POMROY, W. E. (2006). Anthelmintic resistance in New Zealand: A perspective on recent findings and options for the future. *New Zealand Veterinary Journal*, 54, 265–270.

PRICHARD, R. (1994). Anthelmintic resistance. *Veterinary Parasitology*, 54, 259–268.

PRICHARD, R. K. (2001). Genetic variability following selection of *Haemonchus contortus* with anthelmintics. *Trends in Parasitology*, 17, 445–453.

PRICHARD, R. K., HALL, C. A., KELLY, J. D., MARTIN, I. C. & DONALD, A. D. (1980). The problem of anthelmintic resistance in nematodes. *Australian Veterinary Journal*, 56, 239–251.

PRICHARD, R. K., VON SAMSON-HIMMELSTJERNA, G., BLACKHALL, W. J. & GEARY, T. G. (2007). Foreword: Towards markers for anthelmintic resistance in helminths of importance in animal and human health. *Parasitology*, **134**, 1073–1076.

SANGSTER, N. C., RILEY, F. L. & WILEY, L. J. (1998). Binding of [3H]m-aminolevamisole to receptors in levamisole-susceptible and -resistant *Haemonchus contortus*. *International Journal for Parasitology*, **28**, 707–717.

SUTHERLAND, I. A., BROWN, A. E., LEATHWICK, D. M. & BISSET, S. A. (2003). Resistance to prophylactic treatment with macrocyclic lactone anthelmintics in *Teladorsagia circumcincta*. *Veterinary Parasitology*, **115**, 301–309.

SUTHERLAND, I. A., DAMSTEEGT, A., MILLER, C. M. & LEATHWICK, D. M. (2008). Multiple species of nematodes resistant to ivermectin and a benzimidazole-levamisole combination on a sheep farm in New Zealand. *New Zealand Veterinary Journal*, **56**, 67–70.

SUTHERLAND, I. A., LEATHWICK, D. M. & BROWN, A. E. (1999). Moxidectin: Persistence and efficacy against drug-resistant *Ostertagia circumcincta*. *Journal of Veterinary Pharmacology and Therapeutics*, **22**, 2–5.

SUTHERLAND, I. A., LEATHWICK, D. M., MOEN, I. C. & BISSET, S. A. (2002). Resistance to therapeutic treatment with macrocyclic lactone anthelmintics in *Ostertagia circumcincta*. *Veterinary Parasitology*, **109**, 91–99.

THEODORIDES, V. J., SCOTT, G. C. & LADEMAN, M. S. (1970). Strains of *Haemonchus contortus* resistant against benzimidazole anthelmintics. *American Journal of Veterinary Research*, **31**, 859–863.

VAN WYK, J. A. & MALAN, F. S. (1988). Resistance of field strains of *Haemonchus contortus* to ivermectin, closantel, rafoxanide and the benzimidazoles in South Africa. *Veterinary Record*, **123**, 226–228.

VAN WYK, J. A., STENSON, M. O., VAN DER MERWE, J. S., VORSTER, R. J. & VILJOEN, P. G. (1999). Anthelmintic resistance in South Africa: Surveys indicate an extremely serious situation in sheep and goat farming. *Onderstepoort Journal of Veterinary Research*, **66**, 273–284.

VERMUNT, J. J., WEST, D. M. & POMROY, W. E. (1996). Inefficacy of moxidectin and doramectin against ivermectin-resistant *Cooperia* spp. of cattle in New Zealand. *New Zealand Veterinary Journal*, **44**, 188–193.

VLASSOFF, A. & KETTLE, P. R. (1980). Benzimidazole resistance in *Haemonchus contortus*. *New Zealand Veterinary Journal*, **28**, 23–24.

WAGHORN, T. S., LEATHWICK, D. M., RHODES, A. P. *et al.* (2006). Prevalence of anthelmintic resistance on 62 beef cattle farms in the North Island of New Zealand. *New Zealand Veterinary Journal*, **54**, 278–282.

WALLER, P. J. (1987). Anthelminthic resistance and the future for roundworm control. *Veterinary Parasitology*, **25**, 177–191.

WALLER, P. J. (1994). The development of anthelmintic resistance in ruminant livestock. *Acta Tropica*, **56**, 233–243.

WALLER, P. J., ECHEVARRIA, F., EDDI, C., MACIEL, S., NARI, A. & HANSEN, J. W. (1996). The prevalence of anthelmintic resistance in nematode parasites of sheep in Southern Latin America: General overview. *Veterinary Parasitology*, **62**, 181–187.

WALLER, P. J. & PRICHARD, R. K. (1985). Drug resistance in nematodes. *Chemotherapy of Parasitic Infections*, 339–362, Campbell, W.S. & Rew, R.S. (eds), Phenum, New York.

WINTERROWD, C. A., POMROY, W. E., SANGSTER, N. C., JOHNSON, S. S. & GEARY, T. G. (2003). Benzimidazole-resistant b-tubulin alleles in a population of parasitic nematodes (*Cooperia oncophora*) of cattle. *Veterinary Parasitology*, **117**, 161–172.

WOLSTENHOLME, A. J., FAIRWEATHER, I., PRICHARD, R., VON SAMSON-HIMMELSTJERNA, G. & SANGSTER, N. C. (2004). Drug resistance in veterinary helminths. *Trends in Parasitology*, **20**, 469–476.

WRIGLEY, J., MCARTHUR, M., MCKENNA, P. B. & MARIADASS, B. (2006). Resistance to a triple combination of broad-spectrum anthelmintics in naturally-acquired *Ostertagia circumcincta* infections in sheep. *New Zealand Veterinary Journal*, **54**, 47–49.

7 Drenching and resistance

The previous two chapters have described firstly the different drench families available and then the status of, and mechanisms of resistance to, the various chemical classes. The current chapter will now pull this together to review how different drench types and drenching programmes provide selective advantage (or otherwise) for resistant parasites.

If there was no resistance to any of the commercially available anthelmintic drenches, an individual farmer's choice of product would rely on factors such as price, activity requirements relevant to the prevailing parasitism profile and the effectiveness of marketing strategies and the local pharmaceutical sales staff. To a large extent, this remains the case. However, where the farmer and/or his veterinarian/adviser are aware of the need for effective worm control while minimising selection for resistance, drench choice should include the likely impact on both. Furthermore, of particular relevance to drench choice should be the resistance status of the individual property. This is the only way to ensure the optimal level of worm control while minimising any further selective advantage for resistant worms.

Whatever the reasons, history informs us that drench choice on every property growing livestock should be made with the consideration that resistance is either a current or potential problem. There is, therefore, a requirement to understand how resistance has occurred in the past, as well as the influence of the various drench products and drenching practices on the speed and severity of the reduction in anthelmintic efficacy.

Unfortunately, there are many examples to draw on when attempting to minimise the development of resistance not only in susceptible populations but against novel classes of anthelmintics to which resistance has not yet developed. Given that each of the major broad-spectrum classes has almost complete efficacy against susceptible gastrointestinal nematodes (GIN), it seems sensible to begin with a review of the underlying principles of how drenches in general have been used and to the likely impact of these strategies on the development of resistance. These principles include the frequency of treatment, dose rate, persistence of activity, the rotation of chemical classes and finally the combination of active families in drench treatments.

Frequency of treatment

There is a long-established opinion that the frequency of treatment is not only positively correlated with, but a major driver of, the development of anthelmintic resistance. Underpinning this argument is the rather simplistic statement that in the absence of any drenching at all, resistance could not possibly develop (assuming no associated increase in fitness was conferred by a chance resistance mutation independent of treatment). So, is it not also obvious that drenching more often will result in an increased selection for resistant worms?

The answer is, of course, more complicated. Yes, drenching frequency may increase the selective advantage for resistant worms; however, it is clear that a range of management and epidemiological factors will determine whether this actually occurs. As these factors are dealt with in more detail in other chapters, they will be described here only briefly.

The period of prophylactic activity of any given drench against susceptible worms will affect what operators would consider drenching frequency in terms of the interval between drug administrations. Also, continual exposure to prophylactic drug levels could equally be thought of as equivalent to multiple doses of a transient drug. An example is the use of moxidectin as compared to the more transient ivermectin; while a farmer may use fewer doses of moxidectin per animal over a growing season, the period during which drug selection for resistance occurs may in fact be greater. Indeed, for a drug such as moxidectin, which has a declining tail of activity which may allow resistant but not susceptible parasites to establish, increasing treatment frequency may in fact reduce the selective advantage for resistant worms by removing more resident resistant worms.

A drug treatment administered to animals that are then moved to 'clean' or 'safe' pasture will provide a much greater selective advantage for survivors of the treatment, than the animals remaining on pasture contaminated with predominantly susceptible larvae. A classic example is the observation that strategic summer drenching of sheep in Western Australia, during a period of extremely low pasture contamination, is very highly selective for resistance. In this region, resistance has become a serious issue despite the administration of few drenches/animal per annum. Clearly, the frequency of drenching is not the primary driver of resistance in this situation. Similarly, in New Zealand, a modelling study showed that in a system of drench and move onto clean pasture, two drenches were as selective for resistance as five drenches administered in a rotational grazing system (Leathwick *et al.*, 1995).

Under-dosing

The previous chapter introduced the relationship between under-dosing and the tendency for worm populations to exhibit polygenic resistance, as opposed to selection with full dose treatments which are more likely to select for monogenic resistance. However, this did not explore whether under-dosing is likely to select for resistance *per se*.

The likely influence of under-dosing depends largely on two factors; first, the drug levels present and how effective these are against the various genotypes of worm present at the time of exposure and second, the proportion of susceptible, heterozygote- and homozygous-resistant worms present at the time of treatment. These two factors are inextricably linked to produce the frequency of resistant alleles following drug exposure (Smith *et al.*, 1999).

Under-dosing to the extent that a significant proportion of susceptible genotypes survive treatment is unlikely to confer a significant advantage for resistant worms (Smith *et al.*, 1999); obviously this comes at a cost in terms of poor worm control. A modelling study has examined the impact of under-dosing on selection for resistance in detail (Smith *et al.*, 1999). In the model, a dose which removes all of the susceptible, and perhaps a few of the heterozygote-resistant worms, will select for resistance, but only if the proportion of resistant alleles in the treated population is low; the opposite is the case if the proportion of resistant alleles is high, with no enhanced selection for resistance due to under-dosing (Smith *et al.*, 1999). Over multiple model parameters, the dose most likely to select for resistance was always that which removed all susceptible and/or heterozygote-resistant worms. In practical terms, this implies that under-dosing becomes more critical as the level of resistance alleles in a population increases, and that the severity of resistance is likely to accelerate as more and more worms become capable of surviving treatment.

Worms may be exposed to sub-optimal levels of drug in a variety of ways. Poor drenching practice includes factors such as incorrect calibration of drench guns and poor delivery of drug into the back of the mouth. Also, incorrect estimation of animal live-weight is a common problem (and is just as likely to result in overdosing). Furthermore, poor quality product can be a serious issue in many developing countries and can in itself be due to a variety of reasons. The type of product used will also have a significant impact on the likelihood of under-dosing. As stated in Chapter 5, topical application, either as an injectable or pour-on, can alter the pharmacokinetic profile of drugs, delaying the time to peak plasma concentration while also lengthening the declining tail of activity. The profile of certain persistent anthelmintics, such as moxidectin, which has a declining tail of activity even when administered orally, determines that at some point, heterozygote-resistant parasites are able to establish while susceptible worms are excluded; this is effectively under-dosing.

Persistent anthelmintics

Transient drenches are normally administered orally; the active compound should reach peak levels in the blood relatively quickly, then decline relatively quickly. There is, therefore, a short killing period of 1–3 days. Transient drenches include oral ivermectin, levamisole and the benzimidazoles (Table 7.1).

Table 7.1 Selection of anthelmintic products with either transient or persistent activity. References are provided for studies in which either the period of persistence has been determined or in which the efficacy of the product has been shown.

Transient oral drench	Benzimidazole Levamisole Ivermectin/abamectin Naphthalophos Monepantel*	(Brown *et al.*, 1961) (Kates *et al.*, 1971) (Chabala *et al.*, 1980) (Gibson, 1961) (Kaminsky *et al.*, 2008)
Persistent due to pharmacological properties of molecule	Moxidectin Closantel	(Alvinerie *et al.*, 1996) (Mohammed-Ali & Bogan, 1987)
Persistency increased due to route of administration	Injectable moxidectin Injectable doramectin Pour-on macrocyclic lactones Pour-on benzimidazole Pour-on levamisole	(Kerboeuf *et al.*, 1995) (Ballweber *et al.*, 1999) (Eysker & Eilers, 1995) (Leathwick *et al.*, 1998) (Williams, 1991)
Persistency increased due to mode of delivery	Paratect bolus (morantel tartrate) Controlled-release capsules (CRC) containing albendazole CRC containing ivermectin CRC containing albendazole and ivermectin	(Borgsteede, 1982) (Anderson *et al.*, 1980) (Gogolewski *et al.*, 1997) (Sutherland *et al.*, 2008)

*At the time of writing, monepantel was not commercially available.

Recent years have seen the development and commercialisation of a number of drench products with claims of more persistent activity against parasites than that conferred by transient drenches.

Persistent treatments can be broadly separated into three groups (Table 7.1). First, there are those treatments which are persistent because of some inherent chemical property of the molecule. This group includes the macrocyclic lactone moxidectin and the salicylanilide derivative, closantel.

The second group contains those products whose persistence is increased by altering the route of administration; examples in sheep include formulations of the ML drenches moxidectin and doramectin given as injectable treatments; the claim of persistent activity of these products is significantly extended compared to the oral product (Afzal *et al.*, 1994). Numerous pour-on products are available for use in livestock – most obviously in cattle; it should be noted here that pour-on drenches were developed for ease of application on cattle rather than to increase persistent activity *per se*. It is also notable that there is significant variability in plasma concentrations between individuals administered pour-on drenches; this is thought to result from grooming behaviour in which animals directly ingest drug while licking (Sallovitz *et al.*, 2005).

The third grouping of persistent treatments include those in which the mode of delivery, as opposed to the route of application, extended the period of anthelmintic activity. The controlled-release capsules (CRCs) are in this group (Table 7.1). The morantel tartrate bolus (Paratect), designed to release 150 mg of drug/day over a 90 day period was introduced to enable a single treatment of cattle which provided protection over much of the season. A major driver in the development of this bolus was the relative difficulty in administering oral treatments to large animals.

The original product developed for use in sheep released low doses of albendazole over 100 days and was followed by a product releasing ivermectin, then by a product releasing sequential doses of both drugs. More recently, a CRC was developed in New Zealand that releases a combination of abamectin and albendazole over 100 days, while a further New Zealand development is a bolus which releases the recommended daily dose of abamectin and albendazole for 7 days (D. Leathwick, personal communication). These products are all delivered orally, using specially designed applicator guns.

Why use persistent drenches?

Given that these products have been introduced onto the market subsequent to drenches with more transient activity (often containing the same active ingredient), it is worthwhile to consider the benefits that persistent activity offers to farmers. In other words, why to use persistent drenches?

There are a number of reasons why farmers may use persistent treatments; by increasing the period of protection, the number of drenches administered over a season can be reduced, which means reduced labour input and a reduction in environmental damage and possibly disease transmission resulting from frequent mustering. The use of persistent drenches may also be advisable in areas which, at certain times of the year, are prone to outbreaks of haemonchosis in sheep. In these areas, given a high enough level of larval challenge, significant morbidity and mortality may occur despite a regular monthly drenching regime. Basically, however, all these reasons are encompassed by the fact that persistent treatments are used because they kill parasites for longer. This ability to extend the period of protection has led to the promotion of persistent drenches as a means of significantly reducing pasture contamination – the provision of what is known as 'safe pasture' (Chapter 4). Apparently, the classic protocols for preventive drenching programmes developed by the likes of Brunsdon and Michel (Brunsdon, 1980; Michel, 1969) have been inadvertently misappropriated.

The provision of safe pasture and resistance

As stated in Chapter 4, any attempt to kill all parasites on a given property will almost certainly result in the selection for resistant populations. As compared to the regular application of transient drenches that allow the establishment of some susceptible individuals between treatments, the blanket use of persistent products such as CRCs or moxidectin prevent this re-infection, and therefore reduce the likelihood of the replacement or dilution of drench survivors. Assuming the label claims for these products are correct, then this must surely follow. There is certainly a large amount of information available on the efficacy of persistent drenches against susceptible parasites, some of which implies that the period of protection against re-infection with susceptible parasites may even be significantly longer than the payout of drug (Sutherland *et al.*, 2000). It is not difficult to develop a scenario whereby young stock are administered single or sequential persistent treatments which effectively prevent susceptible parasites from producing progeny over an entire growing season, with obvious implications for the development of resistance.

In addition to the administration of persistent drench treatments to young stock, the unerring drive towards parasite-free safe pasture resulted in a number of products being developed for use in lactating adult ruminants. The contribution of the ewe during the PPRI to pasture contamination is discussed more fully elsewhere in this book. However, it should be noted that egg production during the PPRI, and the subsequent availability of L3 to young lambs, has resulted in recommendations that farmers should drench adult stock over this period, particularly if stock are to be grazed on 'clean pasture' with low levels of L3 contamination (Boag & Thomas, 1973). Unfortunately, if adult stock are considered likely to harbour enough parasites to result in significant levels of pasture contamination, which will subsequently be ingested by young stock, then it follows that drenching these adult animals will provide a strong selective advantage for resistant parasites. It should also be obvious that the level of selective advantage would increase with persistency of drug exposure. Thus, administering a persistent treatment to ewes pre-lambing will reduce contamination of pastures with susceptible, but not resistant GIN. These resistant GIN now have a significantly greater selective advantage as they will be ingested in relatively greater proportions by naïve stock. This hypothesis was tested empirically in a large-scale field trial in New Zealand (Leathwick *et al.*, 2006), in which groups of ewes were either administered CRCs releasing albendazole or remained untreated. All treatments were grazed on separate sets of paddocks for 6 years. At the conclusion of the trial, there was indeed significantly more resistance in the areas/animals in which capsules had been administered (Leathwick *et al.*, 2006).

Persistence and efficacy

Claims have been made that persistent treatments are more effective against parasites than the same active administered as a transient oral drench; this has been particularly true for CRCs releasing either benzimidazoles (Fisher *et al.*, 1992; Le Jambre *et al.*, 1981) or ivermectin (Sutherland *et al.*, 2003). Unfortunately, as stated time and again in this book when considering potential control strategies, the use of persistent drenches to control parasites would be highly effective – if there was no such thing as anthelmintic resistance.

The impetus behind the development of the first CRC, by Australian scientists, was the widespread prevalence of parasites resistant to the benzimidazole active family. In this situation, the effectiveness of one of the mainstays of parasite control for many years had been severely eroded. However, the observation that the drench family had a relatively higher efficacy against larval than adult worms led to the development of a product which released low doses of the drug for 100 days and which prevented the establishment of incoming larvae, including those which were resistant (as adults) to oral drenching (Anderson *et al.*, 1980; Le Jambre *et al.*, 1981; Prichard *et al.*, 1978). The development of the CRC therefore extended the life of the benzimidazoles as a parasite control option. This success almost certainly provided an impetus for the development of subsequent persistent anthelmintic products, some of which at least were not required in order to maintain acceptable levels of control of the drench family utilised.

The initial research into the sustained release of benzimidazoles for the control of resistant parasites was also based on the observation that a drug administered as a single oral dose was subject to first-order kinetics of absorption and elimination (Hennessy, 1997). Thus, if a high dose was administered, the initial level in plasma would be correspondingly high; however, this was followed by a relatively more rapid clearance and therefore a similar period of time when the drug was present at a lethal dose. As an illustration of this effect, increasing the dose of oxfendazole by eightfold provided no greater efficacy against benzimidazole-resistant GIN in goats as compared to the recommended dose (Sangster *et al.*, 1991). Therefore, in order to kill resistant worms more effectively, repeated administration of drug was recommended. This was demonstrated by Sangster *et al.* (1991); administering the recommended dose of oxfendazole three times at 12-hourly intervals increased drug efficacy significantly.

An anthelmintic bolus has been developed more recently, which releases the recommended dose of two active families daily for 7 days. This bolus has proved highly effective against sheep GIN resistant to all currently available anthelmintic classes, including those released from the bolus (Leathwick, personal communication).

In contrast to the CRCs, the higher efficacy of the relatively persistent ML moxidectin, compared to that of the related but more transient ivermectin (Steel, 1993), was not due to the period of persistence *per se* (Sutherland *et al.*, 1999a) but was presumed to be the result of an inherent difference in activity.

The relationship between persistence and efficacy is crucial when considering the likely impact of particular drench products on providing a selective advantage for resistant parasites. First, by increasing the period of drug exposure and second, by determining how many resistant parasites are killed during the period of prophylaxis.

Therapeutic efficacy and resistance – 'head selection'

Head selection refers to the removal of those worms resident in the host at the time of drug administration (Le Jambre *et al.*, 1999) and occurs following administration of any anthelmintic, regardless of family, formulation or route of administration. Considering that all available anthelmintics have excellent efficacy against susceptible parasites, the relevant head selection only occurs against resistant genotypes (Leathwick & Sutherland, 2002). Of these resistant individuals, and assuming that monogenic resistance is present, this refers to heterozygotes (RS) and homozygotes (RR); the majority of the worms containing an R gene will belong to the heterozygote cohort, and it is the ability to remove these worms which has the greatest impact on resistance (Dobson *et al.*, 1996). If most or all of the RS are removed, then the resistance is considered to be effectively recessive, while in the alternative scenario in which most or all RS remain, the resistance is considered to be effectively dominant, and resistance would be expected to develop at a relatively faster rate (Dobson *et al.*, 1996). This is an important distinction; in the previous chapter, it was observed that ivermectin resistance in *Teladorsagia circumcincta* was dominant, but that resistance to moxidectin was incompletely dominant (Dobson *et al.*, 2001). This may be due to the known higher efficacy of moxidectin rather than the involvement of a different mechanism of inheritance of resistance (Leathwick & Sutherland, 2002). Given that the influence of head selection will be directly related to the efficacy of treatment, it is obvious that a product with relatively lower therapeutic efficacy, such as a CRC or a topical application may increase the relative importance of the head on the development of resistance.

Prophylactic efficacy and resistance – 'tail selection'

It is logical that any claim for persistent prophylactic activity for an anthelmintic – in other words, the period in which the presence of drug prevents the establishment of worms susceptible to the particular drug levels they encounter on ingestion – has to go hand in hand with an extended period during which worms resistant to the treatment are able to establish. Again, it is a logical conclusion to make the claim that the longer the period of prophylaxis, the greater the potential for selecting resistant genotypes.

This period can be viewed as two separate processes. First, the prevention of establishment by susceptible genotypes following treatment; this reduces the proportion of susceptible genotypes in the relevant parasite population and confers a period of reproductive advantage for any worms that have survived the head selection (Dobson *et al.*, 1996). Second, if ingested resistant individuals are able to establish during the period of prophylaxis while susceptible worms are not, there will be a further period of reproductive advantage for resistant genotypes (Sutherland *et al.*, 1997, 2003; Vickers *et al.*, 2001). In both cases, resistant worms will be mating with resistant worms and producing resistant offspring. Quite how resistant depends on the mode of inheritance of the resistance.

While tail selection is not an issue with transient oral anthelmintics, it does become significant for treatments with declining drug levels following administration and for treatments such as CRCs which pay out relatively constant, low levels of drug, for extended periods (Sutherland *et al.*, 1997, 1999a, 2000). In the former scenario of declining drug levels, if ingested susceptible larvae can eventually establish when the drug dips below a certain concentration, then it is obvious that worms with resistance genes may establish earlier, and therefore have a period of reproductive advantage. This has been observed with defined populations of *T. circumcincta*, where resistant (but not susceptible) worms were able to establish normally 10 days post-treatment of lambs with moxidectin (Sutherland *et al.*, 1997, 2003). Furthermore, a population known to be a heterozygote RS established just as well as one known to be homozygous RR, establishing the resistance to be effectively dominant (Sutherland *et al.*, 2003). In the same study, the same populations of *T. circumcincta* were given to lambs previously administered CRCs releasing ivermectin. In this case, few of the RS worms but most of the RR worms were able to establish.

Heads or tails?

A number of modelling studies have attempted to compare the relative impact of head and tail selection on the selective advantage for resistant worms. An Australian study (Dobson *et al.*, 1996), assumed that (a) head efficacy was either recessive or dominant (b) the tail was perfect and killed all ingested larvae or (c) imperfect and allowed half of the ingested RS larvae to establish halfway through the tail; RR larvae established regardless of the presence of drug. The outputs of this model established that efficacy against established worm burdens was the primary driver for the development of resistance, followed by the length of the tail. Resistance occurred more rapidly when the resistance was effectively dominant than when effectively recessive. This study also claimed that killing all ingested larvae, regardless of genotype, increased the rate of resistance development. This was based on the premise that remaining, drench-resistant worms have a significant period of reproductive advantage.

It would be dangerous, however, to apply the findings of this study too generally. For example, resistance in *Haemonchus contortus* to ivermectin and moxidectin is a dominant trait, characterised by low efficacy of ivermectin against both RS and RR, and high efficacy of moxidectin against both RS and RR (Dobson *et al.*, 2001). This is not the case for *T. circumcincta*; while resistance to ivermectin was again found to be dominant, resistance to moxidectin treatment was incompletely dominant, with much higher activity observed against the RS than against the RR (Sutherland *et al.*, 2002a). The relative impact of the head and tail on selection for resistance will also depend to a large degree on the size and composition of larval challenge. The more larvae ingested – assuming a low proportion of RS and RR larvae and a majority of susceptible worms are present on pasture – the greater will be the number of resistance alleles able to establish and produce offspring while all susceptible alleles are excluded. This is, in practical terms, analogous to an increase in the period of persistent activity, which has been shown to increase the rate of resistance development (Dobson *et al.*, 1996). It is noted that there is likely to be a significant difference in the weight given to tail selection depending on the size of larval challenge. For example, if animals are treated with moxidectin then moved onto clean pasture with little larval challenge, the importance of tail selection is reduced

(Dobson *et al.*, 2001). This presumably explains differences in opinion between scientists in Australia and New Zealand, as the former country is much less conducive to larval development and survival on pasture, and the importance of tail selection would be expected, in general terms, to be less than in the more temperate New Zealand.

The observation that CRCs releasing ivermectin were able to exclude RS *T. circumcincta* (Sutherland *et al.*, 1997) could imply that the use of these products would select less strongly for resistance than products with tails. However, it must be borne in mind that CRCs are active for approximately 100 days, and even with limited larval challenge, and low numbers of RR ingested, selection pressure would be expected to be high (Sutherland *et al.*, 2000).

A 2002 modelling study (Leathwick & Sutherland, 2002) took a novel approach to the heads vs. tails debate, by including a third ML, abamectin, which displays one of the defining characteristics of each of ivermectin and moxidectin, and compared the impact of all three treatments on selection for resistance in *T. circumcincta*. Abamectin has higher therapeutic potency than ivermectin (Leathwick *et al.*, 2000), although not as great as that of moxidectin (Sutherland *et al.*, 2002a); however, abamectin does not display the persistency of moxidectin (Sutherland *et al.*, 2003). In other words, abamectin could potentially kill more resistant parasites in the 'head' but select less strongly for resistant parasites by having a shorter 'tail'.

The model outputs demonstrated quite clearly that for *T. circumcincta*, using abamectin selected less strongly for resistant worms than either ivermectin or moxidectin. This was a result of abamectin having an effective head and a relatively shorter tail (Leathwick & Sutherland, 2002). In laymen's terms, abamectin has most of the advantages but none of the drawbacks of moxidectin. While this study, and the empirical data that underpinned the work, were confined to ML resistance in *T. circumcincta*, the results support the general principle that an ideal anthelmintic, at least in terms of delaying resistance, is one with high therapeutic efficacy and a low period of persistency.

Persistent activity, immunity and resistance

Just as the presence of a prophylactic level of anthelmintic does not completely remove the impact of parasitism, nor does it completely remove the development of anti-parasite immunity (Sutherland *et al.*, 1999b). An experiment in which lambs were administered CRCs releasing either albendazole of ivermectin and were then challenged with a mixture of resistant and susceptible larvae of either *T. circumcincta* or *Trichostrongylus colubriformis*. This challenge was altered to include only susceptible L3 of either species following the exhaustion of drug release, to simulate a filed situation in which ingested susceptible parasites were no longer exposed to anthelmintic. For both CRCs, and both parasite species, the establishment of the susceptible parasites was significantly delayed and was only a low percentage of L3 administered (Sutherland *et al.*, 2000). This study demonstrated that the significant degree of anti-parasite immunity which had developed in animals with CRCs was likely to increase still further the period of selective advantage to those parasites able to establish during treatment.

Persistent activity, density dependence and resistance

Given the density-dependent nature of parasite establishment in abomasal parasites such as *T. circumcincta* (Callinan & Arundel, 1982; Hong *et al.*, 1987), a study in New Zealand tested the hypothesis that removing susceptible parasites at an early stage following ingestion would enable a greater proportion of resistant parasites to establish (Sutherland *et al.*, 2002b). Sheep administered CRCs releasing ivermectin, or left untreated, were artificially challenged with differing numbers of *T. circumcincta* L3, twice-weekly for 6 weeks. While the number of resistant larvae given was fixed across all of the experimental treatments at 500 twice-weekly, the number of susceptible larvae was either 0, 500 or 3000. In the untreated animals, while the total number of worms increased with challenge, it declined as a percentage of L3 administered, confirming the density dependence of *T. circumcincta* infections. However, this density dependence was significantly reduced by the presence of CRCs, with proportionally more resistant parasites able to establish when the susceptible worms were excluded. This implies that prophylaxis had reduced the relative contribution of the susceptible L3 to what should have been 'normal' population dynamics, and therefore enabled proportionally more resistant L3 to establish. Furthermore, those resistant parasites which established and reached maturity were significantly longer and more fecund (only the females were measured) than the resistant parasites which established in the untreated host animals (Sutherland *et al.*, 2002b).

Drench rotation

Varying the drench family used in an annual rotation strategy appears to be a sensible tactic; by changing the point of attack, so to speak, the chances of resistance building up to any one family should be minimised. For much of the past 30 years, this would have involved the use of a benzimidazole, an imidithiazole derivative and an ML. It is tempting to ponder how the global resistance issue would differ today if annual rotation had begun before resistance had developed to one or more of the three major families.

There are, however, two main aspects of resistance management. The first is preventing it occurring or developing, while the second – of more practical importance – is controlling a resistance problem.

Controlling resistance by drench rotation

The likelihood of controlling resistance by varying drench type relies heavily on at least one of two concepts holding true. First, that there will be a form of counter selection, in which parasites which have developed resistance to one drench family are somehow more susceptible to an alternative treatment, or set of selection pressures (Leathwick *et al.*, 2001).

The second concept is that resistant parasites, regardless of the drench family involved, will be somehow less 'fit' than their susceptible counterparts. So, in the absence of the specific selection pressure exerted by the relevant drench, resistant will be out-bred or out-competed by susceptible. While this is a tempting theory, there is little evidence to suggest it actually occurs. While a correlation between fitness and resistance has been claimed for BZ-resistant parasites when cycled in the laboratory in the absence of drug pressure (Simpkin & Coles, 1978), numerous field studies conducted since have failed to consistently demonstrate a similar effect. Most, if not all of these studies commenced before the introduction of the MLs and concentrated on the effect of sustained use of levamisole on the level of BZ resistance. The level of BZ resistance in *T. circumcincta* did fall after 4 years (Martin, 1987; Waller *et al.*, 1988) and in *T. colubriformis* after 8 years of levamisole use (Waller *et al.*, 1989). In none of these cases, however, did resistance disappear completely, and in fact, in each of the studies, BZ resistance quickly reached similar levels as before when treatment with this active family was re-introduced. Other studies conducted along similar lines saw no reduction in the level of BZ resistance in *T. circumcincta*, even after 15 years of levamisole use (Jackson & Coop, 2000), or following 6 years of levamisole use against BZ-resistant *H. contortus* (Borgsteede & Duyn, 1989).

One study did attempt to determine the level of reversion of levamisole resistance in *T. colubriformis* following sustained BZ use (Waller *et al.*, 1989), and found that susceptibility became slightly greater than would be expected from natural reversion, i.e., in the absence of anthelmintic treatment. As before, however, the effect was small and quickly disappeared on the re-introduction of levamisole.

Neither is there any evidence for reversion of resistance to the ML family, with previous levels of resistance attained rapidly on the re-introduction of IVM after a 5-year absence (Pomroy *et al.*, 1998), while there was no difference in fitness as measured in parasitological parameters between one IVM-resistant and two susceptible isolates of *T. colubriformis* (Gopal, 2000). It has been noted (Leathwick *et al.*, 2001) that field studies normally involve the use of an alternative treatment in the intervening period, and therefore some element of counter selection cannot be dismissed.

It seems unlikely, therefore, that there is any significant reduction in fitness associated with resistance to any of the (at the time of writing) commonly used anthelmintic families. What is often observed is a temporary reduction in the resistance status of the population on a property during the period of no treatment or alternative chemical use. It is presumed this can be explained by dilution of the resistant genes by re-assortment with susceptible genes. It is also presumed that the more resistant genes there are in any given population (this may vary for both drench family and worm species), the slower will be the reduction in the level of resistance. The extremes in such a scenario are that there are too few resistant genes to sustain the phenotype and resistance disappears, or that there are sufficient resistant genes present that no reduction in resistance occurs in the absence of the selective drench.

Drench rotation within seasons

Alternating drench families within season (i.e., between weaning and the development of effective immunity) should, in theory, have no measurable impact on drench efficacy against susceptible worms but should kill more resistant worms, as any individuals surviving drench A may be susceptible to drench B and vice-versa.

The exit drench

One solution to the development of resistance to one or more active families used throughout a typical growing season is the use of a final treatment with an unrelated drench family. This 'exit drench' has the potential to remove any resistant worm burdens which have built up over the previous few months and therefore delay the development of resistance.

While this may be a reasonable argument, it seems to have at least two dangers. The first is that depending on such factors as climate, resistance status and prevailing management practices, there could already be a significant level of pasture contamination with resistant larvae. Second, and less definable, is that the strategy could act as a panacea for farmers, who may then paradoxically pay less attention to resistance management.

Modelling drench rotation

A modelling study (Barnes *et al.*, 1995) simulated the impact of drench rotation on the evolution of resistance. The authors assumed that two drugs were used which had independent genes for resistance; the genes for both were co-dominant and each killed 99%, 50% and 10% of SS, RS and RR genotypes, respectively. When the model was used to compare either rotation at each treatment (i.e. within season) or with annual, 5-yearly and 10-yearly rotation, there was little difference in the development of resistance between the scenarios, although annual rotation did result in the maintenance of susceptibility for longer, and resulted in improved levels of worm control.

How to develop resistance with very little effort

There is anecdotal evidence that resistance can quickly redevelop to an active family which has not been used on a property for many years. The use of controlled-release anthelmintic capsules, for example (whether releasing albendazole or ivermectin), particularly if administered to all stock, effectively screens an overwhelming proportion of parasites on a property. In this situation, the selection pressure for resistant genes, even if present at extremely low levels, is enormous.

Combination anthelmintics

The development of combination therapy has been driven by one of two reasons. First, combining drench families can broaden the spectrum of activity to include e.g. liver fluke or tapeworm in addition to nematodes. There has been general acceptance of the utility of such products and they are widely used where relevant. The second reason for combining drench families in a single treatment is to provide increased activity, originally because of the relatively poor efficacy of the available drugs (Egerton *et al.*, 1963), but later as a means of overcoming the development of anthelmintic resistance. This has proved much more controversial; while combination drenches, for both sheep and cattle, are widely used in Australia and New Zealand, other major markets maintain a refusal to register the products, apparently because of concerns that combining active families increases the likelihood of the development of resistance.

To many people involved in worm control and resistance management in areas where combinations are routinely used, this is rather hard to understand. Perhaps it is straightforward, and the differences in opinion between the regions have diverged due to the history and relative severity of the resistance problems. So what evidence is there that combining active families makes the development of resistance less likely?

Removing resistant worm burdens

Modelling studies have proposed that a major determining factor in how rapidly populations develop observable resistance is the number/proportion of resistant parasites able to survive treatment (Barnes *et al.*, 1995). Working on the premise this theory is correct, attaining the greatest efficacy possible should be the aim of any anthelmintic treatment. The weight of evidence suggests that the best way to do this is to use combination chemotherapy.

Efficacy of single actives vs. combinations

Low doses of levamisole have been shown to potentiate the efficacy of benzimidazole drugs, first in a mouse model (Bennet *et al.*, 1978), then against a benzimidazole-resistant population of *H. contortus* in sheep (Bennet *et al.*, 1980). This increased activity was ascribed to the immunostimulatory properties of levamisole acting in concert with the anthelmintic properties of both drugs. Also, co-administration of a low dose of parbendazole along with a full dose of oxfendazole was more effective than the administration of oxfendazole alone; this was proposed to be a result of parbendazole interfering with hepatic activity responsible for breaking down oxfendazole (Hennessy *et al.*, 1985). The cytochrome P450 inhibitor piperonyl butoxide has been used to synergise the activity of fenbendazole activity against benzimidazole-resistant *T. circumcincta* and *H. contortus* in sheep, presumably by delaying its degradation to oxfendazole and lengthening the period of drug absorption

(Benchaoui & McKellar, 1996). However, with the exception of these examples, there is little evidence to suggest that different anthelmintic classes show any synergy when co-administered (McKenna, 1990). This is hardly surprising given the excellent efficacy of the modern anthelmintic classes, each of which effectively removes all resident worms when administered alone. However, this situation changes significantly if parasites are present which are resistant to treatment with one or more active families; it is either the threat or presence of resistance that highlights the value of combination therapy.

The strategic worm control programme, 'Wormkill', developed in Australia in the early 1980s, utilised a combination treatment of closantel and a broad-spectrum anthelmintic as a means of combating resistance in *T. colubriformis*, while also reducing treatment frequency. The claim was made for this strategy that selection pressure for resistance in GIN would be reduced by switching to combination products (Dash, 1986). Since then, a number of scientists have provided evidence, through empirical and modelling work, which supports the utility of using combinations as a means of (a) removing burdens of resistant populations and (b) delaying the development of resistance.

It is obvious that using a combination containing two or more active families, each of which has high efficacy against susceptible worms, will remove all worms present in an animal, assuming that each individual is susceptible to at least one of the drugs. Where there are no resistant worms present, switching to a combination will have no effect on drug efficacy, as compared to either of the constituent actives. This is the same whether there is only a single or multiple parasite species present. A combination containing two distinct families, e.g. a benzimidazole and levamisole, should therefore be effective against a mixed infection in which some individuals (regardless of species) are resistant to either benzimidazole or levamisole. There should also be excellent control of an established infection if, for example, individuals in one population are resistant to benzimidazole while individuals in another population are resistant to levamisole.

There is a potential pitfall if GIN parasites are not considered as a species complex. In many areas of the world, even where resistance is considered to be widespread, it is certainly not always the case that more than one parasite species is resistant to more than one active family. Therefore, even where there is a high prevalence of resistance to one constituent, the use of a combination often provides sustained efficacy of worm control. An excellent example of this was highlighted following a 2006 survey of resistance in New Zealand in which 64% of sheep farms had detectable resistance; while over 40% of these farms had worms resistant to either benzimidazole or levamisole, less than 10% had worms resistant to a combination comprising both active families (Waghorn *et al.*, 2006).

The odds are against multiple mutations

One of the most powerful arguments supporting the use of combinations as a tool to delay the development of resistance is logic. Logic tells us that it is much more likely that a worm will have gene(s) for resistance to one active family (whether the genes were originally present in the population, or arose

Table 7.2 A simplistic representation of the likelihood of single gene mutations conferring resistance to one or more anthelmintics, in a population in which no resistance is present, and where there is no cross-resistance between the genes. A mutation rate of 10^{-7} is based on an estimate of random mutation events in *Caenorhabditis elegans*.

Number of actives	Likelihood of single gene mutation for every active	Mathematical probability of resistance occurring following a single drench
1	10^{-7}	1 in 10^{-7}
2	$10^{-7} \times 10^{-7}$	1 in 10^{-49}
3	$10^{-7} \times 10^{-7} \times 10^{-7}$	1 in 10^{-343}

by mutation) than to two or more. There is also a powerful logic behind the overly simplistic calculation shown in Table 7.2.

Assuming the gene(s) conferring resistance to distinct active families are independent of each other, then the unlikelihood of resistance suddenly appearing is multiplied (and not added, as has occasionally been erroneously stated). It is again logical, therefore, that the chance of resistance developing to a triple or quadruple combination is vanishingly small. It is noted, however, that should sufficient pressure be exerted for long enough, resistance will eventually develop to any drench, whether it be a single or combination product.

Resistance is already present to one or more constituent active

An objection which is often raised against the use of combination drenches is that resistance has already developed to one or more of the constituent actives, and may in fact be very prevalent. It is accepted that even limited use of a single active, prior to switching to a combination containing that active, is likely to reduce the effectiveness of the combination in future. However, there are a number of reasons why combination therapy should still be used.

First, while resistant worms may already be present on a farm, a switch to combinations may prevent the selection of further resistant populations and reduce the potential for drench failure in the future. Second, effective combinations will kill more parasites than a single active.

The origin of combination drenches

The combining of two or more drench families as a resistance-fighting mechanism only became possible as one or more active families came off patent and pharmaceutical companies were able to produce generic product. To date, there has never been a product introduced onto the global drench market which combined two new, unrelated active families.

References

AFZAL, J., STOUT, S. J., DACUNHA, A. R. & MILLER, P. (1994). Moxidectin: Absorption, tissue distribution, excretion, and biotransformation of 14C-labeled moxidectin in sheep. *Journal of Agricultural and Food Chemistry*, **42**, 1767–1773.

ALVINERIE, M., SUTRA, J. F., LANUSSE, C. & GALTIER, P. (1996). Plasma profile study of moxidectin in a cow and its suckling calf. *Veterinary Research*, **27**, 545–549.

ANDERSON, N., LABY, R. H., PRICHARD, R. K. & HENNESSY, D. (1980). Controlled release of anthelmintic drugs: A new concept for prevention of helminthosis in sheep. *Research in Veterinary Science*, **29**, 333–341.

BALLWEBER, L. R., SIEFKER, C., ENGELKEN, T., WALSTROM, D. J. & SKOGERBOE, T. (1999). Persistent activity of doramectin injectable formulation against experimental challenge with *Haemonchus placei* in cattle. *Veterinary Parasitology*, **86**, 1–4.

BARNES, E. H., DOBSON, R. J. & BARGER, I. A. (1995). Worm control and anthelmintic resistance: Adventures with a model. *Parasitology Today*, **11**, 56–63.

BENCHAOUI, H. A. & MCKELLAR, Q. A. (1996). Interaction between fenbendazole and piperonyl butoxide: Pharmacokinetic and pharmacodynamic implications. *Journal of Pharmacy and Pharmacology*, **48**, 753–759.

BENNET, E. M., BEHM, C. & BRYANT, C. (1978). Effects of mebendazole and levamisole on tetrathyridia of *Mesocestoides corti* in the mouse. *International Journal for Parasitology*, **8**, 463–466.

BENNET, E. M., BEHM, C., BRYANT, C. & CHEVIS, R. A. F. (1980). Synergistic action of mebendazole and levamisole in the treatment of a benzimidazole-resistant *Haemonchus contortus* in sheep. *Veterinary Parasitology*, **7**, 207–214.

BOAG, B. T. & THOMAS, R. J. (1973). Epidemiological studies on gastrointestinal nematode parasites of sheep. The control of infection in lambs on clean pasture. *Research in Veterinary Science*, **14**, 11–20.

BORGSTEEDE, F. H. M. (1982). Experiments with the Paratect® bolus system in calves. *Parasitology*, **84**, xxxiv–xxxv.

BORGSTEEDE, F. H. M. & DUYN, S. P. J. (1989). Lack of reversion of a benzimidazole resistant strain of *Haemonchus contortus* after six years of levamisole usage. *Research in Veterinary Science*, **47**, 270–272.

BROWN, H. D., MATZUK, A. R., ILVES, I. R. *et al.* (1961). Antiparasitic drugs. IV. 2-(4b-thiazolyl)-benzimidazole, a new anthelmintic [5]. *Journal of the American Chemical Society*, **83**, 1764–1765.

BRUNSDON, R. V. (1980). Principles of helminth control. *Veterinary Parasitology*, **6**, 185–215.

CALLINAN, A. P. L. & ARUNDEL, J. H. (1982). Population dynamics of the parasitic stages of *Ostertagia* spp. in sheep. *International Journal for Parasitology*, **12**, 531–535.

CHABALA, J. C., MROZIK, H., TOLMAN, R. L. *et al.* (1980). Ivermectin, a new broad-spectrum antiparasitic agent. *Journal of Medicinal Chemistry*, **23**, 1134–1136.

DASH, K. M. (1986). Control of helminthosis in lambs by strategic treatment with closantel and broad-spectrum anthelmintics. *Australian Veterinary Journal*, **63**, 4–7.

DOBSON, R. J., BESIER, R. B., BARNES, E. H. *et al.* (2001). Principles for the use of macrocyclic lactones to minimise selection for resistance. *Australian Veterinary Journal*, **79**, 756–761.

DOBSON, R. J., LE JAMBRE, L. & GILL, J. H. (1996). Management of anthelmintic resistance: Inheritance of resistance and selection with persistent drugs. *International Journal for Parasitology*, **26**, 993–1000.

EGERTON, J. R., OTT, W. H. & CUCKLER, A. C. (1963). Comparative anthelmintic efficacy of thiabendazole and mixtures of phenothiazine and phenzidole. *Nature*, **198**, 309–310.

EYSKER, M. & EILERS, C. (1995). Persistence of the effect of a moxidectin pour-on against naturally acquired cattle nematodes. *Veterinary Record*, **137**, 457–460.

FISHER, M. A., JACOBS, D. E. & JONES, P. A. (1992). Field evaluation of an albendazole intraruminal capsule against benzimidazole-resistant *Haemonchus contortus*. *Veterinary Record*, **130**, 351–353.

GIBSON, T. E. (1961). Controlled tests with three organic phosphorus compounds as anthelmintics against *Haemonchus contortus* in sheep. *The Veterinary record*, **73**, 230–231.

GOGOLEWSKI, R. P., ALLERTON, G. R., RUGG, D., KAWHIA, D., BARRICK, R. A. & EAGLESON, J. S. (1997). Demonstration of the sustained anthelmintic efficacy of a controlled-release capsule formulation of ivermectin in weaner lambs under field conditions in New Zealand. *New Zealand Veterinary Journal*, **45**, 158–161.

GOPAL, R. M. (2000). Some aspects of ivermectin resistance in gastrointestinal nematodes of goats and sheep. Ph.D. Thesis, Massey University, Palmerston North, New Zealand.

HENNESSY, D. R. (1997). Modifying the formulation or delivery mechanism to increase the activity of anthelmintic compounds. *Veterinary Parasitology*, **72**, 367–390.

HENNESSY, D. R., LACEY, E., PRICHARD, R. K. & STEEL, J. W. (1985). Potentiation of the anthelmintic activity of oxfendazole by parbendazole. *Journal of Veterinary Pharmacology and Therapeutics*, **8**, 270–275.

HONG, C., MICHEL, J. F. & LANCASTER, M. B. (1987). Observations on the dynamics of worm burdens in lambs infected daily with *Ostertagia circumcincta*. *International Journal for Parasitology*, **17**, 951–956.

JACKSON, F. C. & COOP, R.L. (2000). The development of anthelmintic resistance in sheep nematodes. *Parasitology*, **120**, S95–S107.

KAMINSKY, R., GAUVRY, N., SCHORDERET WEBER, S. *et al.* (2008). Identification of the amino-acetonitrile derivative monepantel (AAD 1566) as a new anthelmintic drug development candidate. *Parasitology Research*, **103**, 931–939.

KATES, K. C., COLGLAZIER, M. L., ENZIE, F. D., LINDAHL, I. L. & SAMUELSON, G. (1971). Comparative activity of thiabendazole, levamisole, and parbendazole against natural infections of helminths in sheep. *Journal of Parasitology*, **57**, 356–362.

KERBOEUF, D., HUBERT, J., CARDINAUD, B. & BLOND-RIOU, F. (1995). The persistence of the efficacy of injectable or oral moxidectin against *Teladorsagia*, *Haemonchus* and *Trichostrongylus* species in experimentally infected sheep. *Veterinary Record*, **137**, 399–401.

LEATHWICK, D. M., MILLER, C. M., ATKINSON, D. S. *et al.* (2006). Drenching adult ewes: Implications of anthelmintic treatments pre- and post-lambing on the development of anthelmintic resistance. *New Zealand Veterinary Journal*, **54**, 297–304.

LEATHWICK, D. M., MILLER, C. M. & VICKERS, M. C. (1998). Comparative efficacy of a new oxfendazole pour-on in cattle. *Veterinary Record*, **142**, 463–464.

LEATHWICK, D. M., MOEN, I. C., MILLER, C. M. & SUTHERLAND, I. A. (2000). Ivermectin-resistant *Ostertagia circumcincta* from sheep in the lower North Island and their susceptibility to other macrocyclic lactone anthelmintics. *New Zealand Veterinary Journal*, **48**, 151–154.

LEATHWICK, D. M., POMROY, W. E. & HEATH, A. C. G. (2001). Anthelmintic resistance in New Zealand. *New Zealand Veterinary Journal*, 49, 227–235.

LEATHWICK, D. M. & SUTHERLAND, I. A. (2002). Heads or tails – Which drench do I choose? *Proceedings of the 32nd Annual Seminar of the Society of Sheep and Beef Cattle Veterinarians of the New Zealand Veterinary Association*, 115–127.

LEATHWICK, D. M., VLASSOFF, A. & BARLOW, N. D. (1995). A model for nematodiasis in New Zealand lambs: The effect of drenching regime and grazing management on the development of anthelmintic resistance. *International Journal for Parasitology*, 25, 1479–1490.

LE JAMBRE, L. F., J. DOBSON, R., LENANE, I. J. & BARNES, E. H. (1999). Selection for anthelmintic resistance by macrocyclic lactones in *Haemonchus contortus*. *International Journal for Parasitology*, 29, 1101–1111.

LE JAMBRE, L. F., PRICHARD, P. K., HENNESSY, D. R. & LABY, R. H. (1981). Efficiency of oxfendazole administered as a single dose or in a controlled release capsule against benzimidazole-resistant *Haemonchus contortus*, *Ostertagia circumcincta* and *Trichostrongylus colubriformis*. *Research in Veterinary Science*, 31, 289–294.

MARTIN, P. J. (1987). Development and control of resistance to anthelmintics. *International Journal for Parasitology*, 17, 493–501.

MCKENNA, P. B. (1990). The use of benzimidazole-levamisole mixtures for the control and prevention of anthelmintic resistance in sheep nematodes: An assessment of their likely effects. *New Zealand Veterinary Journal*, 38, 45–49.

MICHEL, J. F. (1969). The epidemiology and control of some nematode infections of grazing animals. *Advances in Parasitology*, 7, 211–282.

MOHAMMED-ALI, N. A. & BOGAN, J. A. (1987). The pharmacodynamics of the flukicidal salicylanilides, rafoxanide, closantel and oxyclosanide. *Journal of Veterinary Pharmacology and Therapeutics*, 10, 127–133.

POMROY, W. E., ADLINGTON, B. A. & GOPAL, R. M. (1998). Re-emergence of ivermectin-resistant *Ostertagia* spp in goats and sheep grazing pasture previously contaminated with ivermectin-resistant *Ostertagia* spp. *Proceedings of the Second International Conference on Novel Approaches to the Control of Helminth Parasites of Livestock*, Baton Rouge, Louisiana, 55–56.

PRICHARD, R. K., HENNESSY, D. R. & STEEL, J. W. (1978). Prolonged administration: A new concept for increasing the spectrum and effectiveness of anthelmintics. *Veterinary Parasitology*, 4, 309–315.

SALLOVITZ, J. M., LIFSCHITZ, A., IMPERIALE, F., VIRKEL, G., LARGHI, J. & LANUSSE, C. (2005). Doramectin concentration profiles in the gastrointestinal tract of topically-treated calves: Influence of animal licking restriction. *Veterinary Parasitology*, 133, 61–70.

SANGSTER, N. C., RICKARD, J. M., HENNESSY, D. R., STEEL, J. W. & COLLINS, G. H. (1991). Disposition of oxfendazole in goats and efficacy compared with sheep. *Research in Veterinary Science*, 51, 258–263.

SIMPKIN, K. G. & COLES, G. C. (1978). Instability of benzimidazole resistance in nematode eggs. *Research in Veterinary Science*, 25, 249–250.

SMITH, G., GRENFELL, B. T., ISHAM, V. & CORNELL, S. (1999). Anthelmintic resistance revisited: Under-dosing, chemoprophylactic strategies, and mating probabilities. *International Journal for Parasitology*, 29, 77–91.

STEEL, J. W. (1993). Pharmacokinetics and metabolism of avermectins in livestock. *Veterinary Parasitology*, 48, 45–57.

SUTHERLAND, I. A., BROWN, A. E. & LEATHWICK, D. M. (2000). Selection for drug-resistant nematodes during and following extended exposure to anthelmintic. *Parasitology*, 121, 217–226.

SUTHERLAND, I. A., BROWN, A. E., LEATHWICK, D. M. & BISSET, S. A. (2003). Resistance to prophylactic treatment with macrocyclic lactone anthelmintics in *Teladorsagia circumcincta*. *Veterinary Parasitology,* **115**, 301–309.

SUTHERLAND, I. A., DAMSTEEGT, A., MILLER, C. M. & LEATHWICK, D. M. (2008). Multiple species of nematodes resistant to ivermectin and a benzimidazole-levamisole combination on a sheep farm in New Zealand. *New Zealand Veterinary Journal,* **56**, 67–70.

SUTHERLAND, I. A., LEATHWICK, D. M. & BROWN, A. E. (1999a). Moxidectin: Persistence and efficacy against drug-resistant *Ostertagia circumcincta*. *Journal of Veterinary Pharmacology and Therapeutics,* **22**, 2–5.

SUTHERLAND, I. A., LEATHWICK, D. M., GREEN, R., BROWN, A. E. & MILLER, C. M. (1999b). The effect of continuous drug exposure on the immune response to *Trichostrongylus colubriformis* in sheep. *Veterinary Parasitology,* **80**, 261–271.

SUTHERLAND, I. A., LEATHWICK, D. M., BROWN, A. E. & MILLER, C. M. (1997). Prophylactic efficacy of persistent anthelmintics against challenge with drug-resistant and susceptible *Ostertagia circumcincta*. *Veterinary Record,* **141**, 120–123.

SUTHERLAND, I. A., LEATHWICK, D. M., MOEN, I. C. & BISSET, S. A. (2002a). Resistance to therapeutic treatment with macrocyclic lactone anthelmintics in *Ostertagia circumcincta*. *Veterinary Parasitology,* **109**, 91–99.

SUTHERLAND, I. A., MOEN, I. C. & LEATHWICK, D. M. (2002b). Increased burdens of drug-resistant nematodes due to anthelmintic treatment. *Parasitology,* **125**, 375–381.

VICKERS, M., VENNING, M., MCKENNA, P. B. & MARIADASS, B. (2001). Resistance to macrocyclic lactone anthelmintics by *Haemonchus contortus* and *Ostertagia circumcincta* in sheep in New Zealand. *New Zealand Veterinary Journal,* **49**, 101–105.

WAGHORN, T. S., LEATHWICK, D. M., RHODES, A. P. *et al.* (2006). Prevalence of anthelmintic resistance on sheep farms in New Zealand. *New Zealand Veterinary Journal,* **54**, 271–277.

WALLER, P. J., DOBSON, R.J. & AXELSON, A. (1988). Anthelmintic resistance in the field: Changes in resistance status of parasitic populations in response to anthelmintic treatment. *Australian Veterinary Journal,* **65**, 376–379.

WALLER, P. J., DONALD, A. D., DOBSON, R. J. *et al.* (1989). Changes in anthelmintic resistance status of *Haemonchus contortus* and *Trichostrongylus colubriformis* exposed to different anthelmintic selection pressures in grazing sheep. *International Journal for Parasitology,* **19**, 99–110.

WILLIAMS, J. C. (1991). Efficacy of albendazole, levamisole and fenbendazole against gastrointestinal nematodes of cattle, with emphasis on inhibited early fourth stage *Ostertagia ostertagi* larvae. *Veterinary Parasitology,* **40**, 59–71.

8 Worm control and resistance management

The development of anthelmintic resistance in gastrointestinal nematodes (GIN) of grazing livestock has been growing at an ever-increasing pace in recent years (Besier & Love, 2003; Jackson & Coop, 2000; Waghorn *et al.*, 2006a, b). While new anthelmintic families may enter the market in the near future, these will provide a valuable tool in minimising the impact of resistance, rather than solving the problem *per se*. Besides, while it is always dangerous to predict what will happen to any new family following a period of sustained use, history suggests that resistance will eventually occur to any active family. It is worth considering that there was no resistance to ivermectin in 1981.

It is necessary, therefore, to develop and utilise recommendations that minimise the selective advantage for resistant worms to the existing anthelmintic families, as well as those to which resistance has not yet been recorded. However, recommendations must be developed which maintain a high, or otherwise acceptable, level of worm control if farmers are to apply them on their properties.

When considering how to balance resistance management and worm control strategies, it is worthwhile revisiting one of the central principles of parasite control which has been practised for decades – namely, minimising the exposure of stock to levels of larval challenge likely to result in loss of productivity (Armour, 1980; Brunsdon, 1980; Michel, 1969). Given the high prevalence of resistance in most areas of the world with significant pastoral livestock industries, it is easy to apportion at least some of the blame to this particular parasite control strategy. However, as explained in the previous chapters, it is the degree and means of application of the 'clean grazing' strategy which have contributed to the development of resistance. Examples of what could be termed extreme worm control include drench and move onto pasture with little or no larval contamination and suppressive drenching in which all stock (and all parasites) are targeted for drug treatment.

As explained in Chapter 4, it is crucial that not all parasites on a property (or parts of a property) are exposed to drug treatment as this provides an increased selective advantage for drench survivors (van Wyk, 2001). It is also crucial that livestock containing those drench survivors ingest susceptible parasites subsequent to treatment as this will dilute or replace the resistant genes passed on to subsequent generations.

In addition to the provision of safe pasture, the sustained use of anthelmintic families over many years has historically resulted in resistance. It is noted, however, that drench rotation has not been proven to be a significant brake on the development of resistance (Barnes *et al.*, 1995). Instead, what evidence there is, whether empirical or from modelling studies, suggests that it is the use of single actives *per se* (as opposed to combinations) which is the risk factor for resistance (Barnes *et al.*, 1995).

Combination drenches are effective in managing resistance for two reasons. First, the risk of worms developing resistance to more than one drench family simultaneously is remote (Barnes *et al.*, 1995) and second, combining more than one drench is likely to make the treatment more effective against resistant parasites (Leathwick, 2005).

If the importance of these two factors in the development of resistance is accepted as accurate, it seems reasonable to presume that some modification of each should result in the mitigation of the risk of developing resistance. Thus, manipulating parasite populations on pasture through grazing management techniques could increase the likelihood that susceptible parasites are available for ingestion by suitable stock. Furthermore, using combination treatments to kill more resistant worms will reduce the risk of resistance genes contributing to subsequent generations of parasites.

Unfortunately, the development and uptake of recommendations to apply these two practices have proved to be difficult. Let us reverse the order for a moment and deal first with the resistance in many parts of the world to the use of combination drenches. As discussed in Chapter 7, there is a prevailing belief in some quarters that using combinations will mask the development of resistance and will result in treatment failure developing more quickly to the constituent active families. Until these concerns are overcome, there seems little prospect of combinations contributing to resistance management in some regions.

The practicalities of providing a level of larval contamination on pasture which can control resistance but not result in unacceptable productivity losses have also proven difficult to apply on a wide scale in the livestock industries. Here, however, the difficulty appears to be less over the acceptance of the underlying principles, but rather is around how to best achieve the correct balance (Waghorn *et al.*, 2008). The result, as always, is conflicting advice to farmers, resulting confusion and subsequent resistance to the application of the principle.

The maintenance of a pool of susceptible parasites to control resistance has played a central role in other agricultural sectors, such as the control of crop pests, for many years (Roush & McKenzie, 1987). The practice is otherwise referred to as maintaining a 'refuge' of susceptible individuals – these individuals therefore comprise the 'refugia'. It is only in recent years, however, that the principle of utilising the refuge has been proposed for GIN in grazing livestock (van Wyk, 2001).

What is refugia?

It is important that the definition of the refuge is precise. Many people work on the assumption that having 'dirty' pastures, contaminated with L3, is sufficient to be considered a refuge. This is not the case and reflects perhaps the confusing nature of the term which implies having a reserve of parasites on pasture.

For parasites to be considered part of a refuge (i.e. in refugia), they must (a) be susceptible to the particular anthelmintic being used at the time (b) be ingested by a suitable host animal and (c) establish and mate with suitable worms.

If we consider these criteria in more detail, the first states that the L3 must be susceptible to the relevant anthelmintic in use at the time. If a property has multiple species present which are highly resistant to benzimidazoles, it would be hoped that the farmer would have switched to an alternative action family (or a combination). In this case, the benzimidazole resistance status of the L3 on pasture becomes largely irrelevant if the refuge is being managed to prevent the development of further resistance. With the second criteria, L3 which are ingested by animals in which they are unable to establish cannot possibly contribute any susceptible genes to subsequent generations. Situations in which this may occur could be when the management practices include mixed grazing of different stock classes or species to clean up pasture. Finally, it is vital that the parasites find and mate with suitable partners. For example, if a farmer considers a pasture to be dirty and contains an adequate potential refuge of worms, it is also vital that these worms belong to the relevant species. This is an important point if a farmer is rotating pasture regularly, given the seasonal variation in worm egg output between the major GIN species.

The vast majority of eggs passed on to pasture do not develop to L3 or meet each of these criteria. These worms are, therefore, not in refugia.

Why do we need a refuge?

A controlled artificial challenge experiment demonstrated that resistance developed more quickly when a larger proportion of the worm population (analogous to less refugia) was exposed to treatment (Martin *et al.*, 1981), while a later study using a mathematical modelling approach (Barnes *et al.*, 1995) suggested that, in Australia, leaving a proportion of lambs undrenched was likely to slow the development of resistance – but was also likely to result in increased parasitism and production losses (Barnes *et al.*,

1995). Furthermore, a relatively recent study in Western Australia showed that leaving 10% of worms (based on FEC) unexposed to anthelmintic, at a strategic pre-summer treatment, resulted in less resistance but more parasitism (Besier, 2001).

Three recent field trials conducted in New Zealand have investigated the effect of deliberately retaining unselected parasites on the development of resistance in large-scale replicated field trials which were designed to reflect real on-farm conditions.

In a trial conducted over five grazing seasons, Leathwick *et al.* (2006) compared the rate of development of albendazole resistance under different drenching regimes. One of the comparisons involved drenching lambs six times at 28-day intervals from weaning with either 0% or the 15% heaviest lambs left untreated each time. At the end of the trial, the level of albendazole resistance in the two treatments was not significantly different in *Trichostrongylus colubriformis,* but tended towards being significantly lower for *Teladorsagia circumcincta* when some lambs remained untreated (Leathwick *et al.*, 2006).

In a subsequent experiment, the same research group artificially infected groups of lambs with cohorts of parasites which included 4% of larvae which were resistant to benzimidazole treatment and then grazed them on clean pastures (previously grazed only by cattle). This experiment compared the impact on resistance status of leaving either 0%, 10% or 20% of lambs untreated at each drench date. The resistance status of the resulting worm populations on pasture was then measured using tracer lambs and *in vitro* egg hatch and larval development assays. The results showed a definite, and significant, impact of leaving animals undrenched on reducing the level of resistance in the worm populations, although there was no observable difference between the 10% and 20% treatments (Waghorn *et al.*, 2008).

A further trial by these researchers compared the effect on the level of resistance in worm populations by infecting lambs with parasites (again containing a small proportion of resistant worms), then drenching and moving the animals on to pastures which had been manipulated to contain either low, medium or high levels of larval contamination (Leathwick *et al.*, 2008). It is important to note that these pastures were contaminated with (at least predominantly) susceptible parasites. Following a period of grazing sufficient to allow ingested parasites to reach maturity, all lambs were drenched and the level of resistance in the eggs passed measured using an *in vitro* egg hatch assay. The results of this trial established that lambs moved onto the low-contamination pasture (i.e. with a low level of refugia) contained parasites with a high level of drug resistance. As in the previous experiment, however, there was no observable difference between the resistance status in the medium and high contamination paddocks (Leathwick *et al.*, 2008). This suggests that even a moderate level of pasture contamination is sufficient to mitigate the risk for resistance development and furthermore that acceptable worm control can coexist with resistance management through the use of the refugia. The likely impact of drenching onto 'clean' or dirty pastures is depicted in Figure 8.1.

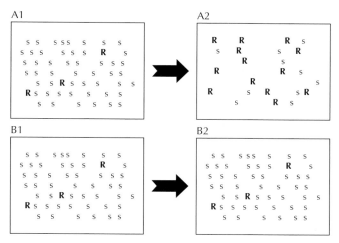

Figure 8.1 A1 to A2 depicts the effect of drench and move to 'safe' or 'clean' pasture, although the assumption has been made that a limited number of susceptible genotypes (s) are present to reduce the proportion of resistant (R) genotypes. B1 to B2 depicts the consequence of drenching and moving onto 'dirty' pasture or alternatively leaving a proportion of stock undrenched.

How to produce and utilise a refuge

There are a number of ways to create a refuge of susceptible parasites on pasture (assuming the problem of resistance has not progressed to a level where susceptible parasites are in the minority). Each of the alternatives, however, should take into account the likely impact of heavy pasture contamination, particularly early in the season, as these parasites will be ingested by susceptible stock, leading to a multiplying effect on contamination later in the year.

Drenching stock only when productivity is significantly depressed or on welfare grounds can reduce drenching intensity and may have applications in older stock which have developed a significant degree of protection against GIN. However, it is doubtful if many farmers, other than those operating organic enterprises, are willing to risk the inevitable production losses in young animals. Extending the interval between drenching to allow ingested parasites to mature and produce offspring without exposure to treatment and the resulting selective advantage to drench survivors can increase the size of the refuge. However, the same problems of heavy pasture contamination may occur if the period extends too far. A preventive drench programme using 28-day intervals should be sufficient to allow some susceptible parasites to get through, assuming that the drench used is not persistent. Drenching several days before a shift to clean pasture should be adopted where possible – this enables susceptible parasites to establish and dilute or replace any drench survivors present. It is obvious that drenching and moving immediately onto clean pasture will provide an enormous selective advantage for the progeny of drench survivors.

While adult sheep and cattle can occasionally harbour relatively large worm burdens, it is normally the case that these animals can be maintained on farm without regular anthelmintic treatment. It is also the case that these stock are net removers of parasites from pasture (Charleston, 1986; Mason *et al.*, 2001), as many of the worms they ingest are rendered non-viable by the immune system. This suggests that utilising adult stock by rotationally grazing them with young animals may provide enough pasture contamination to function as an effective refuge for resistance control while removing enough larvae to control productivity losses. An experiment conducted on farm in New Zealand has empirically measured the impact of this procedure on the development of resistance (Leathwick *et al.*, 2008). The study grazed animals on pastures contaminated with benzimidazole-resistant worm populations and compared whether the level of resistance diverged in groups of lambs which were maintained on lamb-only pastures with those rotationally grazed with ewes. Following a routine five-drench programme using benzimidazole, given at 28-day intervals, the study established that ewes were indeed a source of unselected parasites for lambs and that this could have a beneficial effect on delaying the development of resistance. Furthermore, the study demonstrated that the lambs in the rotationally grazed treatment performed better in terms of productivity than the animals in the lamb-only treatment (Leathwick *et al.*, 2008). An interesting observation to come out of a recent survey of resistance and drenching practices in New Zealand (Lawrence *et al.*, 2006; Waghorn *et al.*, 2006b) was that mixed grazing of sheep and cattle was positively correlated with resistance. While there is no solid evidence supporting why this should be the case, it is reasonable to postulate this while mixed grazing reduces the ingestion of 'suitable' L3 by either host species, thus aiding productivity, the removal of parasites specific for both sheep and cattle is more extreme than rotationally grazing stock classes of the same species, leading to a reduction in the size of the refuge.

Perhaps the simplest approach to preserving a refuge of unselected parasites is to deliberately leave a proportion of animals untreated when drenching – otherwise referred to as 'selective drenching'. As discussed above, there is empirical evidence that this approach can result in the mitigation of the risk for resistance (Waghorn *et al.*, 2008). Questions remain, however, concerning precisely how many animals should be left untreated. Obviously, this is going to vary with many factors such as the genotype of the animals, feed supply/quality, climate and management strategies. The results obtained by Waghorn *et al.* (2008) suggested that, at least in the parasite-friendly conditions found in New Zealand, there was no observable difference between leaving 10% or 20% of animals untreated, implying that even less animals may be required to remain undrenched to provide an adequate refuge.

In some parts of the world, selective drenching is referred to as 'targeted selective treatment' (TST) and has become a cornerstone of research efforts into slowing the development of resistance (van Wyk *et al.*, 2006). The major issues with selective drenching or TST, as already stated, are making sure that the refuge developed is effective in slowing the development of resistance but low enough not to significantly impact on productivity. The key element therein is how to select not only the numbers of animals to remain untreated but also which individuals are chosen. The simplest methods in most situations are selection of animals based on either body-condition scoring or short-term changes in live weight (van Wyk *et al.*, 2006). In most commercial flocks, choosing animals based on FEC would be impractical. In areas where *Haemonchus contortus* is the predominant parasite species, the Famacha© system has been developed as an aid to drench decision-making (van Wyk & Bath, 2002; Vatta *et al.*, 2001). As *H. contortus* is haematophagous, clinical disease can be diagnosed by examining the blood supply in the eyelids of sheep. Those animals which have lost a significant amount of blood can be readily identified and treated, with the corollary that those not requiring treatment on welfare grounds can remain undrenched and act as a source of refugia.

If animals are selected without reference to their egg count, then the level of dilution of resistant survivors achieved by leaving a proportion of a flock untreated can be estimated. A modelling study (Leathwick, personal communication) has calculated the dilution factor, or the proportion of unselected eggs compared to the resistant eggs passed by the whole population when various percentages of animals are left untreated. This study determined that a significant factor in the success of leaving animals undrenched was the efficacy of the drench administered to the treated animals. Where this was 99.9%, or where little resistance was present, leaving 1% of animals untreated was sufficient to provide a 10-fold dilution of drench survivors. As efficacy decreased to 95%, however, 34% of the flock had to remain untreated to achieve a similar dilution.

As an aside, this benefit of minimising the number of resistant worms surviving treatment (i.e. high efficacy) is part of the argument for using combinations of effective actives to delay resistance development.

Importation of resistant parasites

A recent large-scale survey in New Zealand (Lawrence *et al.*, 2006) observed that those farms which routinely bought stock from external sources had a higher prevalence of resistance than those which relied on replacing stock with their own animals. The obvious explanation of this is that these farmers were also purchasing resistant worms. Given the high prevalence of resistance in New Zealand (and many other countries), it is not surprising that this is the case, particularly as farmers may routinely purchase animals sourced from a number of other properties. A related issue is also commonplace in New Zealand and almost certainly contributes to the high prevalence of resistance in cattle parasites; beef and dairy calves are often transported to contract grazing units, where animals from many properties are intensively managed, including the regular application of pour-on single active products, then shipped back to their original farm when they reach a target weight. This is an excellent method of first selecting for resistance and then distributing the worms around the country.

The solution to the problem of the importation of resistant worms is to use an effective quarantine drench before the animals are allowed to graze (and therefore contaminate) pastures. Despite the problem, and profile, of anthelmintic resistance, quarantine drenching is still not common in many livestock enterprises.

The keyword when considering using a quarantine drench is of course 'effective'. The authors have had several conversations with farmers who insist they use quarantine drenching, but who then fail to check whether the anthelmintic they have used is in fact effective. In regions in which combination products are commercially available, it is recommended that a product containing as many different active families as possible be used, and that animals should then be held in a quarantine paddock (if possible) for a few days prior to checking efficacy by FEC.

A twin approach to worm control and resistance management – utilising refugia and combination drenches

The obvious conclusion which can be drawn from the information provided above is that both refugia and the use of effective combination drenches are of value in the management of worms and resistance.

It is worth reiterating that combinations are highly effective in delaying the development of drench resistance. However, in a situation where all animals are drenched with a combination and then moved onto clean pasture, the selective advantage for those parasites able to survive multiple drench families will be high.

References

ARMOUR, J. (1980). The epidemiology of helminth disease in farm animals. *Veterinary Parasitology*, **6**, 7–46.

BARNES, E. H., DOBSON, R. J. & BARGER, I. A. (1995). Worm control and anthelmintic resistance – Adventures with a model. *Parasitology Today*, **11**, 56–63.

BESIER, R. B. (2001). Re-thinking the summer drenching program. *Journal of Agriculture of Western Australia*, **42**, 6–9.

BESIER, R. B. & LOVE, S. C. J. (2003). Anthelmintic resistance in sheep nematodes in Australia: The need for new approaches. *Australian Journal of Experimental Agriculture*, **43**, 1383–1391.

BRUNSDON, R. V. (1980). Principles of helminth control. *Veterinary Parasitology*, **6**, 185–215.

CHARLESTON, W. A. G. (1986). Parasites. In: *Sheep Production. 2. Feeding, Growth and Health* (eds McCutcheon S. N., McDonald M. F. & Wickham G. A.), New Zealand Institute of Agricultural Science and Ray Richards Publisher, Auckland, New Zealand, 204–243.

JACKSON, F. & COOP, R. L. (2000). The development of anthelmintic resistance in sheep nematodes. *Parasitology*, **120** (Suppl), S95–S107.

LAWRENCE, K. E., RHODES, A. P., JACKSON, R., *et al.* (2006). Farm management practices associated with macrocyclic lactone resistance on sheep farms in New Zealand. *New Zealand Veterinary Journal*, **54**, 283–288.

LEATHWICK, D. M. (2005). Anthelmintic resistance in New Zealand: Current status and approaches to management. *Proceedings of the International Conference of the World Association for Advances in Veterinary Parasitology*, **20**, 69.

LEATHWICK, D. M., MILLER, C. M., ATKINSON, D. S., HAACK, N. A., WAGHORN, T. S. & OLIVER, A. M. (2008). Managing anthelmintic resistance: Untreated adult ewes as a source of unselected parasites, and their role in reducing parasite populations. *New Zealand Veterinary Journal*, **56**, 184–195.

LEATHWICK, D. M., WAGHORN, T. S., MILLER, C. M., ATKINSON, D. S., HAACK, N. A. & OLIVER, A. M. (2006). Selective and on-demand drenching of lambs: Impact on parasite populations and performance of lambs. *New Zealand Veterinary Journal*, **54**, 305–312.

MARTIN, P. J., LE JAMBRE, L. F. & CLAXTON, J. H. (1981). The impact of refugia on the development of thiabendazole resistance in *Haemonchus contortus*. *International Journal for Parasitology*, **11**, 35–41.

MASON, P., NOTTINGHAM, R. & MCKAY, C. (2001). A field strain of ivermectin resistant *Ostertagia circumcincta* in sheep in New Zealand. *New Zealand Journal of Zoology*, **28**, 230.

MICHEL, J. F. (1969). The control of some nematode infections in calves. *Veterinary Record*, **85**, 326–329.

ROUSH, R. T. & MCKENZIE, J. A. (1987). Ecological genetics of insecticide and acaricide resistance. *Annual Review of Entomology*, **32**, 361–380.

VAN WYK, J. A. (2001). Refugia – Overlooked as perhaps the most potent factor concerning the development of anthelmintic resistance. *Onderstepoort Journal of Veterinary Research*, **68**, 55–67.

VAN WYK, J. A. & BATH, G. F. (2002). The FAMACHA© system for managing haemonchosis in sheep and goats by clinically identifying individual animals for treatment. *Veterinary Research*, **33**, 509–529.

VAN WYK, J. A., HOSTE, H., KAPLAN, R. M. & BESIER, R. B. (2006). Targeted selective treatment for worm management-How do we sell rational programs to farmers? *Veterinary Parasitology*, **139**, 336–346.

VATTA, A. F., LETTY, B. A., VAN DER LINDE, M. J., VAN WIJK, E. F., HANSEN, J. W. & KRECEK, R. C. (2001). Testing for clinical anaemia caused by *Haemonchus* spp. in goats farmed under resource-poor conditions in South Africa using an eye colour chart developed for sheep. *Veterinary Parasitology*, **99**, 1–14.

WAGHORN, T. S., LEATHWICK, D. M., MILLER, C. M. & ATKINSON, D. S. (2008). Brave or gullible: Testing the concept that leaving susceptible parasites in refugia will slow the development of anthelmintic resistance. *New Zealand Veterinary Journal*, **56**, 158–163.

WAGHORN, T. S., LEATHWICK, D. M., RHODES, A. P., *et al.* (2006a). Prevalence of anthelmintic resistance on 62 beef cattle farms in the North Island of New Zealand. *New Zealand Veterinary Journal*, **54**, 278–282.

WAGHORN, T. S., LEATHWICK, D. M., RHODES, A. P., *et al.* (2006b). Prevalence of anthelmintic resistance on sheep farms in New Zealand. *New Zealand Veterinary Journal*, **54**, 271–277.

9 'Non-chemical' control options

Factors such as the track record of resistance development, some producers' desire to reduce synthetic chemical input, or the unavailability/unaffordability of drenches in certain areas have led some researchers to investigate the administration of so-called 'non-chemical' or 'organic' treatments. The majority of research reports in this area involve two options: either the use of 'anthelmintic' plants (which of course contain chemicals) or the administration of micro-predacious fungi.

Anthelmintic plants

Care must be taken when any plant is claimed to have 'anthelmintic efficacy' as results can easily be confounded by the effect of diet on dry matter intake, the numbers of parasite larvae ingested or a positive impact of improved nutrition on anti-parasite immunity. Thus, while grazing or feeding animals on certain plants may mitigate the impact of parasitism, they may not do so via direct anthelmintic effects on parasite establishment, survival or fecundity the use of an enhanced plane of nutrition on parasitism is described in Chapter 10 and will not be described here.) The administration of a plant extract to combat worms, assuming there was no significant nutritional component, would of course be less open to interpretation than the use of whole plant material. So what would define a plant as having anthelmintic properties? The answer is obvious: there should be an observable, consistent and significant impact on parasite dynamics due to some inherent physical or chemical property of the ingested plant material.

Plants and/or their extracts have been recorded as having anthelmintic properties since the 2nd century AD, when the Greek physician Claudius Galenus developed the system of preparing medicinal treatments from vegetable matter, including those with real or perceived activity against nematode parasites

(Waller, 2001). As Waller (2001) points out, this laid the foundations for centuries of plant-based anthelmintic treatments, which effectively disappeared with the advent of synthetic anthelmintic compounds in the second half of the 20th century. Furthermore, Waller (2001) makes the point that approximately 25% of all medicinal treatments commercially available today are directly produced from, or are based on, plant constituents. Indeed, a number of plants with purported anthelmintic activity were included in the British pharmacopeia until the 1960s, such as oil of chenopodium, used to treat nematode infections in humans. This particular remedy is still used to treat human infections in parts of South America. As far as treating gastrointestinal nematode (GIN) in livestock is concerned, Chapter 5 contained a quote describing the use of a mixture of copper sulphate and nicotine sulphate against a mixed infection of GIN in sheep in the 1940s (Gordon, 1948) – without, it should be said, any striking success.

Traditional or ethnoveterinary medicine has identified a large number of plants with potential anti-parasitic effects. Among the most celebrated is, of course, the bark of the cinchona tree of South America, from which the anti-malarial drug quinine was extracted. Unfortunately, a similar impact, either in efficacy or adoption, has not been described for the various plants listed below in regard to their efficacy against GIN. This should not, however, preclude the possibility this could occur, particularly if traditional remedies provide the basic building block around which synthetic or semi-synthetic treatments could be developed.

The currently available anthelmintic classes do of course contain drugs which have been developed from 'natural products'. The most successful example is not from plants, but from fungi; the avermectin compounds (e.g. ivermectin) were originally identified as fermentation products of actinomycetes.

Technically speaking, anything termed as an anthelmintic must demonstrate a high level of efficacy (>95%) against resident nematode burdens or prevent infection with ingested worms. No traditional plant-based remedies have reached this standard to date; however, demanding such a high efficacy could well be regarded as very 'Western'. It is quite possible that in more traditional, low-intensity livestock systems, traditional plants may have a valuable role to play in maintaining an acceptable level of productivity. This is particularly relevant in a number of developing countries in which animal survival (and other parameters such as reproductive ability) is relatively more important than in intensive systems which demand high levels of meat, wool or milk production.

Considering the drivers for the discovery and use of 'anthelmintic plants' described above, it comes as no surprise, therefore, that most (but not all) originate in developing countries. Many of these plants are reported to have anthelmintic activity when consumed as parts of plants or whole plants, rather than refined or semi-refined extracts. The former will be referred to as 'plant material', as opposed to plant extracts in the following review of both. It should be noted that describing these control options as 'non-chemical' is completely inaccurate but is sufficiently descriptive for the purpose of discussion.

Plant material

The definition of plant material used here covers fresh material as well as preserved (e.g. dried) or ground preparations. Various parts of plants have been used in an attempt to demonstrate activity against GIN infections in grazing livestock – most often, but not exclusively, in small ruminants, which may reflect the fact that most reports of anthelmintic plants are from developing countries.

Examples of various plant parts being used as anthelmintics include the following – leaves of the Fagara plant (*Zanthoxylum zanthoxyloides*), found throughout tropical Africa, have been reported to have significant anthelmintic effects on mixed GIN infections in sheep when consumed over a period of several days (Hounzangbe-Adote *et al.*, 2005). Leaves of the Asian perennial legume, lespedeza (*Sericea lespedeza*), has also been reported as having a significant impact on GIN infections in goats (Min *et al.*, 2004). There have been conflicting reports of the efficacy of leaves of the neem tree (*Azadirachta indica*), a plant with known bioactive properties (including effects on a range of insect pests) (Nisbet *et al.*, 1993) on GIN infections. While no effect was observed against *Haemonchus contortus* infections in some studies (Costa *et al.*, 2006; Githiori *et al.*, 2004), another report indicated the leaves did negatively affect this parasite (Chandrawathani *et al.*, 2006). Various plant materials have been used as anthelmintics in Pakistan (Hussain *et al.*, 2008), including familiar names such as coriander seeds (*Coriandrum sativum*), mango leaves (*Mangifera indica*) and alfalfa (lucerne) stems/leaves (*Medicago sativa*). Quite splendidly, one treatment, administered orally to cattle, consists of 150–200 g of a mixture of plant material including chilli, coriander and garlic, together with a further 60 g of ground red chilli. It is timely to remind ourselves that cattle ruminate and would enjoy the flavour for a lengthy period after treatment. Also of note is the administration to cattle of wheat dough over which an incantation has been performed; unfortunately no efficacy data was available for either of these treatments (Hussain *et al.*, 2008).

Reports of plant material with anthelmintic properties are not completely confined to developing countries. Studies in New Zealand have ascribed a significant effect on GIN infections to forage crops including lotus (*Lotus pedunculatus*) and sulla (*Hedysarum coronarium*) (Niezen *et al.*, 1998a, 2002a). However, as discussed in Chapter 10, there is considerable doubt whether any effects observed on parasites are due to an 'anthelmintic' effect.

Wormwood

The herbaceous perennial *Artemisia absinthium*, or wormwood, is native to temperate regions of Europe (http://en.wikipedia.org/wiki/Europe" \o "Europe"), Asia and northern Africa. The term wormwood presumably results from the use of the leaves and flower-tops as a traditional cure for intestinal worms (as the species name *A. absinthium* suggests, there were other, arguably much more useful properties of the plant than as an anthelmintic). Extract of wormwood can still be purchased, but given some recent case studies, it appears there may be a fine line between killing the parasites and the host.

Plant extracts

By far the greater number of ethnoveterinary reports of anthelmintic plants involve crude or refined plant extracts. This presumably arises from attempts to harness the pharmacological effects of concentrating specific compounds present in whole plants, although it is noted that many plants with anthelmintic properties are not considered as desirable components of animal diets, and as such have to be delivered rather than eaten by choice – something much easier done with an extract than with whole plant material.

Plant extracts have been assessed for their potential effects on intestinal parasites, of animals and humans, in many parts of the world. A brief selection of these, representative of different geographical regions, is presented here.

In Africa, extracts from various components of a range of plants have been assessed and shown to have some effect against GIN, including those from the bark of the African Mahogany tree (*Khaya senegalensis*) (Ademola *et al.*, 2004); extracts from the seeds of leucena (*Leucaena leucocephala*) (Ademola *et al.*, 2005a; Ademola & Idowu, 2006); preparations of whole plants of wormgrass (or wormbush) (*Spigelia anthelmia*) (Ademola *et al.*, 2007), while an extract of crushed leaves of the native South American plant Golden Apple (*Spondias mombin*) has been shown to have some anthelmintic property in a study conducted in West Africa (Ademola *et al.*, 2005b).

There have also been numerous reports of anthelmintic activity in extracts from plants in East Africa, such as from the bark of the weeping wattle (*Peltophorum africanum*) (Bizimenyera *et al.*, 2006), the root bark of the mimosa (*Albizia antihelmintica*) (Gathuma *et al.*, 2004), the roots of the bindweed (*Hilderbrandtia sepalosa*) (Gathuma *et al.*, 2004) and the fruit of two boxwood species (*Myrsine africana* and *Embelia schimperi*) (Bøgh *et al.*, 1996; Gathuma *et al.*, 2004).

Examples of plant extracts from Asia with reported anthelmintic activity (not necessarily against GIN in ruminants) include those prepared from leaves of the neem tree (*A. indica*) (Hordegen *et al.*, 2003), woman's tongue (*Albizia lebbeck*) (El Garhy & Mahmoud, 2002) and tobacco (*Nicotiana tabacum*) (Iqbal *et al.*, 2006).

A number of reportedly anthelmintic plant extracts have traditionally been used in Europe (again, not necessarily against GIN in ruminants). In Turkey, heated juice from cut branches of jasmine (*Jasmimum fruticans*) (Honda *et al.*, 1996), boiled juniper berries (*Juniperus drupacea*) (Yesilada *et al.*, 1993) and pine cones (*Pinus nigra*) (Fujita *et al.*, 1995) have all been assessed and have subsequently been confirmed as having anthelmintic properties against pinworm in mice (Kozan *et al.*, 2006).

It is often the case that claims for the efficacy of traditional remedies as anthelmintics do not survive controlled laboratory investigation. A number of Kenyan remedies, including the perennial herb matungulu (*Afromamum sanguineum*), the hopbush (*Dodonea angustifolia*) and the bindweed (*H. sepalosa*) had no anthelmintic activity against *Heligmosomoides polygyrus* in mice (Githiori *et al.*, 2003), while oil of chenopodium (*Chenopodium ambrosioides*) had no effect against *H. contortus* in goats (Ketzis *et al.*, 2002).

The reason for the disparity between the many claims of anthelmintic activity of plants and the reality – when the plants or plant extracts are subject to controlled laboratory studies – is almost certainly due to unwarranted extrapolation from *in vitro* experiments. Extracting substances from plants for use in tests such as egg hatch or larval development assays will almost always result in parasites being exposed to relatively high levels of at least a single bioactive compound, and can also, unless carefully controlled, subject the parasites to dangerously high levels of e.g. salts. Unfortunately, such *in vitro* results may bear little relevance to the use of the source plant as an anthelmintic *in vivo* (Athanasiadou *et al.*, 2007; Molan *et al.*, 2003a).

Plant secondary metabolites (PSM) as anthelmintics

A wide range of bioactive compounds have been ascribed anthelmintic activity, whether against plant- or animal-parasitic worms. These include fatty acids and tetrahydrofurans (both lipids), phenolics, alkaloids and terpenes (Rochfort *et al.*, 2008). These are designated as PSM, as they are not essential to plant growth and reproduction, but rather to reduce herbivory by vertebrates and invertebrates. One group of PSM which have received considerable attention in recent years are the condensed tannins (CT). The CT are a diverse group of compounds and are polymers consisting of a range of monomers such as flavan-3-ols and their galloyl derivatives (Waterman, 1988). CT may also be referred to as procyanadins (Hoste *et al.*, 2006). The CT have a high affinity for proteins (Asquith & Butler, 1986), particularly those rich in proline such as gelatine and those present in seed-coats; interestingly, browsing animals such as deer can produce high levels of protein in saliva, which may act to bind CT (Robbins *et al.*, 1991) and protect the animal from the resulting adverse effects of eating PSM, which the plant has developed as a defence mechanism (Robbins, 1987). This ability to bind strongly to protein has led to the term 'bypass-protein' being ascribed to CT. This binding protects the proteins from degradation in the rumen, but thereafter conditions distal to the rumen result in dissociation. Considering that this can result in a greater supply of amino acids to the small intestine (Waghorn, 1996), care should be taken in ascribing anthelmintic effects to CT, as the involvement of improved immune function against parasites (should there be a significant reduction in egg output) cannot be ruled out (Min *et al.*, 2003; Waghorn & McNabb, 2003).

The concentration of CT in the diet can have significant impacts on a number of productivity parameters of grazing livestock. When CT concentration is below 6% of the dry matter content of the diet, there are a number of positive effects on live-weight gain and milk and meat production (Douglas *et al.*, 1999; Min *et al.*, 2004). However, and not surprisingly given the role of CT in plant defence, higher levels can have an adverse impact on feed intake and the efficiency of digestion (Athanasiadou *et al.*, 2001; Min *et al.*, 2003; Reed, 1995). It is also likely that the intestinal environment will change markedly with the ingestion of high levels of CT, which may indirectly impact on worms. This is not unique to CT by any means – given that most PSM have a role as anti-feedants or protectants, excessive consumption leads to adverse effects on productivity (Athanasiadou *et al.*, 2007). The evidence for anthelmintic activity of CT is somewhat variable. Numerous *in vitro* studies have reported significant effects on the free-living stages of GIN (Athanasiadou *et al.*, 2001; Molan *et al.*, 2000; Paolini *et al.*, 2004). In addition to crude extracts, purified fractions of plant material containing CT had significant effects on parasites *in vitro* (Barrau *et al.*, 2005; Molan *et al.*, 2003b). As stated above, however, these results do not necessarily translate to similar effects *in vivo*.

When administered as a liquid treatment, quebracho, an extract from the bark of the quebracho tree (*Schinopsis quebracho colorado*), has been shown to reduce FECs and worm burdens in sheep (Athanasiadou *et al.*, 2001; Butter *et al.*, 2001). However, quebracho was observed to affect abomasal worm burdens in one study (Max *et al.*, 2005) but only small intestinal burdens in another (Athanasiadou *et al.*, 2001). Where there were effects on worms, these were reported as either a reduction in establishment of ingested L3 (Paolini *et al.*, 2003) or a reduction in fecundity of established worms (Athanasiadou *et al.*, 2000). In a study which assessed the activity of *Dorycnium rectum* leaves and a grape seed extract preparation, both of which had high levels of CT, against a mixed nematode infection in sheep, failed to show a significant effect on parasite burdens (Waghorn *et al.*, 2006).

Forage legumes

A variety of forage plants containing CT have been tested for their utility as feed for grazing livestock subject to parasitism. As such, the forages not only have to produce a measurable reduction in parasitism but also a greater or similar level of animal productivity than alternative feeds. The most striking conclusion from these studies is the inconsistency of the results. Some studies in which animals have grazed birdsfoot trefoil (lotus) (*Lotus corniculatus*) (Figure 9.1) have demonstrated significant effects on parasitism (Marley *et al.*,

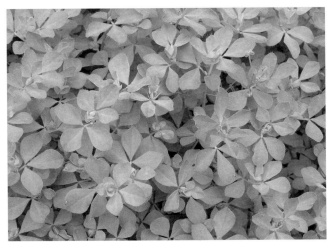

Figure 9.1   Illustration of the forage plant *L. corniculatus*. Image courtesy of Deric Charlton.

Table 9.1 The impact of dietary intake and faecal mass on the number of eggs per gram and total egg production from lambs infected with *T. colubriformis* and fed either a diet sufficient to maintain live-weight or the same dietary components provided *ad libitum*.

Diet	FEC (eggs/g)	Daily faecal mass (g)	Total daily egg output
Maintenance	817	485	395,695
Ad libitum	463	2005	951,131

2003), while others, using the same forage, have not (Niezen *et al.*, 1998b). Similarly, grazing animals on sulla (*Hedysarum coronarium*) resulted in variable effects on parasitism (Niezen *et al.*, 1995, 2002b).

While the variability of results from grazing trials may be influenced by many factors, such as differences in the experimental design, it is also the case that the composition and level of PSM such as CT are themselves inherently variable and are highly climate dependent (Athanasiadou & Kyriazakis, 2004).

There are, however, significant questions still unanswered regarding the antiparasitic properties of forage crops. For example, animals grazing forages that are vertically taller than conventional pasture are almost certain to be ingesting lower numbers of parasite larvae, which, in itself, will impact on parasitism and productivity regardless of the size of the adult worm burden present when the animals are put on to the forage crop. Also, the high nutritive value and excellent palatability of many forages may increase the quantum of dry matter and protein ingested, which may result in improved immune capability and consequent reduction in parasitism (Athanasiadou & Kyriazakis, 2004). Also, it should be noted that ascribing any anthelmintic effect based on FEC must take into account not only eggs per gram of faeces but also the weight of faeces produced by animals on any given food supply (Sutherland, 2003). An example is given in Table 9.1, which compares FEC in animals maintained on different planes of nutrition; while the well-fed animals have significantly lower FEC, total egg output, taking onto account the mass of faeces produced, was actually greater in these animals (Sutherland, unpublished).

Practical applicability on-farm

While there will no doubt continue to be much debate concerning the utility of CT-containing forage crops as anthelmintics, there is no doubt that as forage crops they are extremely effective animal feeds, and may have applicability in, for example, finishing animals more quickly, or for improving the productivity of 'tail-end' stock. As anthelmintics, however, they have to be effective on a consistent and measurable basis. Unless this is the case, most farmers raising stock in intensive management systems would require a high degree of diligence if they were to rely on forage crops to control parasitism.

Other anthelmintic plants

Garlic and vinegar

Some livestock producers advocate the use of garlic/vinegar drenches as an organic alternative to synthetic drenches. However, there appears to be little, if any concrete evidence that this is an effective treatment for GIN of ruminants, neither is there any proven empirical information available on what constituent of garlic is deemed to be anthelmintic. One study which may be of relevance, however, demonstrated that garlic extract caused significant damage to the duodenal epithelium of rats (Amagase *et al.*, 2001). It is possible, therefore, if there is indeed a reduction in parasitism, that the effect could be mediated by an alteration in intestinal physiology, making it a less attractive environment for parasites. This, of course, would be expected to have an equally deleterious effect on the digestive processes.

Micro-predacious fungi

A number of nematophagous fungal species have been shown to have an impact on the free-living larval stages of parasites (Alves *et al.*, 2003; Grønvold, 1989; Larsen & Nansen, 1990; Larsen *et al.*, 1995). These fungi are naturally occurring in the environment, most obviously in soil and are presumed to feed naturally on various soil-dwelling free-living nematode species as parasitic fungi, and on decaying organic matter in the saprophytic phase (Larsen *et al.*, 1997). Fungi are able to migrate into faecal material from the adjacent soil (Hay *et al.*, 2002). Most of the nematophagous fungi affect nematodes in one of two ways; by producing spores which attach to the worm or by constructing traps from the fungal mycelia. Then, once physically attached, the fungi engulf their target.

A trapping fungal species, *Duddingtonia flagrans*, has received the vast majority of attention by researchers, primarily due to the chlamydospores having thick walls and therefore a relatively greater ability to survive passage through the gastrointestinal tract of livestock than other species (Larsen *et al.*, 1992, 1997). This has enabled a wide range of studies into the impact on parasite populations of adding fungal spores directly to faeces *in vitro* (Larsen *et al.*, 1991; Pena *et al.*, 2002) and after oral administration of spores to infected animals (Fontenot *et al.*, 2003; Larsen *et al.*, 1995; Waghorn & McNabb, 2003).

In an experiment conducted in penned sheep, oral administration of 500,000 or 250,000 spores/kg live-weight to lambs infected with a mixture of *Trichostrongylid* nematode species demonstrated a significant effect of *D. flagrans* on the subsequent recovery of larvae, which was reduced by a mean of 78% (Waghorn *et al.*, 2003). On pasture, significant effects have also been observed following oral administration of chlamydospores to sheep and cattle (Githigia *et al.*, 1997; Larsen *et al.*, 1995; Nansen *et al.*, 1995). A reduction in larval development/survival in faeces following oral administration of

D. flagrans, particularly if continued for extended periods, may also reduce pasture contamination and therefore mitigate the effect of parasite challenge on livestock (Fontenot *et al.*, 2003).

There is some evidence of differential activity of the fungus against various target species. With *Teladorsagia circumcincta, Ostertagia ostertagi* and the lungworm *Dictyocaulus viviparus*, for example, efficacy is relatively poor compared to species such as *H. contortus* and *T. colubriformis* (Nansen *et al.*, 1988; Waghorn *et al.*, 2003). It has been postulated that the relative rate of movement within the faecal mass is a determinant in the level of contact between nematodes and trapping fungi, and may therefore explain this differential activity (Waghorn *et al.*, 2003).

Given the success of *D. flagrans* in reducing parasite development/survival in controlled experimental studies, why has the technology not been successfully adapted for a commercial setting? The answer almost certainly involves survival of spores through the gastrointestinal tract. While *D. flagrans* may be more capable than other fungal species in this regard, there is still a significant level of mortality, which requires large numbers of spores to be administered in order for the treatment to have an acceptable level of efficacy.

Some niche markets, in which supplementation is a common practice such as in milking animals, appear to present the most promising for biological control using nematophagous fungi. The situation is more problematic with animals maintained in extensive grazing situations. Here, it seems the development of controlled-release technology such as an intra-ruminal bolus is necessary (Larsen *et al.*, 1997). At the time of writing, however, this has not been developed or commercialised for use in livestock.

It is of course possible that the concentration of research, and therefore resources, on *D. flagrans*, has overlooked another fungal species that may be more suitable for parasite control in livestock, and which may become apparent in future. Another possibility is that technology will be developed which proves both cheap and effective enough in protecting fungal spores during gastrointestinal passage to provide new impetus to the development of biological control using nematophagous fungi.

Homoeopathy

It is debatable whether homoeopathy should be included in any serious review of alternative anti-parasitic control methods. However, it does seem to find favour with some people, so for completeness the evidence will be presented supporting its use. In its favour, of course, is that unlike the use of plant extracts, it can honestly claim to be a method of non-chemical control.

A study conducted in Scotland in 2002 (http://www.abdn.ac.uk/organic/organic_34.php) reported the use of the homoeopathic preparation Blue Merle in lactating ewes during the PPRI and infected with GIN – primarily *T. circumcincta*. This study utilised the FECPAK® system to determine that egg counts were over the company's threshold for anthelmintic intervention of 600 epg. The study determined that two consecutive treatments with the remedy significantly reduced egg output from an average of 373 epg to 72 epg, a reduction of 81%, which was highly significant ($P = 0.002$). Obviously, marvellous stuff. However, even a cursory examination of the methodology reveals a flaw or two in the design. Of particular concern is the lack of any untreated control group. The inclusion of such a group would almost certainly have confirmed the accepted paradigm that the PPRI is a transient phenomenon (particularly when the group of animals given Blue Merle were taken off pasture and housed in pens), and that the results would almost certainly have been similar if not identical regardless of homoeopathic treatment. Only a brave farmer would rely on such a remedy in a commercial situation.

References

ADEMOLA, I. O., AKANBI, A. I. & IDOWU, S. O. (2005a). Comparative nematocidal activity of chromatographic fractions of *Leucaena leucocephala* seed against gastrointestinal sheep nematodes. *Pharmaceutical Biology*, **43**, 599–604.

ADEMOLA, I. O., FAGBEMI, B. O. & IDOWU, S. O. (2005b). Anthelmintic activity of extracts of *Spondias mombin* against gastrointestinal nematodes of sheep: Studies *in vitro* and *in vivo*. *Tropical Animal Health and Production*, **37**, 223–235.

ADEMOLA, I. O., FAGBEMI, B. O. & IDOWU, S. O. (2004). Evaluation of the anthelmintic activity of *Khaya senegalensis* extract against gastrointestinal nematodes of sheep: In vitro and in vivo studies. *Veterinary Parasitology*, **122**, 151–164.

ADEMOLA, I. O., FAGBEMI, B. O. & IDOWU, S. O. (2007). Anthelmintic activity of *Spigelia anthelmia* extract against gastrointestinal nematodes of sheep. *Parasitology Research*, **101**, 63–69.

ADEMOLA, I. O. & IDOWU, S. O. (2006). Anthelmintic activity of *Leucaena leucocephala* seed extract on *Haemonchus contortus* infective larvae. *Veterinary Record*, **158**, 485–486.

ALVES, P. H., ARAUJO, J. V., GUIMARAES, M. P., ASSIS, R. C. L., SARTI, P. & CAMPOS, A. K. (2003). Control of bovine gastrointestinal nematodes using formulation of the nematode-trapping fungus *Monacrosporium thaumasium* (Drechsler, 1937). *Arquivo Brasileiro de Medicina Veterinaria e Zootecnia*, **55**, 568–573.

AMAGASE, H., PETESCH, B. L., MATSUURA, H., KASUGA, S. & ITAKURA, Y. (2001). Intake of garlic and its bioactive components. *Journal of Nutrition*, **131**, 955S–962S.

ASQUITH, T. N. & BUTLER, L. G. (1986). Interactions of condensed tannins with selected proteins. *Phytochemistry*, **25**, 1591–1593.

ATHANASIADOU, S., GITHIORI, J. & KYRIAZAKIS, I. (2007). Medicinal plants for helminth parasite control: Facts and fiction. *Animal*, **1**, 1392–1400.

ATHANASIADOU, S. & KYRIAZAKIS, I. (2004). Plant secondary metabolites: Antiparasitic effects and their role in ruminant production systems. *Proceedings of the Nutrition Society*, **63**, 631–639.

ATHANASIADOU, S., KYRIAZAKIS, I., JACKSON, F. & COOP, R. L. (2000). Effects of short-term exposure to condensed tannins on adult *Trichostrongylus colubriformis*. *Veterinary Record*, **146**, 728–732.

ATHANASIADOU, S., KYRIAZAKIS, I., JACKSON, F. & COOP, R. L. (2001). Direct anthelmintic effects of condensed tannins towards different gastrointestinal nematodes of sheep: In vitro and in vivo studies. *Veterinary Parasitology*, **99**, 205–219.

BARRAU, E., FABRE, N., FOURASTE, I. & HOSTE, H. (2005). Effect of bioactive compounds from Sainfoin (*Onobrychis viciifolia* Scop.) on the *in vitro* larval migration of *Haemonchus contortus*: Role of tannins and flavonol glycosides. *Parasitology*, **131**, 531–538.

BIZIMENYERA, E. S., GITHIORI, J. B., ELOFF, J. N. & SWAN, G. E. (2006). *In vitro* activity of *Peltophorum africanum* Sond. (Fabaceae) extracts on the egg hatching and larval development of the parasitic nematode *Trichostrongylus colubriformis*. *Veterinary Parasitology*, **142**, 336–343.

BØGH, H. O., ANDREASSEN, J. & LEMMICH, J. (1996). Anthelmintic usage of extracts of *Embelia schimperi* from Tanzania. *Journal of Ethnopharmacology*, **50**, 35–42.

BUTTER, N. L., DAWSON, J. M., WAKELIN, D. & BUTTERY, P. J. (2001). Effect of dietary condensed tannins on gastrointestinal nematodes. *Journal of Agricultural Science*, **137**, 461–469.

CHANDRAWATHANI, P., CHANG, K. W., NURULAINI, R. *et al.* (2006). Daily feeding of fresh neem leaves (*Azadirachta indica*) for worm control in sheep. *Tropical Biomedicine*, **23**, 23–30.

COSTA, C. T. C., BEVILAQUA, C. M. L., MACIEL, M. V. *et al.* (2006). Anthelmintic activity of *Azadirachta indica* A. Juss against sheep gastrointestinal nematodes. *Veterinary Parasitology*, **137**, 306–310.

DOUGLAS, G. B., STIENEZEN, M., WAGHORN, G. C., FOOTE, A. G. & PURCHAS, R. W. (1999). Effect of condensed tannins in birdsfoot trefoil (*Lotus corniculatus*) and sulla (*Hedysarum coronarium*) on body weight, carcass fat depth, and wool growth of lambs in New Zealand. *New Zealand Journal of Agricultural Research*, **42**, 55–64.

EL GARHY, M. F. & MAHMOUD, L. H. (2002). Anthelminthic efficacy of traditional herbs on *Ascaris lumbricoides*. *Journal of the Egyptian Society of Parasitology*, **32**, 893–900.

FONTENOT, M. E., MILLER, J. E., PENA, M. T., LARSEN, M. & GILLESPIE, A. (2003). Efficiency of feeding *Duddingtonia flagrans* chlamydospores to grazing ewes on reducing availability of parasitic nematode larvae on pasture. *Veterinary Parasitology*, **118**, 203–213.

FUJITA, T., SEZIK, E., TABATA, M. *et al.* (1995). Traditional medicine in Turkey VII. Folk medicine in middle and west Black Sea regions. *Economic Botany*, **49**, 406–422.

GATHUMA, J. M., MBARIA, J. M., WANYAMA, J., KABURIA, H. F. A., MPOKE, L. & MWANGI, J. N. (2004). Efficacy of *Myrsine africana*, *Albizia anthelmintica* and *Hilderbrandtia sepalosa* herbal remedies against mixed natural sheep helminthosis in Samburu district, Kenya. *Journal of Ethnopharmacology*, **91**, 7–12.

GITHIGIA, S. M., THAMSBORG, S. M., LARSEN, M., KYVSGAARD, N. C. & NANSEN, P. (1997). The preventive effect of the fungus *Duddingtonia flagrans* on trichostrongyle infections of lambs on pasture. *International Journal for Parasitology*, **27**, 931–939.

GITHIORI, J. B., HOGLUND, J., WALLER, P. J. & BAKER, R. L. (2003). Evaluation of anthelmintic properties of extracts from some plants used as livestock dewormers by pastoralist and smallholder farmers in Kenya against *Heligmosomoides polygyrus* infections in mice. *Veterinary Parasitology*, **118**, 215–226.

GITHIORI, J. B., HOGLUND, J., WALLER, P. J. & BAKER, R. L. (2004). Evaluation of anthelmintic properties of some plants used as livestock dewormers against *Haemonchus contortus* infections in sheep. *Parasitology*, **129**, 245–253.

GORDON, H. M. (1948). The epidemiology of parasitic diseases, with special reference to studies with nematode parasites of sheep. *The Australian Veterinary Journal*, **24**, 17–45.

GRØNVOLD, J. (1989). Induction of nematode-trapping organs in the predacious fungus *Arthrobotrys oligospora* (Hyphomycetales) by infective larvae of *Ostertagia ostertagi* (Trichostrongylidae). *Acta Veterinaria Scandinavica*, **30**, 77–87.

HAY, F. S., NIEZEN, J. H., LEATHWICK, D. & SKIPP, R. A. (2002). Nematophagous fungi in pasture: Colonisation of sheep faeces and their potential for control of free-living stages of gastro-intestinal nematode parasites of sheep. *Australian Journal of Experimental Agriculture*, **42**, 7–13.

HONDA, G., YESILADA, E., TABATA, M. *et al.* (1996). Traditional medicine in Turkey VI. Folk medicine in West Anatolia: Afyon, Kutahya, Denizli, Mugla, Aydin provinces. *Journal of Ethnopharmacology*, **53**, 75–87.

HORDEGEN, P., HERTZBERG, H., HEILMANN, J., LANGHANS, W. & MAURER, V. (2003). The anthelmintic efficacy of five plant products against gastrointestinal trichostrongylids in artificially infected lambs. *Veterinary Parasitology*, **117**, 51–60.

HOSTE, H., JACKSON, F., ATHANASIADOU, S., THAMSBORG, S. M. & HOSKIN, S. O. (2006). The effects of tannin-rich plants on parasitic nematodes in ruminants. *Trends in Parasitology*, **22**, 253–261.

HOUNZANGBE-ADOTE, M. S., ZINSOU, F. E., HOUNPKE, V., MOUTAIROU, K. & HOSTE, H. (2005). *In vivo* effects of Fagara leaves on sheep infected with gastrointestinal nematodes. *Tropical Animal Health and Production*, **37**, 205–214.

HUSSAIN, A., KHAN, M. N., IQBAL, Z. & SAJID, M. S. (2008). An account of the botanical anthelmintics used in traditional veterinary practices in Sahiwal district of Punjab, Pakistan. *Journal of Ethnopharmacology*, **119**, 185–190.

IQBAL, Z., LATEEF, M., JABBER, A., GHAYUR, M. N. & GILANI, A. H. (2006). *In vitro* and *in vivo* anthelmintic activity of *Nicotiana tabacum* L. leaves against gastrointestinal nematodes of sheep. *Phytotherapy Research*, **20**, 46–48.

KETZIS, J. K., TAYLOR, A., BOWMAN, D. D., BROWN, D. L., WARNICK, L. D. & ERB, H. N. (2002). *Chenopodium ambrosioides* and its essential oil as treatments for *Haemonchus contortus* and mixed adult-nematode infections in goats. *Small Ruminant Research*, **44**, 193–200.

KOZAN, E., KUPELI, E. & YESILADA, E. (2006). Evaluation of some plants used in Turkish folk medicine against parasitic infections for their *in vivo* anthelmintic activity. *Journal of Ethnopharmacology*, **108**, 211–216.

LARSEN, M. AND NANSEN, P. (1990). Effects of oyster mushroom *Pleurotus pulmonarius* on preparasitic larvae of bovine trichostrongyles. *Acta Veterinaria Scandinavica*, **31**, 509–510.

LARSEN, M., NANSEN, P., GRØNVOLD, J., WOLSTRUP, J. & HENRIKSEN, S. A. (1997). Biological control of gastro-intestinal nematodes – Facts, future, or fiction? *Veterinary Parasitology*, **72**, 479–492.

LARSEN, M., NANSEN, P., WOLSTRUP, J., GRØNVOLD, J., HENRIKSEN, S. A. & ZORN, A. (1995). Biological control of trichostrongyles in calves by the fungus *Duddingtonia flagrans* fed to animals under natural grazing conditions. *Veterinary Parasitology*, **60**, 321–330.

LARSEN, M., WOLSTRUP, J., HENRIKSEN, S. A., DACKMAN, C., GRØNVOLD, J. & NANSEN, P. (1991). *In vitro* stress selection of nematophagous fungi for biocontrol of parasitic nematodes in ruminants. *Journal of Helminthology*, **65**, 193–200.

LARSEN, M., WOLSTRUP, J., HENRIKSEN, S. A., GRØNVOLD, J. & NANSEN, P. (1992). *In vivo* passage through calves of nematophagous fungi selected for biocontrol of parasitic nematodes. *Journal of Helminthology*, **66**, 137–141.

MARLEY, C. L., COOK, R., KEATINGE, R., BARRETT, J. & LAMPKIN, N. H. (2003). The effect of birdsfoot trefoil (*Lotus corniculatus*) and chicory (*Cichorium intybus*) on parasite intensities and performance of lambs naturally infected with helminth parasites. *Veterinary Parasitology*, **112**, 147–155.

MAX, R. A., WAKELIN, D., DAWSON, J. M. *et al.* (2005). Effect of quebracho tannin on faecal egg counts and worm burdens of temperate sheep with challenge nematode infections. *Journal of Agricultural Science*, **143**, 519–527.

MIN, B. R., BARRY, T. N., ATTWOOD, G. T. & MCNABB, W. C. (2003). The effect of condensed tannins on the nutrition and health of ruminants fed fresh temperate forages: A review. *Animal Feed Science and Technology*, **106**, 3–19.

MIN, B. R., POMROY, W. E., HART, S. P. & SAHLU, T. (2004). The effect of short-term consumption of a forage containing condensed tannins on gastro-intestinal nematode parasite infections in grazing wether goats. *Small Ruminant Research*, **51**, 279–283.

MOLAN, A. L., DUNCAN, A. J., BARRY, T. N. & MCNABB, W. C. (2003a). Effects of condensed tannins and crude sesquiterpene lactones extracted from chicory on the motility of larvae of deer lungworm and gastrointestinal nematodes. *Parasitology International*, **52**, 209–218.

MOLAN, A. L., MEAGHER, L. P., SPENCER, P. A. & SIVAKUMARAN, S. (2003b). Effect of flavan-3-ols on *in vitro* egg hatching, larval development and viability of infective larvae of *Trichostrongylus colubriformis*. *International Journal for Parasitology*, **33**, 1691–1698.

MOLAN, A. L., WAGHORN, G. C., MIN, B. R. & MCNABB, W. C. (2000). The effect of condensed tannins from seven herbages on *Trichostrongylus colubriformis* larval migration *in vitro*. *Folia Parasitologica*, **47**, 39–44.

NANSEN, P., GRØNVOLD, J., HENRIKSEN, S. A. & WOLSTRUP, J. (1988). Interactions between the predacious fungus arthrobotrys oligospora and third-stage larvae of a series of animal-parasitic nematodes. *Veterinary Parasitology*, **26**, 329–337.

NANSEN, P., LARSEN, M., GRØNVOLD, J., WOLSTRUP, J., ZORN, A. & HENRIKSEN, S. AA. (1995). Prevention of clinical trichostrongylidosis in calves by strategic feeding with the predacious fungus *Duddingtonia flagrans*. *Parasitology Research*, **81**, 371–374.

NIEZEN, J. H., CHARLESTON, W. A. G., ROBERTSON, H. A., SHELTON, D., WAGHORN, G. C. & GREEN, R. (2002a). The effect of feeding sulla (*Hedysarum coronarium*) or lucerne (*Medicago sativa*) on lamb parasite burdens and development of immunity to gastrointestinal nematodes. *Veterinary Parasitology*, **105**, 229–245.

NIEZEN, J. H., ROBERTSON, H. A., WAGHORN, G. C. & CHARLESTON, W. A. G. (1998a). Production, faecal egg counts and worm burdens of ewe lambs which grazed six contrasting forages. *Veterinary Parasitology*, **80**, 15–27.

NIEZEN, J. H., WAGHORN, G. C. & CHARLESTON, W. A. G. (1998b). Establishment and fecundity of *Ostertagia circumcincta* and *Trichostrongylus colubriformis* in lambs fed lotus (*Lotus pedunculatus*) or perennial ryegrass (*Lolium perenne*). *Veterinary Parasitology*, **78**, 13–21.

NIEZEN, J. H., WAGHORN, G. C., GRAHAM, T., CARTER, J. L. & LEATHWICK, D. M. (2002b). The effect of diet fed to lambs on subsequent development of *Trichostrongylus colubriformis* larvae *in vitro* and on pasture. *Veterinary Parasitology*, **105**, 269–283.

NIEZEN, J. H., WAGHORN, T. S., CHARLESTON, W. A. & WAGHORN, G. C. (1995). Growth and gastrointestinal nematode parasitism in lambs grazing either lucerne (*Medicago sativa*) or sulla (*Hedysarum coronarium*) which contains condensed tannins. *Journal of Agricultural Science*, **125**, 281–289.

NISBET, A. J., WOODFORD, J. A. T., STRANG, R. H. C. & CONNOLLY, J. D. (1993). Systemic antifeedant effects of azadirachtin on the peach-potato aphid *Myzus persicae. Entomologia Experimentalis et Applicata*, **68**, 87–98.

PAOLINI, V., FOURASTE, I. & KOSTE, H. (2004). *In vitro* effects of three woody plant and sainfoin extracts on 3rd-stage larvae and adult worms of three gastrointestinal nematodes. *Parasitology*, **129**, 69–77.

PAOLINI, V., FRAYSSINES, A., DE LA FARGE, F., DORCHIES, P. & HOSTE, H. (2003). Effects of condensed tannins on established populations and on incoming larvae of *Trichostrongylus colubriformis* and *Teladorsagia circumcincta* in goats. *Veterinary Research*, **34**, 331–339.

PENA, M. T., MILLER, J. E., FONTENOT, M. E., GILLESPIE, A. & LARSEN, M. (2002). Evaluation of *Duddingtonia flagrans* in reducing infective larvae of *Haemonchus contortus* in feces of sheep. *Veterinary Parasitology*, **103**, 259–265.

REED, J. D. (1995). Nutritional toxicology of tannins and related polyphenols in forage legumes. *Journal of Animal Science*, **73**, 1516–1528.

ROBBINS, C. T. (1987). Role of tannins in defending plants against ruminants: Reduction in protein availability. *Ecology*, **68**, 98–107.

ROBBINS, C. T., HAGERMAN, A. E., AUSTIN, P. J., MCARTHUR, C. & HANLEY, T. A. (1991). Variation in mammalian physiological responses to a condensed tannin and its ecological implications. *Journal of Mammalogy*, **72**, 480–486.

ROCHFORT, S., PARKER, A. J. & DUNSHEA, F. R. (2008). Plant bioactives for ruminant health and productivity. *Phytochemistry*, **69**, 299–322.

SUTHERLAND, I. A. (2003). Fecal mass and parasite strategies. *Trends in Parasitology*, **19**, 69–69.

WAGHORN, G. C. (1996). Condensed tannins and nutrient absorption from the small intestine. *Animal Science Research and Development, Meeting Future Challenges. Proceedings of the Canadian Society for Animal Production*, 175–194.

WAGHORN, G. C. & MCNABB, W. C. (2003). Consequences of plant phenolic compounds for productivity and health of ruminants. *Proceedings of the Nutrition Society*, **62**, 383–392.

WAGHORN, T. S., LEATHWICK, D. M., CHEN, L. Y. & SKIPP, R. A. (2003). Efficacy of the nematode-trapping fungus *Duddingtonia flagrans* against three species of gastro-intestinal nematodes in laboratory faecal cultures from sheep and goats. *Veterinary Parasitology*, **118**, 227–234.

WAGHORN, T. S., MOLAN, A. L., DEIGHTON, M. *et al.* (2006). *In vivo* anthelmintic activity of *Dorycnium rectum* and grape seed extract against *Ostertagia (Teladorsagia) circumcincta* and *Trichostrongylus colubriformis* in sheep. *New Zealand Veterinary Journal*, **54**, 21–27.

WALLER, P. J., BERNES, G., THAMSBORG, S. M. et al. (2001). Plants as deworming agents of livestock in the Nordic countries: Historical perspective, popular beliefs and prospects for the future. *Acta Veterinaria Scandinavica*, **42**, 31–44.

WATERMAN, P. G. (1988). Tannins-chemical ecology in action. A tribute to the contributions of Professor Tony Swain. *Phytochemistry*, **27**, xii–xiii.

YESILADA, E., HONDA, G., SEZIK, E., TABATA, M., GOTO, K. & IKESHIRO, Y. (1993). Traditional medicine in turkey IV. Folk medicine in the Mediterranean subdivision. *Journal of Ethnopharmacology*, **39**, 31–38.

10 Nutrition and parasitism

The link between gastrointestinal nematode (GIN) parasitism and the nutritional status of the host is well established, to the extent that parasitism has been described as a 'nutritional condition'. This is rather misleading, but perhaps understandably so, given the often-recorded relationship between the plane of nutrition and the symptoms of clinical and sub-clinical parasitism. Not surprisingly, there is enormous variation dependent on worm/host genotype and host phenotype within this relationship. As a gross generalisation, however, well-fed animals appear to suffer less from the effects of parasitism and *vice versa*. This is particularly relevant to most of the major GINs of livestock, as the most common outcome of the infections is not acute and fatal, but rather a chronic state which significantly affects several parameters of animal productivity. In basic terms, continuous challenge with L3 and/or the development of adult worm burdens reduces voluntary feed intake (Sykes & Greer, 2003), disrupts host physiological processes (Hammerberg, 1986; Kyriazakis *et al.*, 1996) and imposes a cost to the animal through the requirement to acquire and express an anti-parasite immune response (Coop & Kyriazakis, 1999).

The physiological relationship between parasites and nutrition can be considered from two angles. First, what are the metabolic costs of parasitism on the host and second, how does the plane of nutrition influence the response to, and impact of, the infection? Then, given the assumption that the availability of improved nutrition is of value in animals under challenge or infected with parasites, what practical steps can be taken by livestock farmers?

Metabolic cost of parasitism

The metabolic cost of parasitism is associated with the extent of damage due to challenge and infection. The direct pathological effects of parasitism are described more fully in Chapter 2, while the aspects of indirect immuno-pathology in response to parasitism are covered in Chapter 12. However, in any discussion of the interaction between nutrition and parasitism, it must be acknowledged that each of these factors carries some degree of metabolic cost to the animals, as indeed does the acquisition and expression of anti-parasite immune responses. An example of this is an estimation of the drain imposed on small ruminants by parasites as approximately 17 g/day of metabolisable protein above maintenance requirement (Liu *et al.*, 2003). In the lack of parasitic infection, this protein would instead be incorporated into muscle, bone, milk and fibre (Knox *et al.*, 2006). It is clear, therefore, that during periods of nutrient scarcity, parasitic infections will have a significant and deleterious effect on animal health.

This cost of 17 g/day protein (Liu *et al.*, 2003) is likely to divert resources from more than one source and will include direct damage caused by parasites as well as indirect pathophysiology, resources allocated to damage repair and resources allocated to the acquisition or expression of anti-parasite immunity. It must be acknowledged that it is extremely difficult, if not impossible, to accurately calculate the costs of each of these factors in isolation. It is for simplicity, therefore, that the metabolic impact of parasites on the nutrient economy of animals will be treated in two sections, the first of which examines the metabolic cost of infection, while the second addresses the metabolic cost of immunity.

Metabolic cost of infection

The 'cost of infection' encompasses the perturbation of nutrient absorption and utilisation as well as the cost of damage to the intestinal tract and other organs and tissues. The gastrointestinal tract has very high metabolic requirements, mainly due to the high rate of protein synthesis and energy expenditure in the small intestine. In sheep, these metabolic activities account for 20–50% of whole body protein turnover and energy expenditure, which is disproportionate to the corresponding contribution to the body mass of only 3–6% (Burrin *et al.*, 1989; Lobley *et al.*, 1992; MacRae *et al.*, 1997). These values indicate that the gastrointestinal tract is a major sink for nutrients which actively competes for amino acids with the remainder of the body, even in the absence of parasite challenge. Indeed, MacRae *et al.* (1997) demonstrated that 80% of the amino acid precursors for gastrointestinal tract protein turnover are derived from the arterial blood supply irrigating the gastrointestinal tract. This highlights the relatively minor contribution of lumen-derived (absorbed) amino acids to total gastrointestinal protein turnover. Consequently, factors that alter the gastrointestinal tract function and/or demand, such as parasite challenge or infection, can have a dramatic impact on nutrient availability for other tissues.

The costs of infection are dependent to a significant extent on the parasite species involved and the degree of damage they cause. Haematophagous worms such as *Haemonchus* spp. are therefore likely to have a relatively greater direct impact on host metabolism than mucosal browsers. As an example, an average *Haemonchus contortus* infection in lambs has been estimated to take around 400 ml of blood/day. The metabolic impact of parasites is also likely to vary depending on the organ they inhabit. For example, abomasal species such as *Teladorsagia circumcincta* in sheep, *Trichostrongylus axei* in sheep/cattle as well as *Haemonchus* spp., result in a temporal, but significant, rise in pH which impacts on the host's digestive efficiency. It remains unclear whether this perturbation of abomasal physiology is a deliberate tactic of the host, of the parasites or an indirect effect of infection; the raised pH is almost certainly responsible for decreased establishment of subsequently ingested larvae (Sutherland, unpublished), which may explain the strong density-dependence observed in species such as *T. circumcincta* (Sutherland *et al.*, 2002). It would also imply, of course, that those parasites able to successfully establish may be indulging, albeit indirectly, in a form of patch protection.

The most detailed observations on the metabolic impact of parasites on grazing livestock have used the small intestinal sheep worm *Trichostrongylus colubriformis*. The response of sheep to a trickle infection with this parasite includes altered protein, carbohydrate, mineral and hormone metabolism (Nielsen, 1982). While nitrogen digestibility in sheep does not appear to be affected by trickle-challenge with *T. colubriformis* (Abbott, 1985; Roseby, 1973; Sykes & Coop, 1976), sub-clinical infection has been shown to decrease whole body protein gain in sheep by more than 40% (Van Houtert *et al.*, 1995). The negative impact of parasite infection on nitrogen retention could be due to reduced nitrogen intake, increased nitrogen flow through the small intestine resulting from increased endogenous nitrogen loss (Rowe *et al.*, 1988) and/or increased urinary nitrogen excretion (Abbott, 1985; Roseby, 1973; Rowe *et al.*, 1988). Any increased urinary nitrogen excretion resulting from parasitism is likely to be due to an increase in amino acid catabolism in the whole animal, most probably in the gastrointestinal tract (Yu *et al.*, 2000) and the liver.

Overall, the change in amino acid and protein metabolism in the gastrointestinal tract resulting from parasitic infection disrupts partitioning of amino acids to other tissues such as the liver (Bermingham *et al.*, 2002; Symons & Jones, 1970, 1975, 1983), muscle (Symons & Jones, 1975) and skin (Jones & Symons, 1982). Consequently, nutrients are diverted from growth to repair of damaged intestinal tissue (Butter *et al.*, 2000) and to mount an immune response to the parasites (Parkins & Holmes, 1989).

Interestingly, recent studies (Bermingham *et al.*, 2008) demonstrate that while larval challenge of sheep with *T. colubriformis* has a significant impact on amino acid absorption and utilisation (Bermingham *et al.*, 2002), the presence of a resident adult worm burden of the same parasite had no significant effect. Changes in gastrointestinal histology, function and secretion have also been observed during infection by *T. colubriformis* (Coop & Angus, 1975; Holmes, 1985; Symons & Jones, 1970) which seem likely to cause further alterations in digestion and in the absorption of nutrients.

Increased mucus production due to a hyperplasia of Goblet cells (Coop & Angus, 1975), increased sloughing of cells and/or plasma leakage of proteins (Poppi *et al.*, 1986), have also been associated with intestinal parasite infection. The proteins that leak into the small intestine are assumed to be mostly resorbed before the terminal ileum and are not therefore considered as lost (Poppi *et al.*, 1986). The flow of non-ammonia nitrogen in digesta at the terminal ileum was estimated to be between 3 and 20 g/day in sheep and has been shown to be elevated during infection (Kimambo *et al.*, 1988a, b; Poppi *et al.*, 1986; Yu *et al.*, 1999). As a result of these endogenous protein secretions, there is an increased demand on amino acids for the synthesis of replacement mucosal proteins or for cell renewal. Increased losses of endogenous protein from the small intestine are transient and can be significantly reduced by week 18 of challenge (Kimambo *et al.*, 1988b). Furthermore, in sheep given a secondary challenge after being free of parasites for 10 weeks, gastrointestinal tract metabolism was not obviously perturbed (Kimambo *et al.*, 1988a).

While no change in the fractional protein synthesis rate of the proximal small intestine was obtained in sheep infected with parasites, the rate was decreased in the terminal part of the organ (Bermingham *et al.*, 2002). These effects were not due to changes in feed intake. Increased protein synthesis in the gastrointestinal tract places an additional energy and amino acid cost on animals; this can be exacerbated if amino acid availability is reduced due to parasitic infection. Decreased amino acids in the small intestine are then reflected in decreased availability of amino acids to peripheral tissues, such as muscle and skin (Poppi *et al.*, 1986; Yu *et al.*, 2000). Peripheral tissues might also be faced with a further metabolic cost if the requirement of the infected small intestine increases and becomes a drain on amino acids currently in the peripheral tissues. Thus, in response to infection, nutrients are re-partitioned from growth and development towards tissue maintenance and repair. The results of this nutrient repartitioning can include an increase in amino acid oxidation and an alteration of protein metabolism in the gut (Bermingham *et al.*, 2002; Yu *et al.* 1999, 2000), increased protein synthesis in the liver (Bermingham *et al.*, 2002) and immune activation (Wakelin, 1996). All of these place additional demands on the animal for amino acids which may not be provided by diet alone, and mobilisation of amino acids from body tissues may occur. It is also possible that particular amino acids are taken in the affected tissues than required by the intestine (MacRae & Lobley, 1991). This could explain the decline in overall growth and wool production which is a characteristic of parasitism (Steel *et al.*, 1982).

Metabolic costs of immunity

In an article which reviewed the likely costs of mobilising resources to mount an immune response against GINs, the author pointed out that immune responses are context specific (Colditz, 2008). That is, a range of factors other than the parasites themselves, such as stress, social status, prior exposure, macro- and micronutrient balance, concurrent infections and, of course, genotype all impact upon the immune phenotype at any given time.

Colditz (2008) suggested that activation of an acute phase response (APR) following parasite challenge will lead to the production of pro-inflammatory cytokines, which in turn induce fever and subsequently perturbations to the anabolic/catabolic balance. Each degree Celsius of fever is estimated to add 5–13% to the metabolic rate, while oxygen consumption and utilisation of glucose and glutamine increases dramatically at a cellular level. However, and as the author states, acute fever is not a characteristic of nematode infections, and while a number of pro-inflammatory cytokines are up-regulated following nematode infection in sheep (Pernthaner *et al.*, 2006) and cattle (Li *et al.*, 2007), it is perhaps dangerous to extrapolate too much from other disease models.

The second cost of immunity proposed by Colditz (2008) was a reduction in nutrient availability due to what is commonly known as parasite-induced inappetance or hypophagia. This is a well-documented phenomenon during nematode infections and can be a major cause for reduced feed intake and therefore live-weight gain in young animals (Fox *et al.*, 2002; Kyriazakis *et al.*, 1996; Sykes & Greer, 2003). The effect of the inappetance varies significantly from 15% to 30% voluntary feed intake and can occur from around 4 to around 10 weeks of age (Sykes, 2008). This is at least coincident with the 'naïve' phase, and it has been proposed that there is a direct link between the end of inappetance and the beginning of the 'mature' phase (Greer, 2008)

Despite the evidence for the phenomenon, and repeated attempts to explain the underlying mechanisms (Roberts *et al.*, 1999), the causes of parasite-induced inappetance remain unclear (Sykes, 2008). Injection of pro-inflammatory cytokines implicated in the APR have been shown to decrease feed intake, while the involvement of Th2-associated cytokines IL-4 and IL-13, CD4+ lymphocytes and cholecystokinin (CCK)-expressing cells in inflamed mucosa have variously been suggested (Sykes, 2008).

A study in New Zealand (Sutherland & Alexander, unpublished) compared the impact of repeated challenge with *T. colubriformis* on voluntary feed intake in lambs. In this case, however, the animals were sourced from divergent genotypes of Romney sheep which had been extensively selected for either resistance or susceptibility, on the basis of FEC, for over 20 years, and a control group which remained unselected over the same period. The resistant-line animals acquire a strong immune response and few if any parasites establish to subsequently produce eggs in faeces. This was the case in the work described here, in which the average FEC over the 2-week experimental period was fourfold lower in the resistant sheep than in the susceptible, and around half that of the control animals. On necropsy, a further 3 weeks later, few if any adult or L4 worms were recovered from the resistant animals. Despite these differences in parasite burdens, there was a similar degree of parasite-induced (or -associated) inappetance between the groups of approximately 15% intake/day (Figure 10.1).

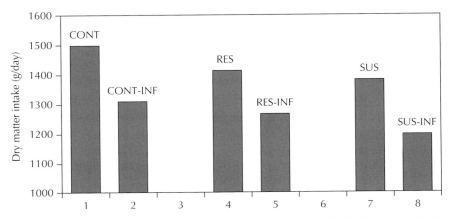

Figure 10.1 The impact of parasitism with *T. colubriformis* on daily dry matter intake in lambs selected either for resistance or susceptibility, or unselected for either trait. Lambs had received larval challenge for 6 weeks post-weaning before measurements were taken (Sutherland & Alexander, unpublished).

While the experiment was not designed to determine the aetiology of inappetance, the results suggest that the development of worms through to mature adults is not required and that larval challenge alone may be sufficient for the effect to occur.

One relationship between animal genotype and parasite-induced inappetance, which has not been explored, is whether a similar magnitude of reduced intake would be observed in animals selectively bred for 'resilience' to infection, i.e. those animals which continue to perform despite the presence of parasites. One theory which may explain the resilient phenotype is a relatively lower impact of parasite-associated intestinal inflammation; as such, it is tempting to postulate that the severity of inappetance may also be reduced.

The hypothesis that larval challenge drives inappetance receives indirect, partial support from grazing studies in lactating dairy cattle. When treated with the ML eprinomectin, cattle grazed for longer periods and there was a significant increase in the production of milk solids (Forbes *et al.*, 2000, 2004, 2007). While the impact of removing the resident adult worm burdens cannot be discounted, it is interesting to note that the greatest effect was recorded 2–3 weeks after treatment, which would be too early for adult worms to be present following the administration of a pour-on anthelmintic product (assuming the drench is effective).

Knowing which facets, i.e. extent of larval challenge and/or adult worm burden, of the host–parasite relationship impact on voluntary feed intake could result in new management strategies to minimise the effect. Such research should be possible in small ruminants, although the cost of conducting properly replicated experiments using cattle, and particularly so in lactating dairy cattle, make similar studies in large ruminants unlikely. A possible alternative to dairy cattle could be the use of milking sheep or goats as cheaper and more practical animal models.

Parasites and nutrition: a nutrient utilisation framework

The development of an adequate or effective immune response to nematodes in grazing livestock occurs over several weeks and is commonly referred to as the period of 'the acquisition of immunity', or 'the period of naivety', although this should be differentiated from the period of suckling in which animals are regarded as hyporesponsive (Sykes, 2008). Regardless of the definition, the direct metabolic impact of parasites is relatively greater during the period of 'naivety' for what may be very sensible reasons. A paper by Coop and Kyriazakis (1999) contained an elegant framework which ranked the major priorities for the allocation of nutrients (assuming these are not plentiful) in animals during both the naïve and mature immune phases. In this framework, the first priority for all animals, whether designated as having naïve or mature immune responses, was the maintenance of body protein, which can also be used as an indicator of the ability to survive (Emmans & Fisher, 1986). In the framework, 'maintenance of body protein' includes repair, replacement and reaction to infection in affected tissues.

The second priority in 'immunologically mature' animals includes those functions responsible for preserving the ability to grow and reproduce, otherwise described as protein gain, while the expression of immunity is prioritised in the third. The fourth and last in the list is the maintenance and gain of body lipid. Coop and Kyriazakis (1999) are careful to note that this is not an absolute framework, with significant overlap occurring within the list of four priorities.

The framework assigned to naïve animals is crucially different from that described above. As stated above, maintenance of body protein has the highest priority regardless of immune status. However, in naïve animals, the second priority is the acquisition of immunity because of its importance in future survival, fitness and reproductive success. Protein gain drops to become the third priority, while the maintenance and gain of body fat remains lowest. As before, it is acknowledged that significant overlap will occur between the priorities.

While this framework may seem confusing at first, it can be simplified as follows: all animals have an absolute need to survive. Animals with a naïve immune response also have to put resources into the development of the mature phenotype, while this is less of a priority for animals which have already attained this mature status. Put another way, improving nutrient availability will enhance the survival of both phenotypes, but will have a proportionally greater impact on the acquisition of immunity by the naïve animals than it will on the expression of that immunity in mature animals.

In practical terms, therefore, an understanding of this framework enables more informed decisions on the value of nutritional status in the different stock classes. It also implies that improving nutrition will have quite different effects on the host–parasite relationship in the naïve and mature animals. In the former, which have not yet acquired effective protection against parasites, nutrition can be used to improve growth but not necessarily immunity – this is often referred to as improving the 'resilience' of the animals. However, in the mature animals, improved nutrition can enhance the protective immunity against parasites – commonly referred to as 'resistance'. As the extent of resilience and resistance of animals will vary continuously through factors such as genotype and environment, independent of nutritional status, these are definitions necessary for ease of explanation and interpretation, as there will be significant overlap in many areas.

While Chapter 11 reviews the concepts of resistance and resilience to GINs more fully, some differences in definition apply when discussing the relationship between parasitism, nutrition and immunity. Briefly, resistance is defined in Chapter 11 as the ability of animals to reduce their parasitic burden, either by preventing larval establishment or by removing established worms more quickly. Within the nutrition partitioning framework, therefore, resistance can be regarded as the time taken to develop a mature immune response and/or as a measure of the effectiveness of that response. However, resilience is defined in Chapter 11 as the ability of animals to maintain acceptable measures of productivity in spite of harbouring 'normal' levels of parasites. When considering nutrition and parasitism, however, much of the literature uses a different definition of resilience in which improved nutrition increases the growth rate of parasitised animals regardless of the extent of parasitism; this definition will be used in the context of the current chapter.

Supplementation for increased resilience to parasites

In young animals with a naïve immune response to parasites, improved nutrition through either supplementation (or greater feed quality/quantity) can have two major functions. First, nutrients become available to the developing immune response and can result in a more rapid acquisition of the mature phenotype in the post-weaning period. (Sykes, 2008). Second, it results in a greater partitioning of nutrients into productivity parameters such as muscle and wool – in what are certainly overly simplistic terms, a high enough quality/quantity of nutrition enables animals to grow regardless of the cost of parasitism. This presents livestock farmers with some complex cost–benefit decisions regarding the importance (and likely effectiveness) of increasing nutrient availability.

Determining what form of supplementation has the greatest benefit for resilience would obviously be an advantage. Given that young animals are prone to direct, parasite-associated damage such as loss of tissue (Holmes, 1993), it has been proposed that increasing protein is the most effective strategy. This theory was shown to be correct in sheep infected with *T. colubriformis* (Bown *et al.*, 1991) in which either protein (in the form of casein) or iso-energetic amounts of energy (in the form of glucose) were infused into the abomasum. Only in the protein treatments was there a significant impact on the resilience of the animals to infection.

A number of subsequent studies have added support to the positive effect of protein supplementation on resilience (Kyriazakis *et al.*, 1994; Van Houtert *et al.*, 1995), although there has been conflicting evidence from studies which were not able to demonstrate a similar effect (Coop *et al.*, 1995; Knox *et al.*, 1994).

Supplementation for increased resistance to parasites

Within the nutrient partitioning framework described above (Coop & Kyriazakis, 1999), there are three distinct opportunities for supplementation to increase the resistance of livestock to parasites. The first of these is in young animals during the 'acquisition' phase of immune development. It has been dogma for some time – supported by research (Coop & Holmes, 1996; Holmes, 1993) – that supplementation increases the rate of immune development, and as such, can be used to make animals resistant more quickly. As Coop and Kyriazakis (1999) correctly state, however, the development of the immune response from completely ineffective to completely functional (i.e. not necessarily completely effective) is a complex continuum and that properly separating the acquisition and mature phases is extremely difficult. Other studies therefore disagree with the dogma and refute the involvement of any appreciable effect of supplementation on the development of resistance in young animals (Coop *et al.*, 1995; Van Houtert & Sykes, 1996).

The situation is somewhat simpler in animals with mature immune responses. Measured directly by its effects on parasites, supplementation with protein and energy can significantly improve the expression of immunity (Coop *et al.*, 1995; Kambara *et al.*, 1993; Mansour *et al.*, 1991, 1992). The study of Bown *et al.* (1991) neatly summarises the distinction between animals in the two immune phases; while infusion of protein had no effect on the establishment of *T. colubriformis* by 6 weeks of challenge, by 12 weeks there was a reduction in worm burden of 55%.

Reproducing animals

The third opportunity for strategic supplementation to increase resistance to parasites is in reproducing animals. In this case, previously 'immune' females undergo PPRI. The mechanisms behind, and impact of, the PPRI are dealt with in other chapters.

It is hardly surprising that livestock, eating what is normally a poor quality/ quantity of feed, have conflicting requirements for available nutrients, or that this situation will be more extreme in reproducing animals in which nutrient requirements are markedly increased. The nutrient partitioning framework of Coop and Kyriazakis (1999) was extended to include reproducing animals and indicated that animals prioritise reproductive success over antiparasite immunity. It is notable that termination of the drain on nutrition (e.g. abortion, weaning) results in an abrupt restoration of immune function

(O'Sullivan & Donald, 1973). Thus, unlike naïve animals, in which immunity is yet to develop, animals in the PPRI have the capability to express a mature phenotype but do not have the resources to do so. It seems reasonable to postulate, therefore, that supplementation of these animals could have a significant impact on anti-parasite immunity.

A study on lactating ewes (Donaldson *et al.*, 1998) elegantly demonstrated this to be the case. Twin-bearing ewes were fed a measured diet of pellets and hay, then were supplemented (or not) with two levels of fish meal (100 or 200 g/kg dry matter of feed/day) from 8 weeks prior to lambing. The ewes were then trickle challenged with L3 of *T. circumcincta* and *T. colubriformis* for 6 weeks until parturition. For both worm species, supplementation enabled the ewes to control worm burdens in a better way and demonstrated that improved nutrient supply could have the positive effect of reducing the severity of the PPRI. While the impact of such targeted supplementation of reproducing animals on parasite epidemiology and economics in whole production systems requires further work, it would be surprising if it was not a significant benefit to farmers.

The observation that immunity is somehow down-regulated in reproducing animals leads on to a related area in which surprisingly little has been published – the effect of reducing nutrient quality/quantity on the acquisition/ expression of immunity.

Undernutrition and parasitism

A study in New Zealand (Sutherland & Alexander, unpublished) examined the impact of poor nutrition on the acquisition and expression of immunity to *T. colubriformis* in sheep. The rationale for these studies was immunological rather than nutritional and was based on the potential risk of poor nutrition to the success of an anti-parasite vaccine. The aim, therefore, was to reach a point at which the acquisition and expression of immunity demonstrated signs of failing.

Groups of weaned lambs were fed on diets designed to be highly divergent – either *ad libitum* lucerne pellets and chaffed lucerne hay vs. the same rations fed in an amount sufficient to maintain a static bodyweight. The animals were kept on these diets for 10 weeks, during which time half of each group were challenged with *T. colubriformis* L3 three times weekly. To more easily differentiate between the naïve and mature phases, all resident infections were terminated by anthelmintic treatment after 8 weeks, while challenge continued. As would be expected from previous studies by Bown *et al.* (1991), there was no significant effect of parasite challenge on weight gain of animals regardless of diet during the 10 weeks of challenge (Figures 10.2a, b).

While this work was not designed to investigate the effect of undernutrition on parasitology *per se* – rather the potential impact on components of anti-parasite immunity – the results support and extend the paradigm that nutrient availability is largely irrelevant to the course of parasite infection in naïve animals.

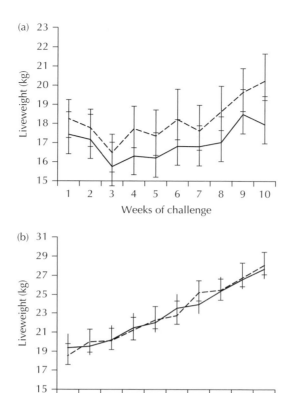

Figure 10.2 (a) Live-weights of lambs either challenged or not with *T. colubriformis* over a 10-week period from weaning: all animals were fed a 'maintenance' diet (Sutherland, Alexander & Leathwick, unpublished). (b) Live-weights of lambs either challenged or not with *T. colubriformis* over a 10-week period from weaning: all animals were provided an *ad libitum* diet (Sutherland, Alexander & Leathwick, unpublished).

Micronutrients and parasitism

While the effect of supplementing with either metabolisable energy or protein, or merely ensuring sufficient feed is available has been dealt with above, there has been no mention yet of the requirements for micronutrients such as minerals. Many of these are essential dietary components for grazing livestock and can severely limit productivity or lead to death if not present in sufficient quantities. A recent review (McClure, 2008) has summarised the significant literature on mineral requirements for productivity and lists iron, iodine, zinc, selenium, manganese, copper, cobalt, chromium and molybdenum as essential, while the lack of members of another lengthy list, including vanadium, silicon, nickel, and somewhat surprisingly arsenic, lithium and lead, can lead to clinical signs. As McClure (2008) states, each of these minerals has a safety range, above which problems may occur.

Minerals fill a number of physiological functions, including as tissue constituents, maintenance of the acid–base balance, osmotic control and oxygen transport, and play key roles in enzyme activity and the regulation of the cell cycle. It is hardly surprising, therefore, that grazing livestock require an adequate intake of key minerals, and these are often made available to animals as components of anthelmintic drenches, or as stand-alone treatments. Neither is it surprising that the key role of immunity within the host–parasite relationship is reliant on the availability of key minerals. As with macronutrients, however, there is an important distinction between the requirements for an adequate mineral supply and whether specific minerals can by utilised to increase resistance or resilience to parasite challenge or infection. Of the many minerals to which specific functions have been described, only cobalt and magnesium are associated with immunity to nematodes in grazing livestock (McClure, 2008), with a deficiency in either decreasing the ability of animals to resist infection (MacPherson *et al.*, 1987; Suttle *et al.*, 1992), with only molybdenum implicated in any increased immune status (Suttle *et al.*, 1992).

Improving nutrient availability

There are some obvious strategies through which farmers can increase the quality or quantity of nutrition available to grazing livestock, some of which are not in the remit of this book such as using improved cultivars, re-sowing pastures or irrigation when required. Optimising grazing management is also crucial to improving nutrition, while improving lambing/calving percentages can reduce the number of adult stock a property has to carry. Finally, and obviously, reducing the stocking density will provide more feed per stock unit, and has the indirect benefit that animals will ingest less L3 per kg dry matter.

As the technology available for managing (ideally automatically) animals improves, the possibilities for manipulating nutrient availability to particular individuals or stock classes also increase. For example, electronically tagged animals could be weighed then, on the basis of this information, be automatically drafted onto pasture with high nutritional value and/or with supplementary feed. Farmers could use this system to boost growth rates to reach a target slaughter weight or to improve the condition of poorly producing animals.

Forage plants and parasitism

While the utility of plants which may have anthelmintic properties is addressed in Chapter 9, farmers do regularly graze stock on forage species to increase productivity (Bagley *et al.*, 1987; Ramírez-Restrepo *et al.*, 2004; Sanderson *et al.*, 2005), and in some cases, this has been associated with a reduction in parasitism (Marley *et al.*, 2005; Min *et al.*, 2004; Niezen *et al.*, 1998; Tzamaloukas *et al.*, 2005, 2006). Care must be taken when associating increases in productivity and/or reductions in the obvious signs of parasitism (principally FEC), as there can often be confounding effects such as a reduction in intake of L3 and increased faecal mass.

Supplementation and immunity: increasing or enabling?

Does supplementary nutrition increase the ability to mount an anti-parasite immune response above and beyond what would be expected to occur in an otherwise healthy animal? Or, does it merely replace one or more limiting factors, thus enabling the animals to express a normal anti-parasite immune response? To some extent, the argument is moot, as in either scenario, supplementation has the potential to quantitatively or qualitatively improve immunity. However, it is important to recognise that while supplementation may result in more productive animals, this does not necessarily reflect any significant reduction in the impact of parasites, but rather that the impact of the parasites is hidden by increased productivity.

References

ABBOTT, E. M., PARKINS, J. J. & HOLMES, P. H. (1985). Influence of dietary protein on the pathophysiology of ovine haemonchosis in Finn Dorset and Scottish Blackface lambs given a single moderate infection. *Research in Veterinary Science*, **38**, 54–60.

BAGLEY, C. P., CARPENTER, J. C., JR, FEAZEL, J. I., HEMBRY, F. G., HUFFMAN, D. C. & KOONCE, K. L. (1987). Effects of forage system on beef cow-calf productivity. *Journal of Animal Science*, **64**, 678–686.

BERMINGHAM, E. N., ROY, N. C., REYNOLDS, G. W. *et al.* (2002). Fractional synthesis rates in lambs infected with *Trichostrongylus colubriformis*. *Journal of Animal Science*, **80**, 207.

BERMINGHAM, E. N., ROY, N. C., SUTHERLAND, I. A. *et al.* (2008). Intestinal amino acid absorption in lambs fed fresh lucerne (*Medicago sativa*) during an established *Trichostrongylus colubriformis* infection. *Animal*, **2**, 1037–1044.

BOWN, M. D., POPPI, D. P. & SYKES, A. R. (1991). The effect of post-ruminal infusion of protein or energy on the pathophysiology of *Trichostrongylus colubriformis* infection and body composition in lambs. *Australian Journal of Agricultural Research*, **42**, 253–267.

BURRIN, D. G., FERRELL, C. L., EISEMANN, J. H., BRITTON, R. A. & NIENABER, J. A. (1989). Effect of level of nutrition on splanchnic blood flow and oxygen consumption in sheep. *British Journal of Nutrition*, **62**, 23–34.

BUTTER, N. L., DAWSON, J. M., WAKELIN, D. & BUTTERY, P. J. (2000). Effect of dietary tannin and protein concentration on nematode infection (*Trichostrongylus colubriformis*) in lambs. *Journal of Agricultural Science*, **134**, 89–99.

COLDITZ, I. G. (2008). Six costs of immunity to gastrointestinal nematode infections. *Parasite Immunology*, **30**, 63–70.

COOP, R. L. & ANGUS, K. W. (1975). The effect of continuous doses of *Trichostrongylus colubriformis* larvae on the intestinal mucosa of sheep and on liver vitamin A concentration. *Parasitology*, **70**, 1–9.

COOP, R. L. & HOLMES, P. H. (1996). Nutrition and parasite interaction. *International Journal for Parasitology*, **26**, 951–962.

COOP, R. L., HUNTLEY, J. F. & SMITH, W. D. (1995). Effect of dietary protein supplementation on the development of immunity to *Ostertagia circumcincta* in growing lambs. *Research in Veterinary Science*, **59**, 24–29.

COOP, R. L. & KYRIAZAKIS, I. (1999). Nutrition-parasite interaction. *Veterinary Parasitology*, **84**, 187–204.

DONALDSON, J., VAN HOUTERT, M. F. J. & SYKES, A. R. (1998). The effect of nutrition on the periparturient parasite status of mature ewes. *Animal Science*, **67**, 523–533.

EMMANS, G. C. & FISHER, C. (1986). Nutrient requirements of poultry and nutritional research. In *Problems in Nutritional Theory* (eds Fisher, C. & Boorman, K. N.), Buttersworth, London, UK, pp. 9–41.

FORBES, A. B., HUCKLE, C. A. & GIBB, M. J. (2004). Impact of eprinomectin on grazing behaviour and performance in dairy cattle with sub-clinical gastrointestinal nematode infections under continuous stocking management. *Veterinary Parasitology*, **125**, 353–364.

FORBES, A. B., HUCKLE, C. A. & GIBB, M. J. (2007). Evaluation of the effect of eprinomectin in young dairy heifers sub-clinically infected with gastrointestinal nematodes on grazing behaviour and diet selection. *Veterinary Parasitology*, **150**, 321–332.

FORBES, A. B., HUCKLE, C. A., GIBB, M. J., ROOK, A. J. & NUTHALL, R. (2000). Evaluation of the effects of nematode parasitism on grazing behaviour, herbage intake and growth in young grazing cattle. *Veterinary Parasitology*, **90**, 111–118.

FOX, M. T., UCHE, U. E., VAILLANT, C., GANABADI, S. & CALAM, J. (2002). Effects of *Ostertagia ostertagi* and omeprazole treatment on feed intake and gastrin-related responses in the calf. *Veterinary Parasitology*, **105**, 285–301.

GREER, A. W. (2008). Trade-offs and benefits: Implications of promoting a strong immunity to gastrointestinal parasites in sheep. *Parasite Immunology*, **30**, 123–132.

HAMMERBERG, B. (1986). Pathophysiology of nematodiasis in cattle. *The Veterinary clinics of North America. Food Animal Practice*, **2**, 225–234.

HOLMES, P. H. (1985). Pathogenesis of trichostrongylosis. *Veterinary Parasitology*, **18**, 89–101.

HOLMES, P. H. (1993). Interactions between parasites and animal nutrition: The veterinary consequences. *Proceedings of the Nutrition Society, UK*, **52**, 113–120.

JONES, W. O. & SYMONS, L. E. (1982). Protein synthesis in the whole body, liver, skeletal muscle and kidney cortex of lambs infected by the nematode *Trichostrongylus colubriformis*. *International Journal for Parasitology*, **12**, 295–301.

KAMBARA, T., MCFARLANE, R. G., ABELL, T. J., MCANULTY, R. W. & SYKES, A. R. (1993). The effect of age and dietary protein on immunity and resistance in lambs vaccinated with *Trichostrongylus colubriformis*. *International Journal for Parasitology*, **23**, 471–476.

KIMAMBO, A. E., MACRAE, J. C. & DEWEY, P. J. S. (1988a). The effect of daily challenge with *Trichostrongylus colubriformis* larvae on the nutrition and performance of immunologically-resistant sheep. *Veterinary Parasitology*, **28**, 205–212.

KIMAMBO, A. E., MACRAE, J. C., WALKER, A., WATT, C. F. & COOP, R. L. (1988b). Effect of prolonged subclinical infection with *Trichostrongylus colubriformis* on the performance and nitrogen metabolism of growing lambs. *Veterinary Parasitology*, **28**, 191–203.

KNOX, M., STEEL, J. W. & LENG, R. A. (1994). The effects of urea supplementation on gastrointestinal parasitism in sheep being fed low quality roughage diets.

Programme and Abstracts of the 13th Annual Scientific Meeting of the Australian Society for Parasitology, Nelson Bay, NSW, p. 28.

KNOX, M. R., BESIER, R. B., CARMICHAEL, I. H. & STEEL, J. W. (2006). Nutrition for parasite management. *International Journal of Sheep and Wool Science*, **54**, 14–21.

KYRIAZAKIS, I., ANDERSON, D. H., COOP, R. L. & JACKSON, F. (1996). The pathophysiology and development of immunity during long-term subclinical infection with *Trichostrongylus colubriformis* of sheep receiving different nutritional treatments. *Veterinary Parasitology*, **65**, 41–54.

KYRIAZAKIS, I., OLDHAM, J. D., COOP, R. L. & JACKSON, F. (1994). The effect of subclinical intestinal nematode infection on the diet selection of growing sheep. *British Journal of Nutrition*, **72**, 665–677.

LI, R. W., SONSTEGARD, T. S., VAN TASSELL, C. P. & GASBARRE, L. C. (2007). Local inflammation as a possible mechanism of resistance to gastrointestinal nematodes in Angus heifers. *Veterinary Parasitology*, **145**, 100–107.

LIU, S. M., MASTERS, D. G. & ADAMS, N. R. (2003). Potential impact of nematode parasitism on nutrient partitioning for wool production, growth and reproduction in sheep. *Australian Journal of Experimental Agriculture*, **43**, 1409–1417.

LOBLEY, G. E., HARRIS, P. M., SKENE, P. A. *et al.* (1992). Responses in tissue protein synthesis to sub- and supra-maintenance intake in young growing sheep: Comparison of large dose and continuous-infusion techniques. *British Journal of Nutrition*, **68**, 373–388.

MACPHERSON, A., GRAY, D., MITCHELL, G. B. & TAYLOR, C. N. (1987). Ostertagia infection and neutrophil function in cobalt-deficient and cobalt-supplemented cattle. *British Veterinary Journal*, **143**, 348–353.

MACRAE, J. C., BRUCE, L. A., BROWN, D. S. & CALDER, A. G. (1997). Amino acid use by the gastrointestinal tract of sheep given lucerne forage. *American Journal of Physiology – Gastrointestinal and Liver Physiology*, **273**, G1200–G1207.

MACRAE, J. C. & LOBLEY, G. E. (1991). Physiological and metabolic implications of conventional and novel methods for the manipulation of growth and production. *Livestock Production Science*, **27**, 43–59.

MANSOUR, M. M., DIXON, J. B., ROWAN, T. G. & CARTER, S. D. (1992). Modulation of calf immune responses by *Ostertagia ostertagi*: The effect of diet during trickle infection. *Veterinary Immunology and Immunopathology*, **33**, 261–269.

MANSOUR, M. M., ROWAN, T. G., DIXON, J. B. & CARTER, S. D. (1991). Immune modulation by *Ostertagia ostertagi* and the effects of diet. *Veterinary Parasitology*, **39**, 321–332.

MARLEY, C. L., FRASER, M. D., FYCHAN, R., THEOBALD, V. J. & JONES, R. (2005). Effect of forage legumes and anthelmintic treatment on the performance, nutritional status and nematode parasites of grazing lambs. *Veterinary Parasitology*, **131**, 267–282.

MCCLURE, S. J. (2008). How minerals may influence the development and expression of immunity to endoparasites in livestock. *Parasite Immunology*, **30**, 89–100.

MIN, B. R., POMROY, W. E., HART, S. P. & SAHLU, T. (2004). The effect of short-term consumption of a forage containing condensed tannins on gastro-intestinal nematode parasite infections in grazing wether goats. *Small Ruminant Research*, **51**, 279–283.

NIELSEN, K. (1982). Pathophysiology of gastrointestinal parasitism. *Parasites – Their World and Ours. Proceedings of the 5th International Congress of Parasitology*, Toronto, pp. 248–251.

NIEZEN, J. H., ROBERTSON, H. A., WAGHORN, G. C. & CHARLESTON, W. A. G. (1998). Production, faecal egg counts and worm burdens of ewe lambs which grazed six contrasting forages. *Veterinary Parasitology*, **80**, 15–27.

O'SULLIVAN, B. M. & DONALD, A. D. (1973). Responses to infection with *Haemonchus contortus* and *Trichostrongylus colubriformis* in ewes of different reproductive status. *International Journal for Parasitology*, **3**, 521–530.

PARKINS, J. J. & HOLMES, P. H. (1989). Effects of gastrointestinal helminth parasites on ruminant nutrition. *Nutrition Research Reviews*, **2**, 227–246.

PERNTHANER, A., COLE, S. A., MORRISON, L., GREEN, R., SHAW, R. J. & HEIN, W. R. (2006). Cytokine and antibody subclass responses in the intestinal lymph of sheep during repeated experimental infections with the nematode parasite *Trichostrongylus colubriformis*. *Veterinary Immunology and Immunopathology*, **114**, 135–148.

POPPI, D. P., MACRAE, J. C., BREWER, A. & COOP, R. L. (1986). Nitrogen transactions in the digestive tract of lambs exposed to the intestinal parasite, *Trichostrongylus colubriformis*. *British Journal of Nutrition*, **55**, 593–602.

RAMÍREZ-RESTREPO, C. A., BARRY, T. N., LÓPEZ-VILLALOBOS, N., KEMP, P. D. & MCNABB, W. C. (2004). Use of *Lotus corniculatus* containing condensed tannins to increase lamb and wool production under commercial dryland farming conditions without the use of anthelmintics. *Animal Feed Science and Technology*, **117**, 85–105.

ROBERTS, H. C., HARDIE, L. J., CHAPPELL, L. H. & MERCER, J. G. (1999). Parasite-induced anorexia: Leptin, insulin and corticosterone responses to infection with the nematode, *Nippostrongylus brasiliensis*. *Parasitology*, **118**, 117–123.

ROSEBY, F. B. (1973). Effects of *Trichostrongylus colubriformis* (Nematoda) on the nutrition and metabolism of sheep. 1. Feed intake, digestion, and utilisation. *Australian Journal of Agricultural Research*, **24**, 947–953.

ROWE, J. B., NOLAN, J. V., DE CHANEET, G. & TELENI, E. (1988). The effect of haemonchosis and blood loss into the abomasum on digestion in sheep. *British Journal of Nutrition*, **59**, 125–139.

SANDERSON, M. A., SODER, K. J., MULLER, L. D., KLEMENT, K. D., SKINNER, R. H. & GOSLEE, S. C. (2005). Forage mixture productivity and botanical composition in pastures grazed by dairy cattle. *Agronomy Journal*, **97**, 1465–1471.

STEEL, J. W., JONES, W. O. & SYMONS, L. E. A. (1982). Effects of a concurrent infection of *Trichostrongylus colubriformis* on the productivity and physiological and metabolic responses of lambs infected with *Ostertagia circumcincta*. *Australian Journal of Agricultural Research*, **33**, 131–140.

SUTHERLAND, I. A., MOEN, I. C. & LEATHWICK, D. M. (2002). Increased burdens of drug-resistant nematodes due to anthelmintic treatment. *Parasitology*, **125**, 375–381.

SUTTLE, N. F., KNOX, D. P., ANGUS, K. W., JACKSON, F. & COOP, R. L. (1992). Effects of dietary molybdenum on nematode and host during *Haemonchus contortus* infection in lambs. *Research in Veterinary Science*, **52**, 230–235.

SYKES, A. R. (2008). Manipulating host immunity to improve nematode parasite control – Quo vadit. *Parasite Immunology*, **30**, 71–77.

SYKES, A. R. & COOP, R. L. (1976). Intake and utilisation of food by growing lambs with parasitic damage to the small intestine caused by daily dosing with *Trichostrongylus colubriformis* larvae. *Journal of Agricultural Science*, **86**, 507–515.

SYKES, A. R. & GREER, A. W. (2003). Effects of parasitism on the nutrient economy of sheep: An overview. *Australian Journal of Experimental Agriculture*, **43**, 1393–1398.

SYMONS, L. E. & JONES, W. O. (1970). *Nematospiroides dubius, Nippostrongylus brasiliensis* and *Trichostrongylus colubriformis*: Protein digestion in infected mammals. *Experimental Parasitology*, **27**, 496–506.

SYMONS, L. E. A. & JONES, W. O. (1975). Skeletal muscle, liver and wool protein synthesis by sheep infected by the nematode *Trichostrongylus colubriformis*. *Australian Journal of Agricultural Research*, **26**, 1063–1072.

SYMONS, L. E. A. & JONES, W. O. (1983). Intestinal protein synthesis in guinea pigs infected with *Trichostrongylus colubriformis*. *International Journal for Parasitology*, **13**, 309–312.

TZAMALOUKAS, O., ATHANASIADOU, S., KYRIAZAKIS, I., HUNTLEY, J. F. & JACKSON, F. (2006). The effect of chicory (*Cichorium intybus*) and sulla (*Hedysarum coronarium*) on larval development and mucosal cell responses of growing lambs challenged with *Teladorsagia circumcincta*. *Parasitology*, **132**, 419–426.

TZAMALOUKAS, O., ATHANASIADOU, S., KYRIAZAKIS, I., JACKSON, F. & COOP, R. L. (2005). The consequences of short-term grazing of bioactive forages on established adult and incoming larvae populations of *Teladorsagia circumcincta* in lambs. *International Journal for Parasitology*, **35**, 329–335.

VAN HOUTERT, M. F. J. & SYKES, A. R. (1996). Implications of nutrition for the ability of ruminants to withstand gastrointestinal nematode infections. *International Journal for Parasitology*, **26**, 1151–1167.

VAN HOUTERT, M. F. J., BARGER, I. A., STEEL, J. W., WINDON, R. G. & EMERY, D. L. (1995). Effects of dietary protein intake on responses of young sheep to infection with *Trichostrongylus colubriformis*. *Veterinary Parasitology*, **56**, 163–180.

WAKELIN, D. (1996). *Immunity to Parasites: How Parasitic Infections are Controlled.* Cambridge University Press, England.

YU, F., BRUCE, L. A., CALDER, A. G. *et al.* (2000). Subclinical infection with the nematode *Trichostrongylus colubriformis* increases gastrointestinal tract leucine metabolism and reduces availability of leucine for other tissues. *Journal of Animal Science*, **78**, 380–390.

YU, F., BRUCE, L. A., COOP, R. L. & MACRAE, J. C. (1999). Losses of non-resorbed endogenous leucine from the intestine of lambs exposed to the intestinal parasite *Trichostrongylus colubriformis*. *Book of Abstracts of the VIIIth International Symposium on Protein Metabolism and Nutrition*, Aberdeen, p. 48.

11 Animal genetics and parasitism

The spectre of anthelmintic resistance has provided the impetus, and indirectly therefore the finance, for numerous long-term studies on the utility of animals which are either more resistant to gastrointestinal nematode (GIN) or maintain an acceptable level of productivity despite carrying significant parasite burdens. In addition to the effect of animal genotype on the pathology associated with the host–parasite relationship, selective breeding for 'host resistance' may offer the further advantage of limiting the success of the parasite life-cycle. In the case of the GIN infecting grazing ruminants, this is primarily through a reduced level of pasture contamination. Thus, not only may animals with a 'resistant genotype' harbour less GIN, but any other genotype present may receive a lower intensity of larval challenge.

Two major factors underpin the manipulation of animal genetics in parasite epizootiology. The first is based on the known variability in the host–parasite relationship between different livestock species or breeds, while the second is based on variability in the same criteria between animals within breeds.

Inter-species variability

Utilising the variability in the response to parasitism by farming particular species can hardly be considered as a perfect example of selective breeding. However, it is a useful, if extreme, example of using genotype to minimise the impact of parasitism on animal productivity. The most common example in livestock farming is mixed grazing of sheep and cattle; in this situation, each species acts as a net remover of L3 from pasture, thus reducing the level of challenge and putatively increasing productivity of the corresponding host species. While mostly regarded as a useful tactic, mixed grazing should still be considered carefully; recent research associates grazing cattle and sheep together with an increased prevalence of anthelmintic resistance (Chapter 8), while some parasite species may adapt to alternate host species or at least cause some degree of pathogenicity if L3 are ingested. It is also noted that the members of some species can be productive in areas unsuitable for others, whether this is due to parasitism or other factors such as climate (these are of course intimately connected). For example, in the far north of New Zealand, livestock farming is heavily dominated by cattle, primarily due to the twin threats of *Haemonchus contortus* and blowfly strike.

Within most farming situations, however, it is the variation in the response to GIN within species or breed, which has been manipulated in the attempts to improve productivity traits and to mitigate the negative consequences of parasitism. This manipulation is made possible because a significant proportion of the variability is genetically determined.

Inter-breed variability

For clarity, by using the term 'breed' we refer to differences between what are normally regarded as distinct populations which are able to reproduce. This is an important distinction as confusion may occur distinguishing between a breed and a species. For example, the two 'species' of cattle, *Bos taurus* and *Bos indicus*, members of which can have highly divergent responses to parasitism (Frisch *et al.*, 2000) are in fact able to inter-breed, and both are breeds of *B. taurus* (Figure 11.1).

Fortunately, there is less confusion amongst breeds of sheep and goats belonging to the same species (respectively, *Ovis aries* and *Capra hircus*). Presumably due to the greater resources available to geneticists in the developed world, by far, the greatest body of work on inter-breed differences in the response to GIN in small ruminants has been performed in sheep. A few examples of breed differences in various geographical regions are described below.

In Africa, the red maasai sheep breed has been demonstrated by a number of researchers to produce lower egg output than other breeds, while maintaining a higher packed cell volume (pcv) under challenge with *H. contortus*

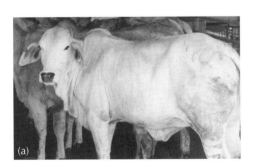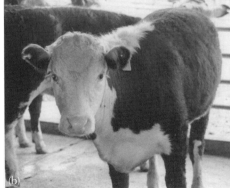

Figure 11.1 Brahmans (a) are typical examples of tropically adapted *Bos indicus* cattle, while the Hereford–Shorthorn (b) are typical examples of a temperate British-breed *Bos taurus*. Photos courtesy of Dave Swain and Tanya Robinson.

(Baker *et al.*, 2003; Mugambi *et al.*, 1996; Wanyangu *et al.*, 1997). However, it is noted, and will become a recurrent theme in this chapter, that this enhanced 'resistance' to GIN infection is associated with relatively depressed productivity (Baker *et al.*, 1999).

In South America, the Santa Ines sheep breed was shown to be relatively more resistant to GIN as reflected by lower egg counts and reduced drenching requirement (Amarante *et al.*, 2004), while the Barbados Blackbelly breed has also evolved the ability to maintain a higher pcv under challenge with *H. contortus* (Yazwinski *et al.*, 1980); in Europe, the Polish long-wool sheep produced three times fewer GIN eggs when compared to other breeds (Nowosad *et al.*, 2003). In terms of the relationship between egg count and productivity traits, a strong correlation has been observed in the Scottish blackface breed (Figure 11.2), implying an excellent potential for selective breeding from these animals (Stear *et al.*, 1996).

One of the more common sheep breeds, the Merino (Figure 11.3), is widely considered to be relatively susceptible to GIN infections, with periparturient ewes, for example, exhibiting a relatively profound and sustained loss of immunity (Donald *et al.*, 1982).

Significant breed differences in the response to GIN have been observed between goat populations. For example, Thai native goats maintained pcv under

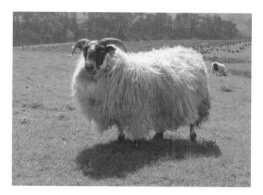

Figure 11.2   Scottish Blackface. Photo courtesy of Chris McComb.

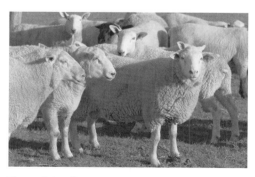

Figure 11.3   Merino. Photo © Mollypix, Dreamstime Royalty Free.

H. contortus challenge relative to Anglo-Nubian animals (and also displayed lower productivity) (Pralomkarn *et al.*, 1997), while the Small East African breed had relatively lower egg counts and higher pcv than other breeds – an effect particularly pronounced over the periparturient (Baker *et al.*, 1998).

As briefly mentioned above, *B. indicus* cattle, often referred to as tropically adapted, display a relatively greater resistance to a range of parasites. While most research has focussed on the reduced impact of ectoparasites such as the cattle tick *Rhipicephalus* (*Boophilus*) *microplus* on animal productivity relative to European or British breeds (Bianchin *et al.*, 2007; Gasparin *et al.*, 2007; Jonsson, 2006), these cattle, derived from Zebu populations, also have relatively lower GIN egg output as compared to temperate breeds (Frisch & O'Neill, 1998; Turner & Short, 1972) though this has not always been a consistent observation. In South America, for example, studies demonstrated that Aberdeen Angus calves appeared to be more resistant to GIN than Santa Gertrudis, a composite breed containing 75% *B. indicus* genetics (Suarez *et al.*, 1995). The use of cross-breeding between Zebu and temperate breeds has been viewed as a potentially fruitful area of research, as the resulting crosses often display increased resistance to disease relative to the temperate parents, while retaining a proportion of their relatively greater productivity (Frisch *et al.*, 2000). The negative correlations often observed between parasite resistance and various productivity parameters is an ongoing concern when selecting or breeding animals and is discussed more in detail below.

Intra-breed variability

The ability to relate the over-dispersion of parasite numbers with a heritable genetic component forms the basis of selective breeding for parasite resistance (Gray & Gill, 1993). However, given the large environmental influence on parameters such as worm burden and FEC, such experiments by necessity involve large numbers of animals and can take place over multiple breeding seasons. As an example, for an accurate estimation of genetic heritability to GIN infection in sheep, it is considered necessary to mate around 60 rams with around 1500 ewes, then follow the progeny to assess the level and impact of parasitism (Falconer, 1989).

The success or failure of any attempt at selective breeding is reliant upon an adequate level of genetic heritability. In basic terms, the higher the heritability of a given trait, the easier should be the process of selective breeding (at least in theory).

Heritability

The heritability of a trait refers to what proportion of the phenotypic variability of the trait (e.g. high vs. low FEC) is due to genetic factors as opposed to environmental factors. Thus, a low heritability indicates a poor correlation between genotype and phenotype, and vice versa.

In sheep and cattle, the heritability of FEC is regarded as moderately heritable and therefore a reasonable candidate for selective breeding. The majority of studies have estimated the heritability of FEC in these species as between 0.2 and 0.4 (Leighton *et al.*, 1989; Mackinnon *et al.*, 1991; Woolaston & Piper, 1996; Woolaston & Windon, 2001). This is deemed sufficiently high that breeding for reduced FEC, which can be considered as breeding for resistance to GIN, becomes a feasible strategy (Gray & Gill, 1993). One potential limiting factor is that heritability is relatively lower in young animals (Vagenas *et al.*, 2002; Woolaston & Piper, 1996); this is unsurprising, as reductions in FEC are at least partially associated with the development of immunity. On the positive side, however, is the observation that the heritability for reduced FEC is similar regardless of parasite species (Gruner *et al.*, 2004; Morris *et al.*, 2004).

Examples of breeding programmes utilising FEC include the Romney sheep selection lines in New Zealand, in which lines of animals were selected on the basis of both high and low egg output (Bisset & Morris, 1996; Morris *et al.*, 2000). The divergence in FEC between these sheep lines continued over a number of years until there was a 21-fold difference in egg output. In Australia, lines of Merino sheep have been selected for reduced FEC under challenge with *Trichostrongylus colubriformis* (Woolaston & Windon, 2001) and *H. contortus* (Woolaston *et al.*, 1990). While these various sheep resources have been primarily utilised for research purposes in both countries, a similar approach has been transferred to a farming context in New Zealand and Australia as the WormFEC (NZ) and Nemesis (Aust) animal breeding programmes.

In cattle, selective breeding experiments have been confined to studies of variability in FEC of individuals within herds subject to natural challenge. Unfortunately, the high cost of cattle relative to sheep (and goats) makes them too expensive for large-scale genetic analysis of artificial infections (Kloosterman *et al.*, 1992). Despite this, a number of studies have estimated heritability of resistance to GIN in cattle and found it to be sufficient for breeding purposes (0.29–0.60) (Frisch *et al.*, 2000; Henshall, 2004; Leighton *et al.*, 1989; Morris *et al.*, 2003; Seifert, 1971).

Resistance vs. productivity

A significant drawback in attempts to selectively breed animals with enhanced resistance is the common observation that associated with the resistance is a cost in another parameter. In the case of production animals, the relevant parameters are of course productivity based such as live-weight gain (Jonsson, 2006), wool (Eady *et al.*, 1998; McEwan *et al.*, 1995) and milk (Walawski, 1999) production. Breeding for resistance, at least in sheep, appears to be linked to an increased inflammatory reaction in the intestine (Bisset *et al.*, 2001; Shaw *et al.*, 1999); the obvious sign of this is greater breech soiling (or dags), which farmers certainly view as a negative association.

In intensive agriculture systems, particularly in areas in which survivability is assumed to be acceptably high, profit margins become the priority, and breeding programmes have to take a multi-trait approach to ensure that disease resistance does not come at too high a cost. Animal populations which have been developed under single-trait selection, such as the Romney sheep lines in New Zealand (Bisset & Morris, 1996), are excellent examples of the negative correlation between traits; selectively breeding from animals on the basis of reduced or increased FEC came at a significant cost in live-weight gain (Bisset & Morris, 1996). It should be noted that these animals were bred for experimental purposes only and as such were not required to remain competitive in a productive sense.

So, while it is possible to include disease resistance as one trait in a multiple-selection programme, it tends to lower the rate of genetic gain of the primary (in this case, disease resistance) trait (Eady *et al.*, 1998; McEwan *et al.*, 1995). One possible solution to this problem was the selection of animals which performed under challenge from parasites – in layman's terms, selecting those animals which were more capable of ignoring the impact of the infection. This trait became known as 'resilience'.

Resilience

What has become referred to as resilience is characterised by animals becoming hosts to 'normal' parasite burdens, while maintaining the ability to be productive in desired parameters (Baker *et al.*, 2003; Behnke *et al.*, 2006; Bisset *et al.*, 1994). A major driver of research into resilience was the observation that 'resistance to infection' did not equate to 'resistance to disease' (Bisset *et al.*, 1996). By testing, over a 3-year period, 14,000 progeny of 213 different Romney rams for resilience, the trait was discovered to have a moderate degree of heritability. The criteria the study took into account were each individual's drench requirements, growth rate, dag-score, FEC and fleeceweight. Overall, the study demonstrated that selecting for resilience would result in animals which had higher growth rates and less problem with dags when left undrenched on infected pasture. Unfortunately, resilience is less heritable (and therefore more difficult to select for) than resistance, and is heavily influenced by environmental factors such as the quantity/quality of available nutrition (Bisset *et al.*, 2001; Knox *et al.*, 2006; Louvandini *et al.*, 2006) and the intensity of larval challenge. The influence of the latter parameter is quite obvious – while in most cases, the heritability is estimated to be between 0.1 and 0.19 (Bisset *et al.*, 1996), under high parasite challenge, the figure increased to between 0.24 and 0.53 (Bisset *et al.*, 2001).

There have been contrasting reports concerning the relationship between resistance and resilience. While an Australian study on the genetics of resistance and resilience to *H. contortus* in Merino sheep detected a positive correlation between the two traits, the NZ study of Bisset and Morris (1996) found no correlation to mixed parasite challenge in Romney sheep. These authors make the point that given the independence of the traits, it is likely that any farmer wishing to breed for both traits would have to do so separately.

It should be noted that resilience and resistance may be more or less valuable depending on the particular farming situation. An obvious example is selecting for animals in areas with a high risk of *H. contortus* infections. With this haematophagous, pathogenic parasite, an ability to remain productive despite the presence of similar worm burdens present in unselected animals is unlikely to confer a significant advantage. The strategy in this situation, therefore, would be to select for resistance.

While breeding for resilience may find a niche in livestock production systems, it does have a significant drawback. While resilient animals may maintain productivity despite harbouring worm burdens, they do continue to produce eggs and therefore contaminate pasture. This, of course, will be more or less relevant depending on epidemiological factors such as climate (Chapter 3).

Pasture contamination, resistance and resilience

The number and viability of L3 on pasture, and the numbers actually ingested by a suitable host, are major factors in the epizootiology of the GIN – not just in terms of pathology but also the development of immunity and subsequent pasture contamination by progeny. Thus, while selective breeding can easily be considered as dealing just with the 'host', this is clearly not the case. As an example, the observation that resilience is more heritable under high larval challenge (Bisset *et al.*, 2001) establishes the fact that the response of the host and the 'parasite' are inextricably linked.

It is useful when determining the impact of increased resistance or resilience on parasite populations to consider the host as being in the middle of a process of larval challenge and subsequent egg production. Within a given population, a relatively 'resistant' host would be expected to ingest an average number of L3 but produce relatively less eggs in faeces than a more 'susceptible' animal. The overall pasture contamination from a flock/herd with a natural distribution of resistance may not change by having a small number of resistant hosts in the population. This would be the expected outcome in any commercial breeding situation and would mask the impact of increased resistance in the selected animals (Bisset *et al.*, 2001). In contrast, when resistant animals are grazed by themselves, pasture contamination and therefore subsequent ingestion of L3 can be significantly reduced, leading to improved productivity (Bisset *et al.*, 1997). By definition, this is unlikely to occur with 'resilient' hosts.

In summary, while both resistance and resilience can have advantages in pastoral livestock management systems, it appears that neither trait is exactly what farmers desire; ideally, what is required are animals which are productive despite parasite challenge and which pass out less eggs to contaminate pasture – or 'resistant + resilient'.

Markers for resistance and resilience

The most common phenotypic measurement used so far in selective breeding for resistance to the GIN is FEC, with, obviously, lower FEC equating to greater resistance and vice versa. As measuring FEC on two occasions during a grazing season provides a higher measure of heritability (e.g. 0.2 vs. 0.35) (Morris *et al.*, 1995), this can be used to accelerate the rate of genetic gain.

Despite its obvious success, there are a number of potential drawbacks with the use of FEC as a phenotypic marker, not least the potential negative associations with productivity parameters. There is a requirement, at least in some conditions, to allow FEC in lambs to reach a trigger level (in New Zealand, a figure of 800 eggs/g faeces is recommended) to ensure robust statistical analysis. This is certainly higher than many farmers would be comfortable with, and there will doubtless be a cost in the lost productivity of the animals. Any selective breeding programme should ideally include all available animals; unfortunately, another drawback of FEC is that a percentage of animals, which may be as high as 10%, have no faeces on any given sampling date. There is a potential, therefore, of missing valuable individuals, although repeat sampling should minimise this risk. Finally, but importantly, many farmers do not like taking faecal samples – regardless of host species. For these various reasons, much research effort in recent years has gone in to finding an adequate, or improved, marker for resistance/resilience to GIN. These have either concentrated on phenotypic markers (like FEC), in which a measurement of a trait can be related to resistance/resilience in animals under challenge with parasites, or to genotypic markers, in which specific portions of DNA can similarly be related to resistance/resilience.

Phenotypic markers

In addition to FEC, a number of potential phenotypic markers have been investigated to assist in selective breeding programmes. Many of these have been related to immune responsiveness, unsurprisingly given the impact of the acquired immune system on parasite resistance (Gray *et al.*, 1992).

A number of anti-parasite antibodies (Ab) have been assessed for their utility as markers. For example, IgG1, IgE and IgM isotypes specific for antigens of *T. colubriformis* were shown to be positively correlated with FEC in the New Zealand Romney selection line sheep (Bisset & Morris, 1996; Douch *et al.*, 1996; Shaw *et al.*, 1999).

It is worth noting, however, that the levels of IgE were negatively correlated with the severity of breech soiling, indicating that while FEC may be lower, this appears to have come at the expense of increased intestinal inflammation (Shaw *et al.*, 1999). In sheep, production of the Ab isotype most intimately associated with intestinal mucosal immune responses, IgA, has also been positively associated with increased resistance to GIN (Martinez-Valladares *et al.*, 2005; Stear *et al.*, 1999; Strain *et al.*, 2002) and has promise as a phenotypic marker (Beraldi *et al.*, 2008). Indeed, recent work in New Zealand has demonstrated that measuring IgA to a nematode antigen in the saliva of lambs is an excellent phenotypic marker for nematode 'resistance' (Shaw, unpublished). This saliva antibody test selects animals which have reduced FEC but which appear to have none of the negative consequences commonly encountered when breeding for resistance. Furthermore, the method overcomes such obstacles associated with FEC such as the requirement to allow egg counts to elevate to significant levels, the return of non-samples and the resistance of farmers to perform faecal sampling.

The potential array of phenotypic markers in cattle is slightly more complex than in sheep. While the levels of IgG1 and IgG2 against *Ostertagia ostertagi* in serum have been shown to be heritable traits, those of anti-*O. ostertagi* IgA and IgM were not (Gasbarre *et al.*, 1990). In contrast, IgA against *C. oncophora* antigens have been shown to be significantly higher in resistant than in susceptible cattle (Bricarello *et al.*, 2008). This apparent contradiction may result from the inherent variability in egg counts from *O. ostertagi*, as opposed to a lack of association between IgA levels and host resistance (Kloosterman *et al.*, 1992).

Genotypic markers

While phenotypic markers reflect the response of animals to parasitism, and may therefore be powerful tools for marker-assisted selection, they do suffer from a requirement that animals are subject to parasitism, with the associated risk of losses in productivity. This would be largely overcome by the identification of changes in the DNA sequence of animals, which could be consistently correlated with the desired trait. As such a difference is 'hard-wired' into the genome, it can be detected in animals at any age. The probability that differences in the genome of phenotypically divergent livestock occur seems likely, given the observed heritability of traits such as FEC.

A number of studies have successfully detected differences in genes from the major histocompatibility complex region on chromosome 20, which are associated with the phenotypic response to GIN parasitism (Buitkamp *et al.*, 1996; Charon *et al.*, 2002; Paterson *et al.*, 1998; Sayers *et al.*, 2005). However, the highly polymorphic nature of this region of the genome, which has over 80 alleles, makes it unlikely that these genes will be suitable markers for GIN resistance (Sayers & Sweeney, 2005).

Given the inherent technical difficulties in identifying individual genes associated with parasite resistance, most research has involved the identification of broader areas of the genome; for obvious reasons, these regions are known as quantitative trait loci (QTL). The search for QTL for parasite resistance utilises known segregation in sires to detect differences in their progeny. For example, a sire produced from a mating of known resistant and susceptible parents is presumed to have genes for both traits. The progeny of this sire are subsequently tested for phenotypic divergence in FEC; this information is then used to detect any associated differences in the genome of divergent animals (Crawford *et al.*, 2006). A number of studies have attempted to identify QTL for GIN resistance in sheep. A study in Merinos derived from crossing divergent selection lines and artificially challenged with *T. colubriformis* failed to detect any QTL associated with the trait of interest, although there were indications of a difference at the chromosome level (Beh *et al.*, 2002). Subsequently, another study in Merinos, this time challenged on two occasions with *H. contortus*, was successful in detecting QTL, although their location could not be determined (Marshall *et al.*, 2004). A similar result was obtained in a study which crossed two sheep breeds with known divergence in their response to parasites (the relatively more resistant Indonesian thin tail and the relatively more susceptible Merino) and challenged twice with *H. contortus*. As before, QTL were identified, but their location was not determined (Raadsma *et al.*, 2002). Two studies on divergent sheep subject to natural challenge in the field were more successful in identifying and locating QTL for GIN resistance. The first was performed in Scottish Blackface sheep and identified a number of QTL on chromosomes 2, 3, 14 and 20 associated with resistance to various GIN species (Davies *et al.*, 2006). The second study used sires derived from crossing rams from resistant and susceptible lines of Romney sheep with Coopworth ewes, and successfully identified six QTL, four of which were associated with FEC and two with aspects of the anti-parasite immune response. However, only one of these QTL, on chromosome 8, was correlated with a measure of parasite resistance (Crawford *et al.*, 2006). The high cost of such studies, and the relatively limited success in locating QTL correlated with GIN resistance, suggest there may be more efficient methods of detecting genotypic differences associated with the desired trait. Recent developments in molecular genetics have enabled high-throughput sequencing of regions of the genome, which enables the detection of single nucleotide changes. These changes are known as single nucleotide polymorphisms (SNP) (Crawford *et al.*, 2006; Slate *et al.*, 2008), and the technology is available to rapidly compare large numbers of SNP in large numbers of divergent phenotypes/genotypes, and may provide a much more efficient method of detecting genotypic markers for GIN resistance.

Genetics, worm control and resistance management

Current, and indeed recent, recommendations which attempt to find an acceptable balance between levels of worm control with little impact on animal productivity while minimising selection or anthelmintic resistance ensure that animals continue to graze contaminated pasture. These include the managed use of refugia and targeted or selective drenching of livestock (Leathwick *et al.*, 2008; Waghorn *et al.*, 2007, 2008). These management options would be helped considerably by the selection of animals which are better able to withstand the effects of ingesting parasites.

References

AMARANTE, A. F. T., BRICARELLO, P. A., ROCHA, R. A. & GENNARI, S. M. (2004). Resistance of Santa Ines, Suffolk and Ile de France sheep to naturally acquired gastrointestinal nematode infections. *Veterinary Parasitology*, **120**, 91–106.

BAKER, R. L., MWAMACHI, D. M., AUDHO, J. O., ADUDA, E. O. & THORPE, W. (1998). Resistance of Galla and small East African goats in the sub-humid tropics to gastrointestinal nematode infections and the peri-parturient rise in faecal egg counts. *Veterinary Parasitology*, 79, 53–64.

BAKER, R. L., MWAMACHI, D. M., AUDHO, J. O., ADUDA, E. O. & THORPE, W. (1999). Genetic resistance to gastrointestinal nematode parasites in Red Maasai, Dorper and Red Maasai × Dorper ewes in the sub-humid tropics. *Animal Science*, 69, 335–344.

BAKER, R. L., NAGDA, S., RODRIGUEZ-ZAS, S. L. *et al.* (2003). Resistance and resilience to gastro-intestinal nematode parasites and relationships with productivity of Red Maasai, Dorper and Red Maasai × Dorper crossbred lambs in the sub-humid tropics. *Animal Science*, 76, 119–136.

BEH, K. J., HULME, D. J., CALLAGHAN, M. J. *et al.* (2002). A genome scan for quantitative trait loci affecting resistance to *Trichostrongylus colubriformis* in sheep. *Animal Genetics*, 33, 97–106.

BEHNKE, J. M., CHIEJINA, S. N., MUSONGONG, G. A. *et al.* (2006). Naturally occurring variability in some phenotypic markers and correlates of haemoncho-tolerance in West African dwarf goats in a subhumid zone of Nigeria. *Veterinary Parasitology*, 141, 107–121.

BERALDI, D., CRAIG, B. H., BISHOP, S. C., HOPKINS, J. & PEMBERTON, J. M. (2008). Phenotypic analysis of host-parasite interactions in lambs infected with *Teladorsagia circumcincta*. *International Journal for Parasitology*, 38, 1567–1577.

BIANCHIN, I., CATTO, J. B., KICHEL, A. N., TORRES, R. A. A. & HONER, M. R. (2007). The effect of the control of endo- and ectoparasites on weight gains in crossbred cattle (*Bos taurus taurus x Bos taurus indicus*) in the central region of Brazil. *Tropical Animal Health and Production*, 39, 287–296.

BISSET, S. A. & MORRIS, C. A. (1996). Feasibility and implications of breeding sheep for resilience to nematode challenge. *International Journal for Parasitology*, 26, 857–868.

BISSET, S. A., MORRIS, C. A., MCEWAN, J. C. & VLASSOFF, A. (2001). Breeding sheep in New Zealand that are less reliant on anthelmintics to maintain health and productivity. *New Zealand Veterinary Journal*, 49, 236–246.

BISSET, S. A., MORRIS, C. A., SQUIRE, D. R., HICKEY, S. M. & WHEELER, M. (1994). Genetics of resilience to nematode parasites in Romney sheep. *New Zealand Journal of Agricultural Research*, 37, 521–534.

BISSET, S. A., VLASSOFF, A., DOUCH, P. G. C., JONAS, W. E., WEST, C. J. & GREEN, R. S. (1996). Nematode burdens and immunological responses following natural challenge in Romney lambs selectively bred for low or high faecal worm egg count. *Veterinary Parasitology*, 61, 249–263.

BISSET, S. A., VLASSOFF, A., WEST, C. J. & MORRISON, L. (1997). Epidemiology of nematodosis in Romney lambs selectively bred for resistance or susceptibility to nematode infection. *Veterinary Parasitology*, 70, 255–269.

BRICARELLO, P. A., ZAROS, L. G., COUTINHO, L. L. *et al.* (2008). Immunological responses and cytokine gene expression analysis to *Cooperia punctata* infections in resistant and susceptible Nelore cattle. *Veterinary Parasitology*, 155, 95–103.

BUITKAMP, J., FILMETHER, P., STEAR, M. J. & EPPLEN, J. T. (1996). Class I and class II major histocompatibility complex alleles are associated with faecal egg counts following natural, predominantly *Ostertagia circumcincta* infection. *Parasitology Research*, 82, 693–696.

CHARON, K. M., MOSKWA, B., RUTKOWSKI, R., GRUSZCZYNSKA, J. & SWIDEREK, W. (2002). Microsatellite polymorphism in DRB1 gene (MHC class II) and its relation to nematode faecal egg count in Polish Heath Sheep. *Journal of Animal and Feed Sciences*, **11**, 47–58.

CRAWFORD, A. M., PATERSON, K. A., DODDS, K. G. *et al.* (2006). Discovery of quantitative trait loci for resistance to parasitic nematode infection in sheep: I. Analysis of outcross pedigrees. *BMC Genomics*, **7**, 178.

DAVIES, G., STEAR, M. J., BENOTHMAN, M. *et al.* (2006). Quantitative trait loci associated with parasitic infection in Scottish Blackface sheep. *Heredity*, **96**, 252–258.

DONALD, A. D., MORLEY, F. H. W. & WALLER, P. J. (1982). Effects of reproduction, genotype and anthelmintic treatment of ewes on *Ostertagia* spp. populations. *International Journal for Parasitology*, **12**, 403–411.

DOUCH, P. G. C., GREEN, R. S., MORRIS, C. A., MCEWAN, J. C. & WINDON, R. G. (1996). Phenotypic markers for selection of nematode-resistant sheep. *International Journal for Parasitology*, **26**, 899–911.

EADY, S. J., WOOLASTON, R. R., LEWER, R. P., RAADSMA, H. W., SWAN, A. A. & PONZONI, R. W. (1998). Resistance to nematode parasites in Merino sheep: Correlation with production traits. *Australian Journal of Agricultural Research*, **49**, 1201–1211.

FALCONER, D. S. (1989). *An Introduction to Quantitative Genetics*, 3rd edition, Longman, Harlow.

FRISCH, J. E. & O'NEILL, C. J. (1998). Comparative evaluation of beef cattle breeds of African, European and Indian origins. 2. Resistance to cattle ticks and gastrointestinal nematodes. *Animal Science*, **67**, 39–48.

FRISCH, J. E., O'NEILL, C. J. & KELLY, M. J. (2000). Using genetics to control cattle parasites – The Rockhampton experience. *International Journal for Parasitology*, **30**, 253–264.

GASBARRE, L. C., LEIGHTON, E. A. & DAVIES, C. J. (1990). Genetic control of immunity to gastrointestinal nematodes of cattle. *Veterinary Parasitology*, **37**, 257–272.

GASPARIN, G., MIYATA, M., COUTINHO, L. L. *et al.* (2007). Mapping of quantitative trait loci controlling tick [*Rhipicephalus (Boophilus) microplus*] resistance on bovine chromosomes 5, 7 and 14. *Animal Genetics*, **38**, 453–459.

GRAY, G. D., BARGER, I. A., LE JAMBRE, L. F. & DOUCH, P. G. C. (1992). Parasitological and immunological responses of genetically resistant Merino sheep on pastures contaminated with parasitic nematodes. *International Journal for Parasitology*, **22**, 417–425.

GRAY, G. D. & GILL, H. S. (1993). Host genes, parasites and parasitic infections. *International Journal for Parasitology*, **23**, 485–494.

GRUNER, L., BOUIX, J. & BRUNEL, J. C. (2004). High genetic correlation between resistance to *Haemonchus contortus* and to *Trichostrongylus colubriformis* in Inra 401 sheep. *Veterinary Parasitology*, **119**, 51–58.

HENSHALL, J. M. (2004). A genetic analysis of parasite resistance traits in a tropically adapted line of *Bos taurus*. *Australian Journal of Agricultural Research*, **55**, 1109–1116.

JONSSON, N. N. (2006). The productivity effects of cattle tick (*Boophilus microplus*) infestation on cattle, with particular reference to *Bos indicus* cattle and their crosses. *Veterinary Parasitology*, **137**, 1–10.

KLOOSTERMAN, A., PARMENTIER, H. K. & PLOEGER, H. W. (1992). Breeding cattle and sheep for resistance to gastrointestinal nematodes. *Parasitology Today*, **8**, 330–335.

KNOX, M. R., TORRES-ACOSTA, J. F. J. & AGUILAR-CABALLERO, A. J. (2006). Exploiting the effect of dietary supplementation of small ruminants on resilience and resistance against gastrointestinal nematodes. *Veterinary Parasitology*, **139**, 385–393.

LEATHWICK, D. M., MILLER, C. M., ATKINSON, D. S., HAACK, N. A., WAGHORN, T. S. & OLIVER, A. M. (2008). Managing anthelmintic resistance: Untreated adult ewes as a source of unselected parasites, and their role in reducing parasite populations. *New Zealand Veterinary Journal*, **56**, 184–195.

LEIGHTON, E. A., MURRELL, K. D. & GASBARRE, L. C. (1989). Evidence for genetic control of nematode egg-shedding rates in calves. *Journal of Parasitology*, **75**, 498–504.

LOUVANDINI, H., VELOSO, C. F. M., PALUDO, G. R., DELL'PORTO, A., GENNARI, S. M. & MCMANUS, C. M. (2006). Influence of protein supplementation on the resistance and resilience on young hair sheep naturally infected with gastrointestinal nematodes during rainy and dry seasons. *Veterinary Parasitology*, **137**, 103–111.

MACKINNON, M. J., MEYER, K. & HETZEL, D. J. S. (1991). Genetic variation and covariation for growth, parasite resistance and heat tolerance in tropical cattle. *Livestock Production Science*, **27**, 105–122.

MARSHALL, K., VAN DER WERF, J. H. J., MADDOX, J. F. *et al.* (2004). A genome scan for quantitative trait loci for resistance to the gastrointestinal parasite *Haemonchus contortus* in sheep. *Proceedings Association for the Advancement of Animal Breeding and Genetics*, **16**, 115–1118.

MARTINEZ-VALLADARES, M., VARA-DEL RIO, M. P., CRUZ-ROJO, M. A. & ROJO-VAZQUEZ, F. A. (2005). Genetic resistance to *Teladorsagia circumcincta*: IgA and parameters at slaughter in Churra sheep. *Parasite Immunology*, **27**, 213–218.

MCEWAN, J. C., GREEN, R. S., DOUCH, P. G. C. *et al.* (1995). Genetic estimates for parasite resistance traits in sheep and their correlations with production traits. *New Zealand Journal of Zoology*, **22**, 177.

MORRIS, C. A., BISSET, S. A., VLASSOFF, A., WEST, C. J. & WHEELER, M. (2004). Genetic parameters for *Nematodirus* spp. egg counts in Romney lambs in New Zealand. *Animal Science*, **79**, 33–39.

MORRIS, C. A., GREEN, R. S., CULLEN, N. G. & HICKEY, S. M. (2003). Genetic and phenotypic relationships among faecal egg count, anti-nematode antibody level and live weight in Angus cattle. *Animal Science*, **76**, 167–174.

MORRIS, C. A., VLASSOFF, A., BISSET, S. A. *et al.* (2000). Continued selection of Romney sheep for resistance or susceptibility to nematode infection: Estimates of direct and correlated responses. *Animal Science*, **70**, 17–27.

MORRIS, C. A., WATSON, T. G., BISSET, S. A., VLASSOFF, A. & DOUCH, P. G. C. (eds). (1995). *Breeding Sheep in New Zealand for Resistance or Resilience to Nematode Parasites*, Australian Centre for International Agricultural Research, Canberra.

MUGAMBI, J. M., WANYANGU, S. W., BAIN, R. K., OWANGO, M. O., DUNCAN, J. L. AND STEAR, M. J. (1996). Response of Dorper and red Maasai lambs to trickle *Haemonchus contortus* infections. *Research in Veterinary Science*, **61**, 218–221.

NOWOSAD, B., GRUNER, L., SKALSKA, M., FUDALEWICZ-NIEMCZYK, W., MOLENDA, K. & KORNAS, S. (2003). Genetic difference in natural resistance to gastrointestinal nematodes in Polish long-wool, Blackface and Weisses Alpenschaf sheep. *Acta Parasitologica*, **48**, 131–134.

PATERSON, S., WILSON, K. & PEMBERTON, J. M. (1998). Major histocompatibility complex variation associated with juvenile survival and parasite resistance in a large unmanaged ungulate population (*Ovis aries* L.). *Proceedings of the National Academy of Sciences of the United States of America*, **95**, 3714–3719.

PRALOMKARN, W., PANDEY, V. S., NGAMPONGSAI, W. *et al.* (1997). Genetic resistance of three genotypes of goats to experimental infection with *Haemonchus contortus*. *Veterinary Parasitology*, **68**, 79–90.

RAADSMA, H. W., MARGAWATI, E. T., PIEDRAFITA, D. *et al.* (2002). Towards molecular genetic characterisation of high resistance to internal parasites in Indonesian thin tail sheep. *Proceedings of the 7th World Congress of Genetic Applications to Livestock Production*, 13–19, Montpellier, INRA France.

SAYERS, G., GOOD, B., HANRAHAN, J. P., RYAN, M., ANGLES, J. M. & SWEENEY, T. (2005). Major histocompatibility complex DRB1 gene: Its role in nematode resistance in Suffolk and Texel sheep breeds. *Parasitology*, **131**, 403–409.

SAYERS, G. & SWEENEY, T. (2005). Gastrointestinal nematode infection in sheep – A review of the alternatives to anthelmintics in parasite control. *Animal Health Research Reviews/Conference of Research Workers in Animal Diseases*, **6**, 159–171.

SEIFERT, G. W. (1971). Ecto- and endoparasitic effects on the growth rates of Zebu crossbred and British cattle in the field. *Australian Journal of Agricultural Research*, **22**, 839–850.

SHAW, R. J., MORRIS, C. A., GREEN, R. S. *et al.* (1999). Genetic and phenotypic relationships among *Trichostrongylus colubriformis*-specific immunoglobulin E, anti-*Trichostrongylus colubriformis* antibody, immunoglobulin G1, faecal egg count and body weight traits in grazing Romney lambs. *Livestock Production Science*, **58**, 25–32.

SLATE, J., GRATTEN, J., BERALDI, D., STAPLEY, J., HALE, M. & PEMBERTON, J. M. (2009). Gene mapping in the wild with SNPs: Guidelines and future directions. *Genetica*, **136**, 1–11.

STEAR, M., PARK, M. & BISHOP, S. (1996). The key components of resistance to *Ostertagia circumcincta* in lambs. *Parasitology Today*, **12**, 438–441.

STEAR, M. J., STRAIN, S. AND BISHOP, S. C. (1999). How lambs control infection with *Ostertagia circumcincta*. *Veterinary Immunology and Immunopathology*, **72**, 213–218.

STRAIN, S. A. J., BISHOP, S. C., HENDERSON, N. G. *et al.* (2002). The genetic control of IgA activity against *Teladorsagia circumcincta* and its association with parasite resistance in naturally infected sheep. *Parasitology*, **124**, 545–552.

SUAREZ, V. H., BUSETTI, M. R. & LORENZO, R. M. (1995). Comparative effects of nematode infection on *Bos taurus* and *Bos indicus* crossbred calves grazing on Argentina's Western Pampas. *Veterinary Parasitology*, **58**, 263–271.

TURNER, H. G. & SHORT, A. J. (1972). Effects of field infestations of gastrointestinal helminths and of the cattle tick (*Boophilus microplus*) on growth of three breeds of cattle. *Australian Journal of Agricultural Research*, **23**, 177–193.

VAGENAS, D., JACKSON, F., RUSSEL, A. J. F., MERCHANT, M., WRIGHT, I. A. & BISHOP, S. C. (2002). Genetic control of resistance to gastrointestinal parasites in crossbred cashmere-producing goats: Responses to selection, genetic parameters and relationships with production traits. *Animal Science*, **74**, 199–208.

WAGHORN, T. S., LEATHWICK, D. M., MILLER, C. M. & ATKINSON, D. S. (2008). Brave or gullible: Testing the concept that leaving susceptible parasites in refugia will slow the development of anthelmintic resistance. *New Zealand Veterinary Journal*, **56**, 158–163.

WAGHORN, T. S., LEATHWICK, D. M., MILLER, C. M. & ATKINSON, S. (2007). Strategies for management of anthelmintic resistance in New Zealand. *New Zealand Journal of Zoology*, **34**, 156–156.

WALAWSKI, K. (1999). Genetic aspects of mastitis resistance in cattle. *Journal of Applied Genetics*, **40**, 117–128.

WANYANGU, S. W., MUGAMBI, J. M., BAIN, R. K., DUNCAN, J. L., MURRAY, M. AND STEAR, M. J. (1997). Response to artificial and subsequent natural infection with *Haemonchus contortus* in Red Maasai and Dorper ewes. *Veterinary Parasitology*, **69**, 275–282.

WOOLASTON, R. R., BARGER, I. A. & PIPER, L. R. (1990). Response to helminth infection of sheep selected for resistance to *Haemonchus contortus*. *International Journal for Parasitology*, **20**, 1015–1018.

WOOLASTON, R. R. & PIPER, L. R. (1996). Selection of Merino sheep for resistance to *Haemonchus contortus*: Genetic variation. *Animal Science*, **62**, 451–460.

WOOLASTON, R. R. & WINDON, R. G. (2001). Selection of sheep for response to *Trichostrongylus colubriformis* larvae: Genetic parameters. *Animal Science*, **73**, 41–48.

YAZWINSKI, T. A., GOODE, L., MONCOL, D. J., MORGAN, G. W. & LINNERUD, A. C. (1980). *Haemonchus contortus* resistance in straightbred and crossbred Barbados Blackbelly sheep. *Journal of Animal Science*, **51**, 279–284.

12 The immune response to parasites

Manipulating the host immune response to reduce the impact of parasites on productivity or disease state has been a major research objective for many years. Leaving aside the selection of animals with relatively greater immunity to infection/disease, which was addressed in Chapter 11, such immune manipulation is traditionally thought of in terms of vaccine development. Most animals are capable of mounting an effective acquired anti-parasite immune response to most nematode infections, which provides the assumption that such immunity can be artificially stimulated (Emery *et al.*, 1993; Miller, 1996).

Despite significant effort over many years, there are currently no suitable vaccines available for use against gastrointestinal nematodes (GINs). The reasons for this are many and varied. Certainly, the success of various anthelmintic families and the relatively small size of any potential commercial market are contributing factors. We would argue, however, that by far, the greatest contributing factor is a lack of understanding of the host–parasite relationship, and therefore its effective manipulation.

There are many obstacles to overcome, if a fuller and more fundamental understanding of the interaction between GINs and the host immune system is to become possible. Firstly, there is the apparent lack of track record of the scientific establishment, which is a significant disadvantage to obtaining enough funding to address the many unanswered questions. In no particular order of importance, and by no means exhaustive, these include the following.

1   How do worms know which host species they have been ingested by (and which organ they are in)?
2   How does the invaded, potential host recognise the parasite?
3   Does the parasite alter its environment within the host? There is limited evidence that this is the case for GINs of livestock, although there is a significant body of work pointing to parasite-induced alterations of immunity in filarial infections.

4 How do parasites survive and/or replicate in such a potentially hostile environment?

Finally, and perhaps of greatest relevance is:

5 How do hosts kill parasites?

There are a number of valid excuses for the relative lack of progress in defining the relevant host–parasite relationships.

First, the field has to encompass several species of both host and parasite. Second, individual parasite species inhabit significantly different niches in any given host species. Third, wide divergence in immune status arises due to both host genotype and phenotype (Pernthaner *et al.*, 2005). Fourth, which of the vast array of host responses to infection are actually protective and which are merely associated with either infection or damage – or both? Fifth, any proper investigation of the host–parasite relationship (regardless of host or parasite species) requires a truly multi-disciplinary approach to long-term studies of alterations in both host and parasite from before first exposure through the period of immune acquisition to the expression of a protective response. Such studies should utilise the skills of, at least, parasitologists, statisticians, immunologists, physiologists and molecular biologists. Sixth, overriding all these factors is the enormously complex continuum of host–parasite interactions, and the severe technical and financial limitations inherent in the study of parasites inhabiting the gastrointestinal tract of large animals. Seventh, the array of reagents available to researchers working on livestock parasites is limited as compared to those, e.g., mice, or indeed humans. It is possible that this problem may be overcome in the near future with the rapid changes occurring in molecular techniques and bioinformatics.

Despite so many unanswered questions, there is an enormous and complex body of literature which describes the effect of parasite challenge on the development of the vast array of immune phenotypes. In addition to the impact of the development of resistance to infection as mediated by immune responses, there are very many accounts of the effect of parasite challenge or infection on individual components of the immune system.

It would be impossible to do justice to this extensive literature, and research effort, in one chapter of this book. However, what has been attempted is an overview of immunoparasitology research, and comments on key findings, past failures and future opportunities.

Evolution of the host–parasite relationship

Alterations in grazing strategies resulting from domestication may have significantly affected the way animals see and therefore respond to GIN challenge. For example, the difference between goats and sheep is informative: while goats are commonly considered to be highly susceptible to GINs, this may in fact not be strictly correct. These animals, which evolved as browsers, and would therefore have had little contact with parasite larvae on pasture, can harbour relatively large worm burdens with little evident pathology (Hoste *et al.*, 2008). However, there does appear to be a threshold over which serious pathology occurs. Together, these characteristics suggest that goats have evolved a resilient, rather than susceptible phenotype.

Grazing ruminants, however, have evolved in a much closer association with GIN, although the extent of the parasite challenge has changed dramatically since the introduction of broad-spectrum anthelmintics. This development resulted in two major changes to livestock farming. First, stocking density could be increased significantly as a result of improved parasite control and second, animals could now be selectively bred, whether deliberately or not, for increased productivity, with an associated loss in immune capability. While this is almost certainly occurring in cattle, the effect of breeding for live-weight gain is most obviously seen in sheep. As an example, it is suggested that in the New Zealand national sheep flock, 'resistance to parasites' is decreasing on an annual basis (http://www.sil.co.nz/Latest-reports/ACE-reports.aspx). In a relatively short period of time, intensive grazing practices have resulted in production systems in which regular drenching is necessary on production if not welfare grounds.

Despite the shift in balance between productivity and immunity, it is obvious that grazing animals in most cases continue to develop an effective immunity to GIN. Not surprisingly, however, there is no 'one size fits all' process through which this occurs, given both host and parasite variability.

Immunity and GIN population dynamics

As a general rule, the rate of development of acquired immunity depends to a significant degree on the intensity of larval challenge (Dobson *et al.*, 1990b). There are, however, significant differences between parasite species. For example, in sheep, an effective sterile immunity develops following continued challenge with the sheep's small intestinal species *Trichostrongylus colubriformis*. This process occurs in reasonably discrete steps: after 5–7 weeks, incoming larvae become unable to establish; worm fecundity is then depressed by 10–12 weeks; and resident adult worms are expelled by 16–20 weeks (Dobson *et al.*, 1992). The immunity to *T. colubriformis*, described somewhat simplistically, develops against larval challenge first, before expelling or killing the established adult worm burden. The opposite appears to be true, e.g., the abomasal parasite *Teladorsagia circumcincta*, in which immunity develops first against the resident adults that are expelled after a period of residence, which allows the maturation of ingested or arrested L3 and L4; this is followed by the development of a significant, if not necessarily sterile, immunity to ingested larvae (Dobson *et al.*, 1992).

Larval challenge alone, in animals treated with prophylactic anthelmintics to prevent further worm development, results in a reduced but observable level of immunity to subsequent challenge. Two experiments were conducted in which L3 of either *T. circumcincta* (Sutherland *et al.*, 2000) or *T. colubriformis* (Sutherland *et al.*, 1999a) were given to lambs previously administered CRCs. After several weeks of challenge, exposure to L3 in the presence of drug either reduced subsequent establishment of larvae (Sutherland *et al.*, 2000) or resulted in an increase in immunological parameters intermediate between unchallenged and immune animals (Sutherland *et al.*, 1999a).

The immune phenotype

Most of the remainder of this chapter is devoted to immune responses against GIN in sheep; this is largely due to the greater volume of work performed in this particular host species. The research that has been performed in cattle infected with GIN, primarily in *Cooperia oncophora* infections (Kanobana *et al.*, 2002, 2003), largely agrees with the major findings in sheep–GIN systems. An exception is the immune response of cattle to infection with *Ostertagia ostertagi*. A separate section below addresses the immune phenotype of cattle during infections with this species.

Immunological unresponsiveness

The development of protective immunity to GIN is, not surprisingly, highly variable. There are, however, some common characteristics, not least of which is the relatively lengthy period of exposure to either larval challenge or the presence of adult worms required for immunity to develop.

Lambs younger than 6 months of age are less able than adults to resist parasite establishment or remove existing burdens of *T. colubriformis* (Dobson *et al.*, 1990a; Gibson & Parfitt, 1972), *T. circumcincta* (Smith *et al.*, 1985), *Nematodirus* spp. and *Haemonchus contortus* (Manton *et al.*, 1962). This tends to be regarded as a problem of hypo-responsiveness of the immune system, associated with decreased magnitude of the relevant immune responses. The reasons for this hypo-responsiveness remain unclear. A number of differences in the proportions of immune components have been reported between young 'naïve' and older 'immunocompetent' animals; the young stock have lower proportions of CD4+ and CD8+ lymphocytes, produce less interferon-γ and cannot produce the levels of antibody observed in older animals (Colditz *et al.*, 1996). These observations, however, do not provide any obvious means through which the hypo-responsiveness could be overcome, thereby reducing the susceptibility of younger animals.

In sheep, protective immunity (with some variability between parasite species) generally develops by 10–12 months of age (Vlassoff *et al.*, 2001), while in cattle effective immunity has developed to some species by 12 months of age (e.g. *C. oncophora* and *Trichostrongylus axei*) and immunity to others (e.g. *O. ostertagi*) may not develop until the following year (Williams *et al.*, 1993). Indeed, the continued ability of *O. ostertagi* L3 to establish and then be arrested as inhibited L4 in older cattle suggests a limited immune response develops against this stage/species (Armour & Duncan, 1987).

The reasons for this extended period during which immunity is not effective at either resisting larval establishment or expelling resident parasites, despite sustained parasite challenge, remain unclear.

Exposure to parasite antigen shortly after birth may lead to the generation of inappropriate responses which are not protective and which may result in pathogenic intestinal inflammation (Paalangara *et al.*, 2003). These authors delivered crude either *T. colubriformis* L3 extract or saline orally to lambs *in utero*, then challenged the animals 4–6 weeks after birth with live *T. colubriformis* L3. There were a number of significant effects of exposure to parasite antigen *in utero* observed following challenge. For example, the numbers of goblet cells, eosinophils, antigen-presenting cells, CD4+ and CD5+ cells were lower in the exposed group. This reduction in the numbers of immune-associated cells was not reflected in any developmental advantage to the parasites on subsequent challenge, suggesting that while the lambs challenged *in utero* are capable of responding to immunological challenge, the result is not in any way protective. Furthermore, the ability of parasite antigen to down-regulate immune responses in the intestine persists for a significant period after which the remainder of the immune system fails to respond to immune induction. The authors did note, however, that *in utero* exposure to antigen resulted in the loss of approximately half of the fetuses, which they postulated as owing to the generation of an inappropriate inflammatory response (Paalangara *et al.*, 2003).

Components of host responses to GI parasites

Natural resistance – refraction to parasitic infection

Individual GIN species fit particular niches within given host animals, breeds or species. *T. circumcincta*, as an example, has evolved to inhabit the hostile environment of the abomasum, while *T. colubriformis* requires the proximal small intestine. It is debatable whether the inability of either species to survive in the other's organ can be defined as immune related. Presumably, the host developed an acidic environment in the abomasum for nutritional reasons and not as a mechanism to prevent the establishment of a particular parasite species. Within particular organs, however, many changes occur in response to infection which impact on parasite populations. It is possible that these changes may be physiological in nature and not reflect a host immune response *per se*. An example of this is a reduction in establishment of *T. circumcincta* larvae in abomasa with a resident adult worm population. In this case, an increase in luminal pH due to parasite infection (McKellar, 1993) appears to inhibit the ability of ingested larvae to either recognise its site of predilection or to develop successfully. Removing the resident worm burden by drenching immediately results in reduced pH and a correspondingly greater parasite establishment, at least in naïve animals (Sutherland, unpublished).

Innate immune responses to GINs

The innate, or non-adaptive, immune response to GIN infections has received much less attention than acquired immunity. Recently, however, the importance of innate immunity to a wide range of infectious agents, including GINs, has become increasingly recognised. Of particular relevance here are (a) innate barriers to the establishment and survival of parasites and (b) the process by which the host animal recognises the presence of parasites and subsequently activates a response.

Mucus

The surface of the GI tract is covered with a layer of mucus, mainly produced by epithelial goblet cells and comprised mostly of highly glycosylated mucin molecules (Deplancke & Gaskins, 2001). Mucus also contains an array of bioactive molecules, many of which are known to be anti-microbial, such as defensins (Gibson *et al.*, 1996; Tjabringa *et al.*, 2005). Other bioactive molecules have paracrine or chemotactic roles which stimulate inflammation and may contribute to subsequent acquired responses (Dimaline & Varro, 2007; Holzer, 2001). Mucus derived from sheep which had been selected for either elevated or depressed egg output from parasites was compared for its effect on L3 using an *in vitro* LMI assay (Douch *et al.*, 1984). In this experiment, low egg production *in vivo* was associated with a greater inhibitory effect on larval movement *in vitro*. The implication here was that some substance or substances in the mucus had a direct inhibitory effect on larvae.

Lectins

Carbohydrate-binding proteins, or lectins, are released into mucus from epithelial cells soon after parasite infection, and the peak of secretion can be associated with parasite expulsion. It has been proposed that these lectins may recognise and bind to surface epitopes of parasites, and that they may assist in parasite expulsion by either binding to mucins (thus increasing the viscosity of mucus – known to be associated with expulsion), or by forming a bridge between the mucins and the parasites, leading to reduced mobility and/or expulsion.

In recent years, a family of calcium-dependent galactose binding lectins was described (Chang *et al.*, 2004; Komiya *et al.*, 1998; Lee *et al.*, 2001; Tsuji *et al.*, 2001), which were postulated to play a role in protection against bacterial infection (Tsuji *et al.*, 2001). Otherwise known as the intelectins, these molecules have since been observed to be produced from goblet cells in sheep airways, and their synthesis can be up-regulated *in vitro* following the addition of the Th2 cytokine interleukin-4 (IL-4) (French *et al.*, 2007, 2008). Considering the involvement of IL-4 and other known components of the Th2 response to nematode infection in sheep (see below), it is possible that these lectins may play an important role in the recognition not only of bacteria but of nematodes in the gastrointestinal tract.

Eosinophils

Eosinophils have long been associated with nematode infections in the gastrointestinal tract (Buddle *et al.*, 1992; Henderson & Stear, 2006; Kanobana *et al.*, 2002;

Smith *et al.*, 1983). This eosinophilia has been observed both in peripheral blood and intestinal tissue. While parasite infection has been classically associated with elevated numbers of eosinophils, one study, in which peripheral eosinophils were measured during challenge of lambs with *T. circumcincta*, cell numbers were significantly lower over the period of primary infection (Sutherland *et al.*, 1999b); it was proposed this may have resulted from the recruitment of cells into the intestinal epithelium. Peripheral eosinophilia, at least in *T. colubriformis* in lambs, is elevated after several weeks of challenge – and rapidly drops then rises following anthelmintic treatment – which implies that larval challenge alone is insufficient to stimulate the response (Sutherland, unpublished) (Figure 12.1).

Elevated eosinophilia has also been observed in association with inflammation, and protection against infection, with *H. contortus* (Balic *et al.*, 2006; Rainbird *et al.*, 1998), *T. circumcincta* (Henderson & Stear, 2006), *Nematodirus battus* (Winter *et al.*, 1997) and in *C. oncophora* in calves (Kanobana *et al.*, 2002). The increase in cell numbers is associated with elevated production of Th2 cytokines produced by CD4+ cells, such as IL-4 (Finkelman *et al.*, 2004), IL-5 (Rainbird *et al.*, 1998) and IL-13 (Finkelman *et al.*, 2004), while the cells release a cocktail of pro-inflammatory mediators, including cytotoxic granule proteins, cytokines and chemokines (Walsh, 2001).

Mast cells

There is conflicting evidence for the involvement of mast cells in the immune response to GIN. Kanobana *et al.* (2002) found no correlation between cell numbers in the intestinal epithelium and infection with *C. oncophora* in calves, while a number of other studies have by contrast demonstrated a positive correlation between mast cell numbers of immunity to infection (Huntley *et al.*, 1995; Stevenson *et al.*, 1994; Winter *et al.*, 1997), while in *T. colubriformis* infections in sheep, Douch *et al.* (1986) determined that mast cell numbers increased 10-fold in the mucosa of immunised animals.

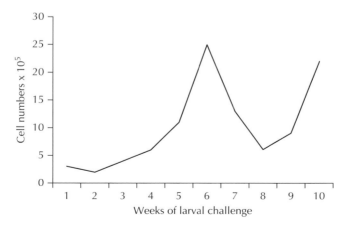

Figure 12.1 Peripheral eosinophil numbers in sheep, challenged twice weekly with *T. colubriformis* L3. Anthelmintic treatment was administered at week 6.

Globule leucocytes

The origin of globule leucocytes has been the subject of some debate, with conflicting reports on whether they are derived from lymphocytes (Douch *et al.*, 1986; Kent, 1952) or from mucosal mast cells (Huntley *et al.*, 1984). The numbers of globule leucocytes is positively correlated with the effect of *ex vivo* mucus on the movement of L3 *in vitro* (Douch *et al.*, 1986), while the same study observed a 30-fold increase in cell numbers in the mucosa of sheep immunised against *T. colubriformis*. The distribution of the cells in the intestinal mucosa closely followed the physical proximity of parasites, leading the authors to conclude that it was these cells which were most responsible for immunity to parasites (Douch *et al.*, 1986).

Figure 12.2 demonstrates the difference in numbers of mast cells/globule leucocytes in lines of Romney sheep selected for either 'resistance' or 'susceptibility' to parasitism following challenge with *T. colubriformis*; while it is accepted there may be a difference in effect or mechanisms between 'resistant' and 'immune' sheep, there was a strong correlation between cell numbers and worm burdens.

Adaptive immune responses to GINs

T helper-1 and -2 type immune responses

The so-called Th1/Th2 dichotomy is used to differentiate, in broad terms, between 'acute' (Th1) and 'chronic' (Th2) infections. Again speaking very broadly, acute Th1-inducing infections, typically viruses and bacteria, are often debilitating or fatal but are resolved relatively quickly. By contrast, Th2-inducing infections (in which there is often an initial Th1 type response) are characteristically chronic, and typify the types of responses induced in response to more complex parasitic infections, including those due to intestinal nematodes (Jankovic *et al.*, 2001). The Th2-like phenotype is therefore associated with protection to infection, and a Th1-like phenotype is viewed as unsuccessful and associated with survival of the parasites (Lacroux *et al.*, 2006).

While the Th1/Th2 dichotomy has not yet been proven to exist in sheep, numerous components of what could be described as typical of a Th2-type response have been implicated in the acquired immune response to GIN infection. For example, immunity is associated with increased numbers of gastrointestinal mast cells, peripheral and tissue eosinophilia, the production of Th2-associated cytokines and the elevated production of multiple antibody isotypes (Gill *et al.*, 2000).

What follows is a brief review of the major components on the acquired immune responses to GIN; it should be borne in mind that most if not all of these components have been observed during the continuum of an immune

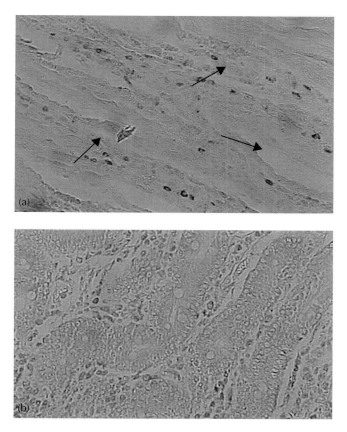

Figure 12.2   Mast cells/globule leucocytes in sections of small intestine from 6-month-old lambs challenged with *T. colubriformis* L3 for 9 weeks prior to necropsy. (a) sample from an animal selected for 'resistance' based on FEC. (b) sample from an animal selected for 'susceptibility' based on FEC. While numerous mast cells/globule leucocytes are obvious in 'a' as indicated by arrows, none were observed in 'b'. Results were consistent across multiple animals (group size = 6) (Sutherland & Alexander, unpublished).

cascade, and many are interdependent. Unless specifically stated, no claims are made on the timing of production and impact of specific components.

T-lymphocytes

In line with the generation of a Th2-type immune response, the numbers of CD4+ cells is correlated with resistance to parasites. In sheep infected with *H. contortus*, the administration of anti-CD4+ antibody resulted in an abrogation of anti-parasite immunity (Gill *et al.*, 1993; Miller & Horohov, 2006), while increased numbers of CD4+ cells have been detected in the abomasal mucosa of sheep infected with *T. circumcincta* (Balic *et al.*, 2006) and in the intestinal lamina propria of sheep infected with *T. colubriformis* (Gorrell *et al.*, 1988).

B-lymphocytes

The major role of B-cells in immunity is the production of antibodies (Ab) in response to the presence of an antigen. Antibody production associated with GIN infection is discussed briefly below. However, B-cells may also play a role in the development of Th-2 type reactions by acting as antigen-presenting cells and stimulating the production of IL-4 from CD4+ T-cells in mice (Lenschow *et al.*, 1996). Perhaps not surprisingly given the complexity of cell-mediated immune responses, B-cells can also fulfil an opposite function by down-regulating T-cell activity (Tivol *et al.*, 1995; Waterhouse *et al.*, 1995).

Cytokines

Like many other 'compartments' of immunity, a complete review of the literature on cytokine responses during GIN infections would take up several volumes. However, there are some cytokines which appear to be key components of anti-GIN immunity (and immunopathology). In particular, these have implicated the increased production of IL-4, IL-5 and IL-13, all nominally Th2-type cytokines. This has been observed in sheep infected with *T. circumcincta* (Craig *et al.*, 2007), *H. contortus* (Lacroux *et al.*, 2006) and *T. colubriformis* (Hein *et al.*, 2004). The involvement of a Th2-like phenotype is further supported by the down-regulation of nominally Th1-type cytokines during GIN infection, including IL-12 (Craig *et al.*, 2007). Whilst it is dangerous to assign definitive functions to individual cytokines during such a complex cascade, it is worthwhile noting that IL-4 and IL-13 are associated with mast cell proliferation (Finkelman *et al.*, 2004) and switching from IgE to IgG1 production (Snapper, 1988) in mice.

Antibodies

Increased levels of IgG, IgA and IgE are associated with GIN infections. The literature describing antibody (Ab) responses to GIN is extensive. Levels of IgG1 are positively correlated with immunity of sheep to *H. contortus* (Gill *et al.*, 1993, 1994; Vervelde *et al.*, 2003) and *T. colubriformis* (Pernthaner *et al.*, 2006). Levels of IgG2 also increase as animals develop immunity to GIN (Douch *et al.*, 1994; Pernthaner *et al.*, 2006). Interestingly, sheep selected for both resistance and resilience to parasite infection had higher levels of anti-L3 IgG2 as compared to controls and sheep selected for susceptibility to infection (Pernthaner *et al.*, 2006) (Figure 12.3).

Increased production of IgE has also been reported in sheep following infection with *T. colubriformis* (Shaw *et al.*, 1999), *H. contortus* (Kooyman *et al.*, 1997) and *T. circumcincta* (Huntley *et al.*, 1998) and was negatively correlated with worm burdens.

The correlation between levels of IgA in serum and intestinal mucosa is strong enough to presume some functional role of this antibody in anti-parasite

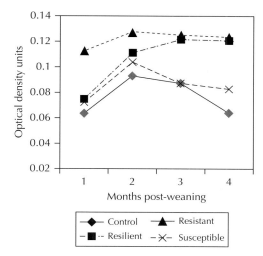

Figure 12.3 Levels of IgG2 specific for adult *T. colubriformis* antigen in the plasma of either unselected lambs or in lambs selected for resilience, resistance or susceptibility to parasitism. Samples were assayed monthly from weaning (Sutherland, Green, Alexander & Leathwick, unpublished).

immunity. In particular, a negative correlation has been observed between abomasal mucosal IgA levels and the length of adult female *T. circumcincta* (Stear *et al.*, 1996; Strain & Stear, 1999). Furthermore, the levels of circulating IgA have been correlated with the propensity of larvae to arrest as L4 (Stear *et al.*, 2004), although doubts were raised by the authors concerning a causative role for IgA in this phenomenon.

More recently, a negative correlation has been observed between the levels of serum and mucosal (salivary) IgA and reduced GIN egg output from sheep; this work has also established that those animals with reduced egg output tend to maintain relatively high levels of productivity (Shaw, personal communication).

The anti-GIN immune response in cattle to *O. ostertagi*

There is significant variability in the development of protective immunity to the various GIN species infecting cattle. While protection develops relatively quickly to *Oesophagostomum radiatum* (Gasbarre & Canals, 1989) and less so to *Cooperia* spp. and *Haemonchus placei*, immunity to *O. ostertagi* tends to develop much more slowly, with animals often remaining susceptible until over 2 years of age (Gasbarre *et al.*, 2001; Michel *et al.*, 1979). For this reason, *O. ostertagi* causes productivity losses for much longer than other species, making it the pre-eminent GIN in cattle in many parts of the world.

Unlike other systems discussed above, repeated challenge with *O. ostertagi* results in the down-regulation of IL-4 production (Almería *et al.*, 1998), which is not typical of a classic Th2 phenotype. However, a more recent study established that *O. ostertagi* infection did in fact induce a Th2-like response in abomasal lymph nodes (Claerebout *et al.*, 2005), but that this response appeared to have no relationship to the up-regulation of effect or mechanisms in the abomasal mucosa. One possible solution to the enigma of why there is such a limited protection against *O. ostertagi* has been proposed, and involves the immunomodulation of protective responses by the parasite itself (Gasbarre *et al.*, 2001). Clearly, there is still much to be defined in this particular host–parasite relationship.

Impact of immunity on parasites

The development of immunity affects the population dynamics of GIN species in various ways. Ingested L3 may be stimulated to enter a state of arrested development as L4 – a phenomenon observed in many species, but most commonly associated with the abomasal species *T. circumcincta* (Hong *et al.*, 1986) and *H. contortus* in sheep (Blitz & Gibbs, 1972) and *O. ostertagi* in cattle (Michel, 1974). Maintaining this pool of arrested larvae appears to be at least partially immune-mediated (Dunsmore, 1963). Ingested L3 may also be rapidly expelled from animals which have developed protective immunity (McClure *et al.*, 1992), or may be displaced from their site of predilection to a more distal and presumably less hostile (and also presumably less favourable) region of the gastrointestinal tract (Roy *et al.*, 2004). Interestingly, incubating exsheathed *T. colubriformis* L3 with an antibody – raised against a carbohydrate antigen found on the surface of all GIN species – caused the larvae to either be expelled immediately or to establish distal to their site of predilection, implying some role of the surface antigen in the ability of the worms to establish (Harrison *et al.*, 2003). It is further implied that the production of an antibody against this antigen *in vivo* may affect parasite establishment.

The initial effect of a developing immunity against adult worms is a reduction in adult female worm length and fecundity (Stear *et al.*, 1997), which is correlated with a reduction in faecal egg output (Stear *et al.*, 1999). In addition to this impact on the size and fecundity of adult female worms, presumably caused by factors in an increasingly hostile environment such as a reduction in the quality of food supply, the sex ratio of worms also alters with the development of protective immunity, with the proportion of males gradually increasing (Sutherland, unpublished) – again, this may be due to the greater mortality of females which are likely to have a higher metabolic requirement and therefore a higher intake of immune components. The death rate of adult worms in animals under parasite challenge is assumed to increase with immunity, particularly for species such as *T. circumcincta* and *O. ostertagi*. A study using *T. circumcincta* established that this was indeed the case, with death rates under challenge of 5%/day in naïve lambs rising to 10%/day by the second month of challenge with L3 (Sutherland, unpublished).

Immunopathology

Protection against challenge and/or adult worm burdens of GINs is generally associated with a degree of immunopathology – most obviously parasite-associated intestinal inflammation. The pathophysiological aspects of immune responses are addressed in Chapter 2, while the physiological cost of immunity is discussed in Chapter 10. However, it is relevant in this chapter on immune manipulation to discuss which components of the immune response to parasites are responsible for pathology, which are responsible for protection, and to what degree, if at all, these components can be distinguished. In other words, is there 'good' and 'bad' immunity?

An example of the delineation between what can be described as good and bad immunity can be seen in recent unpublished research in New Zealand that compares the use of FECs for the selection of resistant sheep as compared to the application of an immunological-based test, which measures the levels of IgA in saliva that is specific to an antigen found only on the surface of GIN larvae. While FEC, which is an indirect measure of the ability of sheep to resist or repulse GIN infection, can indeed select well for resistant sheep, this can be associated with negative consequences of host selection, such as scouring (and associated breech-soiling) and losses in productivity. The antibody test, by contrast, provides an indication of which individuals develop the most rapid/strongest IgA response to challenge; this 'high-responder' phenotype is not associated with any increase in scouring or any loss in productivity (Shaw, personal communication). It is proposed, therefore, that the use of FEC may select for those animals with bad, or a combination of bad and good immunity, while at the very least, the antibody test selects more strongly for the good component (or less strongly for the bad).

Separating out the components of good and bad immunity will be difficult in any experimental situation, but should be considered as a research priority.

Periparturient rise

The decrease in resistance during the PPRI is assumed to have an immunological basis, related to the re-distribution of nutrients to milk production (Houdijk *et al.*, 2001). In both cattle and sheep, there appears to be a general reduction in many elements of immunity, including neutrophil function, antibody and complement production (Detilleux *et al.*, 1994) and the functional capacity of lymphocytes (Kimura *et al.*, 2002), while the intensity of cell-mediated immune responses in the gut mucosa are reduced (O'Sullivan & Donald, 1973).

Utilising immune responses to control GIN

As discussed above, a major limiting factor in the manipulation of 'natural immunity' to GINs is the lack of conclusive evidence of precisely which parasite and host factors are involved in the 'natural' process. Many studies have tried to define parasite proteins that invoke particular immune responses, and then to create and deliver recombinant versions of these proteins as artificial vaccines. This has met with little or no success so far.

The majority of the economically important GIN present peculiar difficulties regarding vaccination strategies. As mucosal browsers on the gastrointestinal epithelium, delivery of a vaccine will be extremely challenging, given the inherent difficulty in inducing a significant mucosal immune response. This is not a problem unique to GIN – protective vaccines against a range of intestinal pathogens, including typhus and polio, most often requires the use of attenuated or killed organisms (Holmgren & Czerkinsky, 2005). So, scientists are not only faced with designing effective vaccines, but also how to deliver the vaccine in such a way as to stimulate effective mucosal immunity.

In a quirk of evolution, the species of GIN which, at least in sheep, is the most damaging economically and physically, has made itself most available to the host immune system by feeding directly on blood. Given its importance and relative availability to immune effectors, it is no surprise that *H. contortus* has dominated global vaccination efforts among the GIN (Newton & Munn, 1999; Peacock & Poynter, 1980).

Vaccination studies to protect hosts against GIN have concentrated on two strategies. First, the use of natural antigens, against which the host responds during infection and second, the utilisation of a 'hidden' antigen approach, in which a molecule not normally presented to the immune system is used to stimulate a protective response.

Natural antigens

The use of a natural antigen approach has proved useful against some parasite species, notably the lungworm *Dictyocaulus viviparus* (Peacock & Poynter, 1980) and the tapeworm *Taenia ovis* (Harrison *et al.*, 1996). In the case of the former, the immunity is induced by the administration of irradiated larvae, while the latter uses defined oncosphere antigens. However, despite many attempts to use either irradiated larvae, crude or purified antigens of various GIN species as vaccines, few have induced a level of protection sufficient to be pursued as a commercial product. These have included a range of parasite extracts and ES antigens from all of the major GIN infecting sheep (Emery *et al.*, 1991; Greenhalgh *et al.*, 1999; Jacobs *et al.*, 1995; O'Donnell *et al.*, 1989a, b; Raleigh *et al.*, 1996). Excellent levels of protection were obtained in controlled laboratory experiments using a glycosylated protein (glycoprotein or glycan) antigen present on the surface of *H. contortus* L3 (Jacobs *et al.*, 1995) and a pair of low molecular weight E/S antigens from adults of the same species (Schallig *et al.*, 1997). It is not known whether any of these candidates have been considered as suitable for commercialisation, and, if they have not, why? A polyprotein allergen found in *O. ostertagi* E/S product (OPA) protected calves against homologous challenge, although only the native protein stimulated any protective immunity (Vercauteren *et al.*, 2004); this failure of a recombinant version of a protective antigen to elicit protective immunity has been observed previously, in what has now become the flag bearer of hidden antigens from GIN – *H. contortus* H11.

Hidden antigens

The H11 molecule (actually H110D) is an integral membrane glycoprotein found only in the intestinal microvilli of the parasitic life cycle stages (Newton & Munn, 1999). Numerous studies using a variety of preparations of H11, and with a variety of adjuvants, have been tested in sheep, with many proving highly effective against homologous challenge (Jasmer *et al.*, 1993; Smith & Smith, 1996; Smith *et al.*, 1993, 1994).

The successful protection of lambs against *H. contortus* challenge conferred following the administration of the gut membrane antigen H11 gave rise to considerable excitement and raised expectations that a commercially-viable vaccine against this worm species was imminent. Unfortunately, this has proved to be overly optimistic. While the success of the initial trial has been replicated on a number of occasions, – each time protection required the use of native antigen, extracted from adult worms that were in turn derived from donor animals. Not surprisingly, this did not seem to be a sensible approach to worm control. Each subsequent attempt to produce a recombinant version of the H11 protein which conferred a significant level of protection against challenge has been unsuccessful.

A number of other hidden antigens have provided some measure of protection against GIN. The *H. contortus* galactose-containing glycoprotein complex (H-*gal*-GP) and a thiol sepharose binding protein (TSBP) from the same GIN species have both shown some promise (Knox *et al.*, 2005). Common to all of these candidate antigens, however, is an inability to replicate results from native through to recombinant antigens. While the reasons for this remain unclear, is it just a coincidence that recombinant proteins are unable to replicate the immunogenic effects of native glycoproteins?.

Continuing attempts to utilise proteins as vaccines is understandable, given the ability to produce large quantities of recombinant antigens in the laboratory. However, it is conceivable that other classes of potential antigens, particularly carbohydrates, may actually be more suitable as vaccine candidates. The surface of GINs is almost entirely consistituted of carbohydrates or glycans, and it is these molecules that are almost certainly in the earliest, most intimate and enduring contact with elements of the host immune system. It seems logical, therefore, that parasite glycans would be a valuable resource when investigating potential protective antigens.

In addition to the glycans from GIN mentioned above, a fucosylated lacdiNAc is present in excretory–secretory preparations from adult *H. contortus* and has been shown to provide significant protection against homologous challenge (Vervelde *et al.*, 2003). A glycan antigen has also been identified on the surface of L3 (sheathed and exsheathed) which invokes a strong antiparasite antibody response, which can protect against infection (Harrison *et al.*, 2003). The antigen, designated CarLA, has been detected, in various versions, on all GIN of grazing livestock investigated thus far, raising the possibility that a pan-species vaccine may be possible. The authors are unaware of current developments regarding this candidate antigen.

What next for immunoparasitology research?

Given the economic impact of GIN worldwide, and the increasing constraints on anthelmintic use due to cost and a desire in many markets to minimise chemical applications in the livestock sectors, there will continue to be valid reasons for pursuing the Holy Grail of an effective pan-nematode vaccine. It is encouraging that research efforts are now moving towards other potential targets such as carbohydrates and lipids, although the technical difficulties of working with these classes of molecules should not be ignored.

One step behind from anti-parasite vaccine production is the development of treatments which modulate the host response to infection in some way. Such immunomodulators may reduce the severity of immunopathology or increase the relative impact of the protective components of the immune system. Such an approach has the potential to significantly mitigate the costs associated with GIN in livestock.

The intimate association between hosts and nematode parasites throughout mammalian evolution, including the development of mucosal immune mechanisms, leads to a potentially fruitful area of research – one which has become widely known as 'the hygiene hypothesis' (Koloski *et al.*, 2008; Maizels, 2005). Given the expertise of many researchers in the intestinal immune response to GIN infections, surely immunoparasitologists could play a central role in what increasingly is a high profile area, particularly given the availability of large animal models of intestinal inflammation.

A further topic that has been largely ignored by GIN immunoparasitologists – with apologies due to those actively researching in the area – is the inter-relationship between GIN and other infections such as Johne's Disease (*Mycobacterium paratuberculosis*), another common and important productivity constraint on grazing livestock (Davies, 1997; Kennedy & Benedictus, 2001). Evidence from other systems indicates there is likely to be a substantial level of interaction between the responses to this and other infections, with ramifications for pathology and the ability of animals to become immune, either naturally or artificially (Bell *et al.*, 1984; Chiejina & Wakelin, 1994; Madwar *et al.*, 1989).

References

ALMERÍA, S., CANALS, A., GÓMEZ-MUÑOZ, M. T., ZARLENGA, D. S. & GASBARRE, L. C. (1998). Characterization of protective immune responses in local lymphoid tissues after drug-attenuated infections with *Ostertagia ostertagi* in calves. *Veterinary Parasitology*, **80**, 53–64.
ARMOUR, J. & DUNCAN, M. (1987). Arrested larval development in cattle nematodes. *Parasitology Today*, **3**, 171–176.

BALIC, A., CUNNINGHAM, C. P. & MEEUSEN, E. N. T. (2006). Eosinophil interactions with *Haemonchus contortus* larvae in the ovine gastrointestinal tract. *Parasite Immunology*, 28, 107–115.

BELL, R. G., ADAMS, L. S. & OGDEN, R. W. (1984). *Trypanosoma musculi* and *Trichinella spiralis*: Concomitant infections and selection for resistance genotypes in mice. *Experimental Parasitology*, 58, 19–26.

BLITZ, N. M. & GIBBS, H. C. (1972). Studies on the arrested development of *Haemonchus contortus* in sheep 1. The induction of arrested development. *International Journal for Parasitology*, 2, 5–12.

BUDDLE, B. M., JOWETT, G., GREEN, R. S., DOUCH, P. G. C. & RISDON, P. L. (1992). Association of blood eosinophilia with the expression of resistance in Romney lambs to nematodes. *International Journal for Parasitology*, 22, 955–960.

CHANG, B. Y., PEAVY, T. R., WARDRIP, N. J. & HEDRICK, J. L. (2004). The *Xenopus laevis* cortical granule lectin: cDNA cloning, developmental expression, and identification of the eglectin family of lectins. *Comparative Biochemistry and Physiology – A Molecular and Integrative Physiology*, 137, 115–129.

CHIEJINA, S. N. & WAKELIN, D. (1994). Interactions between infections with blood protozoa and gastrointestinal nematodes. *Helminthologia*, 31, 17–21.

CLAEREBOUT, E., VERCAUTEREN, I., GELDHOF, P. *et al.* (2005). Cytokine responses in immunized and non-immunized calves after *Ostertagia ostertagi* infection. *Parasite Immunology*, 27, 325–331.

COLDITZ, I. G., WATSON, D. L., GRAY, G. D. & EADY, S. J. (1996). Some relationships between age, immune responsiveness and resistance to parasites in ruminants. *International Journal for Parasitology*, 26, 869–877.

CRAIG, N. M., MILLER, H. R. P., SMITH, W. D. & KNIGHT, P. A. (2007). Cytokine expression in naive and previously infected lambs after challenge with *Teladorsagia circumcincta*. *Veterinary Immunology and Immunopathology*, 120, 47–54.

DAVIES, H. L. (1997). Ovine Johne's disease. *Australian Veterinary Journal*, 75, 799.

DEPLANCKE, B. & GASKINS, H. R. (2001). Microbial modulation of innate defense: Goblet cells and the intestinal mucus layer. *American Journal of Clinical Nutrition*, 73, 1131S–1141S.

DETILLEUX, J. C., KOEHLER, K. J., FREEMAN, A. E., KEHRLI, M. E., JR, & KELLEY, D. H. (1994). Immunological parameters of periparturient Holstein cattle: Genetic variation. *Journal of Dairy Science*, 77, 2640–2650.

DIMALINE, R. & VARRO, A. (2007). Attack and defence in the gastric epithelium – A delicate balance. *Experimental Physiology*, 92, 591–601.

DOBSON, R. J., BARNES, E. H. & WINDON, R. G. (1992). Population dynamics of *Trichostrongylus colubriformis* and *Ostertagia circumcincta* in single and concurrent infections. *International Journal for Parasitology*, 22, 997–1004.

DOBSON, R. J., WALLER, P. J. & DONALD, A. D. (1990a). Population dynamics of *Trichostrongylus colubriformis* in sheep: The effect of host age on the establishment of infective larvae. *International Journal for Parasitology*, 20, 353–357.

DOBSON, R. J., WALLER, P. J. & DONALD, A. D. (1990b). Population dynamics of *Trichostrongylus colubriformis* in sheep: The effect of infection rate on the establishment of infective larvae and parasite fecundity. *International Journal for Parasitology*, 20, 347–352.

DOUCH, P. G. C., GREEN, R. S. & RISDON, P. L. (1994). Antibody responses of sheep to challenge with *Trichostrongylus colubriformis* and the effect of dexamethasone treatment. *International Journal for Parasitology*, 24, 921–928.

DOUCH, P. G. C., HARRISON, G. B. L., BUCHANAN, L. L. & BRUNSDON, R. V. (1984). Relationship of histamine in tissues and antiparasitic substances in gastrointestinal mucus to the development of resistance to trichostrongyle infections in young sheep. *Veterinary Parasitology*, **16**, 273–288.

DOUCH, P. G. C., HARRISON, G. B. L. & ELLIOTT, D. C. (1986). Relationship of gastrointestinal histology and mucus antiparasite activity with the development of resistance to trichostrongyle infections in sheep. *Veterinary Parasitology*, **20**, 315–331.

DUNSMORE, J. D. (1963). Effect of the removal of an adult population of *Ostertagia* on concurrently existing arrested larvae. *Australian Veterinary Journal*, **39**, 459–463.

EMERY, D. L., BENDIXSEN, T. & MCCLURE, S. J. (1991). The use of electroblotted antigens of *Trichostrongylus colubriformis* to induce proliferative responses in sensitized lymphocytes from sheep. *International Journal for Parasitology*, **21**, 179–185.

EMERY, D. L., MCCLURE, S. J. & WAGLAND, B. M. (1993). Production of vaccines against gastrointestinal nematodes of livestock. *Immunology and Cell Biology*, **71**, 463–472.

FINKELMAN, F. D., SHEA-DONOHUE, T., MORRIS, S. C. *et al.* (2004). Interleukin-4- and interleukin-13-mediated host protection against intestinal nematode parasites. *Immunological Reviews*, **201**, 139–155.

FRENCH, A. T., BETHUNE, J. A., KNIGHT, P. A. *et al.* (2007). The expression of intelectin in sheep goblet cells and upregulation by interleukin-4. *Veterinary Immunology and Immunopathology*, **120**, 41–46.

FRENCH, A. T., KNIGHT, P. A., SMITH, W. D. *et al.* (2008). Up-regulation of intelectin in sheep after infection with *Teladorsagia circumcincta*. *International Journal for Parasitology*, **38**, 467–475.

GASBARRE, L. C. & CANALS, A. (1989). Induction of protective immunity in calves immunized with adult *Oesophagostomum radiatum* somatic antigens. *Veterinary Parasitology*, **34**, 223–238.

GASBARRE, L. C., LEIGHTON, E. A. & SONSTEGARD, T. (2001). Role of the bovine immune system and genome in resistance to gastrointestinal nematodes. *Veterinary Parasitology*, **98**, 51–64.

GIBSON, P. R., ANDERSON, R. P., MARIADASON, J. M. & WILSON, A. J. (1996). Protective role of the epithelium of the small intestine and colon. *Inflammatory Bowel Diseases*, **2**, 279–302.

GIBSON, T. E. & PARFITT, J. W. (1972). The effect of age on the development by sheep of resistance to *Trichostrongylus colubriformis*. *Research in Veterinary Science*, **13**, 529–535.

GILL, H. S., ALTMANN, K., CROSS, M. L. & HUSBAND, A. J. (2000). Induction of T helper 1- and T helper 2-type immune responses during *Haemonchus contortus* infection in sheep. *Immunology*, **99**, 458–463.

GILL, H. S., GRAY, G. D., WATSON, D. L. & HUSBAND, A. J. (1993). Isotype-specific antibody responses to *Haemonchus contortus* in genetically resistant sheep. *Parasite Immunology*, **15**, 61–67.

GILL, H. S., HUSBAND, A. J., WATSON, D. L. & GRAY, G. D. (1994). Antibody-containing cells in the abomasal mucosa of sheep with genetic resistance to *Haemonchus contortus*. *Research in Veterinary Science*, **56**, 41–47.

GORRELL, M. D., WILLIS, G., BRANDON, M. R. & LASCELLES, A. K. (1988). Lymphocyte phenotypes in the intestinal mucosa of sheep infected with *Trichostrongylus colubriformis*. *Clinical and Experimental Immunology*, **72**, 274–279.

GREENHALGH, C. J., LOUKAS, A. & NEWTON, S. E. (1999). The organization of a galectin gene from *Teladorsagia circumcincta*. *Molecular and Biochemical Parasitology*, **101**, 199–206.

HARRISON, G. B. L., HEATH, D. D., DEMPSTER, R. P. *et al.* (1996). Identification and cDNA cloning of two novel low molecular weight host-protective antigens from *Taenia ovis* oncospheres. *International Journal for Parasitology*, **26**, 195–204.

HARRISON, G. B. L., PULFORD, H. D., HEIN, W. R. *et al.* (2003). Immune rejection of *Trichostrongylus colubriformis* in sheep; a possible role for intestinal mucus antibody against an L3-specific surface antigen. *Parasite Immunology*, **25**, 45–53.

HEIN, W. R., BARBER, T., COLE, S. A., MORRISON, L. & PERNTHANER, A. (2004). Long-term collection and characterization of afferent lymph from the ovine small intestine. *Journal of Immunological Methods*, **293**, 153–168.

HENDERSON, N. G. & STEAR, M. J. (2006). Eosinophil and IgA responses in sheep infected with *Teladorsagia circumcincta*. *Veterinary Immunology and Immunopathology*, **112**, 62–66.

HOLMGREN, J. & CZERKINSKY, C. (2005). Mucosal immunity and vaccines. *Nature Medicine*, **11**, S45–S53.

HOLZER, P. (2001). Gastroduodenal mucosal defense: Coordination by a network of messengers and mediators. *Current Opinion in Gastroenterology*, **17**, 489–496.

HONG, C., MICHEL, J. F. & LANCASTER, M. B. (1986). Populations of *Ostertagia circumcincta* in lambs following a single infection. *International Journal for Parasitology*, **16**, 63–67.

HOSTE, H., TORRES-ACOSTA, J. F. J. & AGUILAR-CABALLERO, A. J. (2008). Nutrition-parasite interactions in goats: Is immunoregulation involved in the control of gastrointestinal nematodes? *Parasite Immunology*, **30**, 79–88.

HOUDIJK, J. G. M., KYRIAZAKIS, I., JACKSON, F. & COOP, R. L. (2001). The relationship between protein nutrition, reproductive effort and breakdown in immunity to *Teladorsagia circumcincta* in periparturient ewes. *Animal Science*, **72**, 595–606.

HUNTLEY, J. F., NEWLANDS, G. & MILLER, H. R. (1984). The isolation and characterization of globule leucocytes: Their derivation from mucosal mast cells in parasitized sheep. *Parasite Immunology*, **6**, 371–390.

HUNTLEY, J. F., PATTERSON, M., MACKELLAR, A., JACKSON, F., STEVENSON, L. M. & COOP, R. L. (1995). A comparison of the mast cell and eosinophil responses of sheep and goats to gastrointestinal nematode infections. *Research in Veterinary Science*, **58**, 5–10.

HUNTLEY, J. F., SCHALLIG, H. D. F. H., KOOYMAN, F. N. J., MACKELLAR, A., JACKSON, F. & SMITH, W. D. (1998). IgE antibody during infection with the ovine abomasal nematode, *Teladorsagia circumcincta*: Primary and secondary responses in serum and gastric lymph of sheep. *Parasite Immunology*, **20**, 565–571.

JACOBS, H. J., ASHMAN, K. & MEEUSEN, E. (1995). Humoral and cellular responses following local immunization with a surface antigen of the gastrointestinal parasite *Haemonchus contortus*. *Veterinary Immunology and Immunopathology*, **48**, 323–332.

JANKOVIC, D., LIU, Z. & GAUSE, W. C. (2001). Th1- and Th2-cell commitment during infectious disease: Asymmetry in divergent pathways. *Trends in Immunology*, **22**, 450–457.

JASMER, D. P., PERRYMAN, L. E., CONDER, G. A., CROW, S. & MCGUIRE, T. (1993). Protective immunity to *Haemonchus contortus* induced by immunoaffinity isolated antigens that share a phylogenetically conserved carbohydrate gut surface epitope. *Journal of Immunology*, **151**, 5450–5460.

KANOBANA, K., KOETS, A., KOOYMAN, F. N. J., BAKKER, N., PLOEGER, H. W. & VERVELDE, L. (2003). B cells and antibody response in calves primary-infected or re-infected with *Cooperia oncophora*: Influence of priming dose and host responder types. *International Journal for Parasitology*, 33, 1487–1502.

KANOBANA, K., PLOEGER, H. W. & VERVELDE, L. (2002). Immune expulsion of the trichostrongylid *Cooperia oncophora* is associated with increased eosinophilia and mucosal IgA. *International Journal for Parasitology*, 32, 1389–1398.

KENNEDY, D. J. & BENEDICTUS, G. (2001). Control of *Mycobacterium avium* subsp. paratuberculosis infection in agricultural species. *OIE Revue Scientifique et Technique*, 20, 151–179.

KENT, J. F. (1952). The origin, fate and cytochemistry of the globule leucocyte of the sheep. *Anatomical Record*, 112, 91–115.

KIMURA, K., GOFF, J. P., KEHRLI, M. E., JR, HARP, J. A. & NONNECKE, B. J. (2002). Effects of mastectomy on composition of peripheral blood mononuclear cell populations in periparturient dairy cows. *Journal of Dairy Science*, 85, 1437–1444.

KNOX, D. P., SMITH, S. K., REDMOND, D. L. & SMITH, W. D. (2005). Protection induced by vaccinating sheep with a thiol-binding extract of *Haemonchus contortus* membranes is associated with its protease components. *Parasite Immunology*, 27, 121–126.

KOLOSKI, N. A., BRET, L. & RADFORD-SMITH, G. (2008). Hygiene hypothesis in inflammatory bowel disease: A critical review of the literature. *World Journal of Gastroenterology*, 14, 165–173.

KOMIYA, T., TANIGAWA, Y. & HIROHASHI, S. (1998). Cloning of the novel gene intelectin which is expressed in intestinal Paneth cells in mice. *Biochemical and Biophysical Research Communications*, 251, 759–762.

KOOYMAN, F. N. J., VAN KOOTEN, P. J. S., HUNTLEY, J. F., MACKELLAR, A., CORNELISSEN, A. W. C. A. & SCHALLIG, H. D. F. H. (1997). Production of a monoclonal antibody specific for ovine immunoglobulin E and its application to monitor serum IgE responses to *Haemonchus contortus* infection. *Parasitology*, 114, 395–406.

LACROUX, C., NGUYEN, T. H. C., ANDREOLETTI, O. *et al.* (2006). *Haemonchus contortus* (Nematoda: Trichostrongylidae) infection in lambs elicits an unequivocal Th2 immune response. *Veterinary Research*, 37, 607–622.

LEE, J. K., SCHNEE, J., PANG, M. *et al.* (2001). Human homologs of the *Xenopus* oocyte cortical granule lectin XL35. *Glycobiology*, 11, 65–73.

LENSCHOW, D. J., WALUNAS, T. L. & BLUESTONE, J. A. (1996). CD28/B7 system of T cell costimulation. *Annual Review of Immunology*, 14, 233–258.

MADWAR, M. A., EL TAHAWY, M. & STRICKLAND, G. T. (1989). The relationship between uncomplicated schistosomiasis and hepatitis B infection. *Transactions of the Royal Society of Tropical Medicine and Hygiene*, 83, 233–236.

MAIZELS, R. M. (2005). Infections and allergy – Helminths, hygiene and host immune regulation. *Current Opinion in Immunology*, 17, 656–661.

MANTON, V. J. A., PEACOCK, R., POYNTER, D., SILVERMAN, P. H. & TERRY, R. J. (1962). The influence of age on naturally acquired resistance to *Haemonchus contortus* in lambs. *Research in Veterinary Science*, 3, 308–314.

MCCLURE, S. J., EMERY, D. L., WAGLAND, B. M. & JONES, W. O. (1992). A serial study of rejection of *Trichostrongylus colubriformis* by immune sheep. *International Journal for Parasitology*, 22, 227–234.

MCKELLAR, Q. A. (1993). Interactions of *Ostertagia* species with their bovine and ovine hosts. *International Journal for Parasitology*, 23, 451–462.

MICHEL, J. F. (1974). Arrested development of nematodes and some related phenomena. *Advances in Parasitology*, 12, 279–366.

MICHEL, J. F., LANCASTER, M. B. & HONG, C. (1979). The effect of age, acquired resistance, pregnancy and lactation on some reactions of cattle to infection with *Ostertagia ostertagi*. *Parasitology*, **79**, 157–168.

MILLER, H. R. P. (1996). Prospects for the immunological control of ruminant gastrointestinal nematodes: Natural immunity, can it be harnessed? *International Journal for Parasitology*, **26**, 801–811.

MILLER, J. E. & HOROHOV, D. W. (2006). Immunological aspects of nematode parasite control in sheep. *Journal of Animal Science*, **84** (Suppl), E124–E132.

NEWTON, S. E. & MUNN, E. A. (1999). The development of vaccines against gastrointestinal nematode parasites, particularly *Haemonchus contortus*. *Parasitology Today*, **15**, 116–122.

O'DONNELL, I. J., DINEEN, J. K., WAGLAND, B. M. *et al.* (1989a). Characterization of the major immunogen in the excretory-secretory products of exsheathed third-stage larvae of *Trichostrongylus colubriformis*. *International Journal for Parasitology*, **19**, 793–802.

O'DONNELL, I. J., DINEEN, J. K., WAGLAND, B. M., LETHO, S., WERKMEISTER, J. A. & WARD, C. W. (1989b). A novel host-protective antigen from *Trichostrongylus colubriformis*. *International Journal for Parasitology*, **19**, 327–335.

O'SULLIVAN, B. M. & DONALD, A. D. (1973). Responses to infection with *Haemonchus contortus* and *Trichostrongylus colubriformis* in ewes of different reproductive status. *International Journal for Parasitology*, **3**, 521–530.

PAALANGARA, R., MCCLURE, S. & MCCULLAGH, P. (2003). Intestinal exposure to a parasite antigen *in utero* depresses cellular and cytokine responses of the mucosal immune system. *Veterinary Immunology and Immunopathology*, **93**, 91–105.

PEACOCK, R. & POYNTER, D. (1980). Field experience with a bovine lungworm vaccine. *Vaccines Against Parasites*, **18**, 141–148.

PERNTHANER, A., COLE, S. A., MORRISON, L., GREEN, R., SHAW, R. J. & HEIN, W. R. (2006). Cytokine and antibody subclass responses in the intestinal lymph of sheep during repeated experimental infections with the nematode parasite *Trichostrongylus colubriformis*. *Veterinary Immunology and Immunopathology*, **114**, 135–148.

PERNTHANER, A., COLE, S. A., MORRISON, L. & HEIN, W. R. (2005). Increased expression of interleukin-5 (IL-5), IL-13, and tumor necrosis factor alpha genes in intestinal lymph cells of sheep selected for enhanced resistance to nematodes during infection with *Trichostrongylus colubriformis*. *Infection and Immunity*, **73**, 2175–2183.

RAINBIRD, M. A., MACMILLAN, D. & MEEUSEN, E. N. T. (1998). Eosinophil-mediated killing of *Haemonchus contortus* larvae: Effect of eosinophil activation and role of antibody, complement and interleukin-5. *Parasite Immunology*, **20**, 93–103.

RALEIGH, J. M., BRANDON, M. R. & MEEUSEN, E. (1996). Stage-specific expression of surface molecules by the larval stages of *Haemonchus contortus*. *Parasite Immunology*, **18**, 125–132.

ROY, E. A., HOSTE, H. & BEVERIDGE, I. (2004). The effects of concurrent experimental infections of sheep with *Trichostrongylus colubriformis* and *T. vitrinus* on nematode distributions, numbers and on pathological changes. *Parasite*, **11**, 293–300.

SCHALLIG, H. D. F. H., VAN LEEUWEN, M. A. W. & CORNELISSEN, A. W. C. A. (1997). Protective immunity induced by vaccination with two *Haemonchus contortus* excretory secretory proteins in sheep. *Parasite Immunology*, **19**, 447–453.

SHAW, R. J., MORRIS, C. A., GREEN, R. S. *et al.* (1999). Genetic and phenotypic relationships among *Trichostrongylus colubriformis*-specific immunoglobulin E, anti-*Trichostrongylus colubriformis* antibody, immunoglobulin G1, faecal egg count and body weight traits in grazing Romney lambs. *Livestock Production Science*, **58**, 25–32.

SMITH, S. K. & SMITH, W. D. (1996). Immunisation of sheep with an integral membrane glycoprotein complex of *Haemonchus contortus* and with its major polypeptide components. *Research in Veterinary Science*, **60**, 1–6.

SMITH, T. S., MUNN, E. A., GRAHAM, M., TAVERNOR, A. S. & GREENWOOD, C. A. (1993). Purification and evaluation of the integral membrane protein H11 as a protective antigen against *Haemonchus contortus*. *International Journal for Parasitology*, **23**, 271–280.

SMITH, W. D., JACKSON, F., JACKSON, E. & WILLIAMS, J. (1983). Studies on the local immune response of the lactating ewe infected with *Ostertagia circumcincta*. *Journal of Comparative Pathology*, **93**, 295–305.

SMITH, W. D., JACKSON, F., JACKSON, E. & WILLIAMS, J. (1985). Age immunity to *Ostertagia circumcincta*: Comparison of the local immune responses of 4 1/2 - and 10-month-old lambs. *Journal of Comparative Pathology*, **95**, 235–245.

SMITH, W. D., SMITH, S. K. & MURRAY, J. M. (1994). Protection studies with integral membrane fractions of *Haemonchus contortus*. *Parasite Immunology*, **16**, 231–241.

SNAPPER, C. M., FINKELMAN, F.D. & PAUL, W.E. (1988). Regulation of IgG1 and IgE production by interleukin 4. *Immunological Reviews*, **102**, 591–601.

STEAR, M., PARK, M. & BISHOP, S. (1996). The key components of resistance to *Ostertagia circumcincta* in lambs. *Parasitology Today*, **12**, 438–441.

STEAR, M. J., BAIRDEN, K., DUNCAN, J. L. *et al.* (1997). How hosts control worms. *Nature*, **389**, 27.

STEAR, M. J., BAIRDEN, K., INNOCENT, G. T., MITCHELL, S., STRAIN, S. & BISHOP, S. C. (2004). The relationship between IgA activity against 4th-stage larvae and density-dependent effects on the number of 4th-stage larvae of *Teladorsagia circumcincta* in naturally infected sheep. *Parasitology*, **129**, 363–369.

STEAR, M. J., STRAIN, S. & BISHOP, S. C. (1999). How lambs control infection with *Ostertagia circumcincta*. *Veterinary Immunology and Immunopathology*, **72**, 213–218.

STEVENSON, L. M., HUNTLEY, J. F., SMITH, W. D. & JONES, D. G. (1994). Local eosinophil- and mast cell-related responses in abomasal nematode infections of lambs. *FEMS Immunology and Medical Microbiology*, **8**, 167–174.

STRAIN, S. A. J. & STEAR, M. J. (1999). The recognition of molecules from fourth-stage larvae of *Ostertagia circumcincta* by IgA from infected sheep. *Parasite Immunology*, **21**, 163–168.

SUTHERLAND, I. A., BROWN, A. E., GREEN, R. S., MILLER, C. M. & LEATHWICK, D. M. (1999a). The immune response of sheep to larval challenge with *Ostertagia circumcincta* and *O. ostertagi*. *Veterinary Parasitology*, **84**, 125–135.

SUTHERLAND, I. A., BROWN, A. E. & LEATHWICK, D. M. (2000). Selection for drug-resistant nematodes during and following extended exposure to anthelmintic. *Parasitology*, **121**, 217–226.

SUTHERLAND, I. A., BROWN A. E. & LEATHWICK, D. M. The development of immunity to *Teladorsagia circumcincta*. *The New Zealand Journal of Zoology*, in press.

SUTHERLAND, I. A., LEATHWICK, D. M., GREEN, R., BROWN, A. E. & MILLER, C. M. (1999b). The effect of continuous drug exposure on the immune response to *Trichostrongylus colubriformis* in sheep. *Veterinary Parasitology*, **80**, 261–271.

TIVOL, E. A., BORRIELO, F., SCHWEITZER, A. N., LYNCH, P. W., BLUESTONE, J. A. & SHARPE, A. H. (1995). Loss of CTLA-4 leads to massive lymphoproliferations and fetal multiorgan tissue destruction, revealing a critical negative regulatory role of CTLA-4. *Immunity*, **3**, 542.

TJABRINGA, G. S., VOS, J. B., OLTHUIS, D. *et al.* (2005). Host defense effector molecules in mucosal secretions. *FEMS Immunology and Medical Microbiology*, **45**, 151–158.

TSUJI, S., UEHORI, J., MATSUMOTO, M. *et al.* (2001). Human intelectin is a novel soluble lectin that recognizes galactofuranose in carbohydrate chains of bacterial cell wall. *Journal of Biological Chemistry*, **276**, 23456–23463.

VERCAUTEREN, I., GELDHOF, P., VERCRUYSSE, J. *et al.* (2004). Vaccination with an *Ostertagia ostertagi* polyprotein allergen protects calves against homologous challenge infection. *Infection and Immunity*, **72**, 2995–3001.

VERVELDE, L., BAKKER, N., KOOYMAN, F. N. J. *et al.* (2003). Vaccination-induced protection of lambs against the parasitic nematode *Haemonchus contortus* correlates with high IgG antibody responses to the LDNF glycan antigen. *Glycobiology*, **13**, 795–804.

VLASSOFF, A., LEATHWICK, D. M. & HEATH, A. C. G. (2001). The epidemiology of nematode infections of sheep. *New Zealand Veterinary Journal*, **49**, 213–221.

WALSH, G. M. (2001). Eosinophil granule proteins and their role in disease. *Current Opinion in Hematology*, **8**, 28–33.

WATERHOUSE, P., PENNINGER, J. M., TIMMS, E. *et al.* (1995). Lymphoproliferative disorders with early lethality in mice deficient in Ctla-4. *Science*, **270**, 985–988.

WILLIAMS, J. C., KNOX, J. W. & LOYACANO, A. F. (1993). Epidemiology of *Ostertagia ostertagi* in weaner-yearling cattle. *Veterinary Parasitology*, **46**, 313–324.

WINTER, M. D., WRIGHT, C. & LEE, D. L. (1997). The mast cell and eosinophil response of young lambs to a primary infection with *Nematodirus battus*. *Parasitology*, **114**, 189–193.

Postscript

Speaking as people who considered themselves to have a broad and detailed understanding of the subject area, writing this book has proven to be unexpectedly interesting, if not humbling. In particular, stepping back far enough to consider both the genesis and evolution of whole subject areas has been a revelation. For the most part, unfortunately, the revelation points to a dire shortfall in progress over the last 30 years. The real groundbreaking work was, in many areas, carried out decades ago by the likes of John Michel at the Central Veterinary Laboratories in England and Ron Brunsdon at the Wallaceville Animal Research Centre in New Zealand. An honourable mention goes to Peter Waller (amongst a generation of high-profile Australian veterinary parasitologists), and of course, many others around the globe who have contributed significantly to this area of study.

It is tempting to propose that the slowing of progress in the field in recent years has coincided with a global shift in research funding priorities which, in many cases, have changed from maximising and/or maintaining productivity from pastoral agriculture to the short-term focus on developing technologies. That said, there continues to be exciting research opportunities into the GIN of grazing ruminants – certainly as long as there is a desire for protein and other products such as fibre and leather. As subjects for studies of evolutionary biology, intestinal immunity/physiology, etc., GIN parasites and their hosts provide wonderful large animal models. Compare, for example, the practicalities of performing laboratory-based studies on *ex vivo* cells from rodents with those derived from sheep or goats. Furthermore, marrying such models with the exciting and recent developments in high-throughput 'omics' technologies promises significant rewards – assuming, of course, that these studies take note of parasite biology and the host–parasite relationship.

While the impact of broad-spectrum anthelmintics, which transformed the pastoral industries, cannot be denied, it is important we do not focus solely on drug development and application in the future – yes, we must embrace chemotherapy, but we must also look beyond it and beside it. There are very significant questions which remain unanswered; for example, millions of dollars are spent annually by agronomists to improve the performance of pasture species in an attempt to boost animal productivity: has anyone ever asked a veterinary parasitologist how to improve feed efficiency by 2%? Or, has anyone funded work which properly explained the aetiology of parasite-induced inappetance? Perhaps, one day we may define exactly how each of the GIN species decides on its site of predilection, or how worms manage to survive for extended periods in extremely hostile environments. We may determine how anti-GIN immunity works, as well as how their own immune system defends them in the gastrointestinal tract.

Ian Sutherland
Ian Scott
New Zealand, 2009

Index